Selected Papers on the Pathogenic Rickettsiae

Selected Papers
on the
Pathogenic Rickettsiae

Edited by Nicholas Hahon

Harvard University Press

Cambridge Massachusetts

1968

To my mother and father

Preface

The purpose of this volume is to present a collection of original papers that have significantly advanced our comprehension of the microorganisms known as rickettsiae and the diseases they produce. The knowledge that has been gained, under hazardous and difficult conditions through bold and brilliant investigations, has been applied recently to the successful control of rickettsial diseases in the civilized world. In the light of the past history of epidemic rickettsial diseases, this culmination of clinical, laboratory, and field studies represents an imposing achievement in medical microbiology that deserves to be recorded. Because rickettsiae have the potential to evoke epidemics and recurrent outbreaks of disease in the world populace whenever living standards decline as a consequence of natural or manmade catastrophes, they still remain a threat to world health. From a fundamental standpoint, rickettsiae are important because they possess certain unique features that make them suitable as prototypes in studies relating to the understanding of intracellular parasitism. Their importance and usefulness in this capacity has not been fully realized or exploited. For these reasons, interest in, and the importance of, rickettsial diseases needs to be reaffirmed.

This collection of papers on rickettsiae is limited to those agents that are pathogenic for man, although the majority of rickettsiae are nonpathogenic for man and are symbiotic with a variety of arthropods. Much of our knowledge and understanding of the nature, behavior, and complex ecologic relations of rickettsiae, however, has been derived directly from investigations on the pathogenic rickettsiae.

Several of the selections originally published in a foreign language appear in English translation for the first time. Some of the papers that compose the collection are classics of scientific investigation, inference, and reporting. The text of each paper is preceded by a preface to orient the reader unfamiliar with the rickettsioses. These introductory comments help to place the papers in proper perspective by providing pertinent background information, stressing the significance of the contribution, and noting the influence of the work on the direction of subsequent research and developments. In deference to the many papers that were worthy of inclusion but were omitted owing to the necessity to keep the volume within reasonable bounds, references to some of these papers are made in the commentaries. The selected papers span the period from the earliest recorded clinical description of a rickettsial disease in the sixteenth century to modern times and are arranged chronologically in the text. As a consequence, a historical theme pervades the volume. The collection, however, is not intended to be a history of the rickettsioses.

This volume may seem parochial in being confined to a genus of microorganisms and specifically to the pathogenic rickettsiae. But the existing knowledge on the subject is the result of concerted efforts by researchers representing a diversity of disciplines, e.g., physicians, microbiologists, pathologists, biologists, immunologists, entomologists, biochemists, and epidemiologists. For this reason, I hope that the collection will appeal to the many disciplines that compose the scientific community. For students the volume may serve as a general review of the pathogenic rickettsiae and may also enrich their appreciation and comprehension of scientific inquiry by providing examples of outstanding historical and current reports on the manifold facets of research. For the general reader it may exemplify man's determination and progress in understanding, controlling, and eradicating infectious diseases. Lastly, may the volume stand as a tribute to the memory of those early workers who gave their lives to advance our knowledge of rickettsial infections.

I am most grateful to the authors of the papers, the editors, and the copyright owners of the different journals for graciously granting me permission to reprint the original articles. Specific acknowledgments are listed on pages ix and x. To the authors who supplied reprints of their papers, my sincere appreciation is extended.

Frederick, Maryland   Nicholas Hahon

Acknowledgements

Hieronymi Fracastorii, "The Fever Called Lenticulae or Puncticulae" is reprinted from Fracastorius's *De contagione et contagiosis morbis et eorum curatione*, III (1546), trans. W. C. Wright (Putnam, 1930).

W. W. Gerhard, "On the Typhus Fever . . ." is abridged and reprinted from *Am. J. Med. Sci.*, *19* (1837), 289–322.

H. T. Ricketts, "Further Experiments with the Wood Tick in Relation to Rocky Mountain Spotted Fever" is reprinted from *JAMA*, *49* (1907), 1278–1281.

Charles Nicolle *et al.*, "Experimental Transmission of Exanthematic Typhus through Body Lice" is reprinted from *C. R. Acad. Sci.*, *149* (1909), 486–489, by permission of Gauthier-Villars, the publisher.

H. T. Ricketts and R. M. Wilder, "The Etiology of the Typhus Fever (Tabardillo) of Mexico City" is reprinted from *JAMA*, *54* (1910), 1373–1375 by permission of the publisher.

A. Conor and A. Bruch, "An Eruptive Fever Observed in Tunisia" is reprinted from *Bull. Soc. Path. Exot.*, *3* (1910), 492–496 by permission of the publisher.

Nathan E. Brill, "An Acute Infectious Disease of Unknown Origin" is reprinted from *Am. J. Med. Sci.*, *139* (1910), 484–502, by permission of Lea & Febiger, the publisher.

H. da Rocha-Lima, "On the Etiology of Typhus Fever" is reprinted from *Berl. klin. Wschr.*, *53* (1916), 567–569, by permission of Springer-Verlag, the publisher.

E. Weil and A. Felix, "On Serological Diagnosis of Spotted Fever" is reprinted from *Wien. klin. Wschr.*, *13* (1916), 33–35, by permission of Springer-Verlag, the publisher.

Hans Zinsser, "Varieties of Typhus Virus and the Epidemiology of the American Form of European Typhus Fever (Brill's Disease)," *Am. J. Hyg.*, *20* (1934), 513–532; and Herbert L. Ley, Jr., *et al.*, "Immunization against Scrub Typhus . . .," *Am. J. Hyg.*, *56* (1952), 313–319, are reprinted by permission of the publisher and (latter article) of the authors.

E. H. Derrick, "'Q' Fever, a New Fever Entity . . ." is reprinted from *Med. J. Austral.*, *2* (1937), 281–299, by permission of the Australasian Medical Publishing Company Ltd., the publisher, and of the author.

R. Lewthwaite and S. R. Savoor, "Rickettsia Diseases of Malaya . . ." is reprinted from *The Lancet*, February 10 and 17, 1940, pp. 255 and 305, by permission of the publisher and the authors.

E. Gildemeister and E. Haagen, "Typhus Fever Studies . . " is reprinted from *Dtsch. med. Wschr.*, *66* (1940), 878–880, by permission of Georg Thieme Verlag, the publisher.

Acknowledgements

Norman H. Topping and M. J. Shear, "Studies of Typhus Fever Vaccines . . ." is reprinted from National Institute of Health Bulletin No. 183 (1945), 13–17 by permission of the authors.

James H. Gilford and Winston H. Price, "Virulent-Avirulent Conversions of *Rickettsia rickettsii* in Vitro" is reprinted from *Proc. Nat. Acad. Sci.*, *41* (1955), 870–873, by permission of the publisher and the authors.

M. G. P. Stoker and P. Fiset, "Phase Variation of the Nine Mile and Other Strains of *Rickettsia burneti*" is reprinted from *Canad. J. Microbiol.*, *2* (1956), 310–321 by permission of the National Research Council, Canada, the publisher, and of the authors.

M. Schaecter *et al.*, "Study on the Growth of Rickettsiae . . ." is reprinted from *Virology*, *3* (1957), 160–172, by permission of Academic Press, the publisher, and of the authors.

Marianna R. Bovarnick, "Incorporation of Acetate-l-C^{14} into Lipid by Typhus Rickettsiae" is reprinted from *J. Bact.*, *80* (1960), 508–512, by permission of the American Society for Microbiology, the publisher, and of the author.

J. W. Vinson and H. S. Fuller, "Studies on Trench Fever . . ." is reprinted from *Pathologia et Microbiologia*, 24 Supp. (1961), 152–166 by permission of S. Karger-Basel/New York, the publisher, and of the authors.

The following articles are reprinted from *J. Exp. Med.* by permission of the Rockefeller Institute Press, the publisher, and of the authors: Clara Nigg and K. Landsteiner, "Studies on the Cultivation of the Typhus Fever Rickettsia in the Presence of Live Tissue," 55 (1932), 681–686; Harry Plotz *et al.*, "Morphological Structure of Rickettsiae," 77 (1943), 355–358; Donald Greiff *et al.*, "Effect of Enzyme Inhibitors and Activators on the Multiplication of Typhus Rickettsiae . . .," *80* (1944), 561–574; Marianna R. Bovarnick and John C. Snyder, "Respiration of Typhus Rickettsiae," *89* (1949), 561–565; Hans Ris and John P. Fox, "The Cytology of Rickettsiae," *89* (1949), 681–686.

The following articles are reprinted from *Public Health Reports* by permission of the authors when appropriate: M. H. Neill, "Experimental Typhus Fever in Guinea Pigs," *32* (1917), 1105–1108; Kenneth F. Maxcy, "Typhus Fever in the United States," *44* (1929), 1735–1742; Herald R. Cox, "Use of Yolk Sac of Developing Chick Embryo as Medium for Growing Rickettsiae of Rocky Mountain Spotted Fever and Typhus Groups," *53* (1938), 2241–2247; Robert J. Huebner *et al.*, "Rickettsial-pox—A Newly Recognized Rickettsial Disease . . . ," *61* (1946), 1605–1614.

Contents

Contents

Selected Papers on the Pathogenic Rickettsiae

Introduction

Rickettsiae comprise a group of pleomorphic, coccobacillary micro-organisms that have been regarded as intermediate between viruses and bacteria. There is no evidence, however, to indicate that rickettsiae represent a direct evolutionary link between the two groups. Although they are usually obligatory intracellular parasites and require a living host cell for replication, a feature held in common with viruses, this characteristic is not unconditional. There is evidence that some rickett-siae multiply at the surface of cells lining the intestinal tract of arthro-pods, and recently the etiological agent of trench fever, *Rickettsia quintana*, has been grown in cell-free medium. Rickettsiae possess certain mor-phological and tinctorial characteristics and can perform physiological activities that are similar to those of bacteria. In thin sections rickettsiae show almost all the structural features of bacteria; by histochemical techniques the presence of both deoxyribonucleic and ribonucleic acids has also been demonstrated. In chemical composition rickettsiae cell walls resemble those of bacteria in being composed mainly of poly-saccharides and amino acids. That muramic acid has been detected in rickettsial cell walls is a highly relevant finding because this constituent has not been found except in bacteria and certain algae. Binary fission is now generally considered to be the mode of reproduction of rickett-siae, such fission having been observed in a number of species. A feature that markedly differentiates rickettsiae from viruses is the possession of metabolic systems by the former that permit them to carry out certain physiological functions independent of the host cell. It has been suggested that host cells act as suppliers of substrates for the metabolic machinery of rickettsiae. The sensitivity of rickettsiae to broad-spectrum antibiotics is another feature shared with bacteria. The increasing body of evidence strongly suggests that rickettsiae are true bacteria. Because rickettsiae infect both invertebrate and verte-brate hosts, exhibit varied degrees of pathogenicity, and closely resemble bacteria, they constitute a unique biological group well suited for exploring the evolution of parasitism at the microbial level.

Most rickettsiae are nonpathogenic for man and exist as natural inhabitants of arthropods with which they maintain a symbiotic rela-tionship. A small portion of the rickettsiae assume practical importance because they are responsible for a number of specific infections of man and animals called rickettsioses. It has been from exigent and intensive studies of the pathogenic rickettsiae that most of our knowledge of the general nature and behavior of the rickettsiae has been attained. The pathogenic rickettsiae are transmitted to man by a variety of arthropods, e.g., ticks, mites, fleas, and lice. Generally, these infectious agents live in various degrees of symbiosis with the affected arthropod. In ticks and mites the rickettsiae exist as symbionts, in mutual harmony with the vector, and are maintained in the host from generation to generation by transovarial passage, e.g., the Rocky Mountain spotted fever and the scrub typhus rickettsiae. Murine typhus rickettsiae also appear to be well adapted to fleas, wherein they multiply without noticeable harm to the host. The relation between the epidemic typhus fever rickettsia and the body louse is not one of symbiosis. The rickettsiae are lethal for the host: their pathogenicity for lice arises from their destructive action on the stomach epithelium, resulting in the loss of its functional properties. This circumstance constitutes the basis for the prevailing belief that the relation between the epidemic typhus fever rickettsia and lice is a more recent adaptation in comparison to that of other rickettsiae-vector hosts.

In nature both wild and domestic animals may form a reservoir of rickettsial infection and act as the source of infection for blood-sucking arthropods. The majority of rickettsial diseases have an epidemiological pattern that mainly involves the spread of infection to man and animals through arthropods which either secrete rickettsiae from their salivary glands or excrete the infectious agent in their feces. Though some rickettsial infections are essentially human diseases, others are clearly accidental infections of man. The latter are the consequence of man's intrusion into the "silent" cycle of infection between vector and animal, e.g., scrub typhus. The epidemiology of epidemic typhus fever and trench fever assumes a different form: infection is spread from man to man by lice and does not involve an intermediate animal host; man appears to be the reservoir for the infectious agents. Q fever is unique in that the infection, among other means, can be transmitted in nature to man by inhalation of the etiological agent in an airborne state. The ability to adapt to new hosts and surroundings to insure their survival and spread in nature, an inherent characteristic of biological entities, is also exhibited by rickettsiae. New ecological cycles of infection continue to be found in nature, and outbreaks of disease occur in environments far removed from primitive locales. The outbreaks of rickettsialpox that occurred in modern apartments of New York City exemplify rickettsial ecological adaptability. From the preceding brief review of some of the salient features of the rickettsiae it is apparent that because of their kaleidoscopic and paradoxical behavior rickettsiae constitute a group of microorganisms about which it is difficult to generalize.

The development of our knowledge on the nature and behavior of the pathogenic rickettsiae and the evolvement of effective preventive, control, and chemotherapeutical measures against the diseases that these microorganisms produce in man have been attained in the relatively short span of the past 50 years. This remarkable achievement assumes singular importance in the light of experiences of past centuries, when man had to endure the ravages of recurrent outbreaks and epidemics of rickettsial disease without recourse and without the vaguest notion of what caused the diseases or how they were spread.

The first rickettsial disease to be established as a clinical entity was epidemic typhus fever. The history of this disease, foremost in notoriety of the rickettsioses, is a record of man's tribulations in the wake of this reappearing pestilence. Epidemics of typhus fever probably occurred for many centuries prior to its recognition as a distinct disease entity by Girolamo Fracastoro in the sixteenth century. Hans Zinsser in his book *Rats, Lice and History* provided an excellent biographical treatise of typhus fever and its epidemic exploits. The disease was an active participant, usually on both sides, in such major military conflicts as the Thirty Years War, Seven Years War, Napoleonic campaigns, Crimean War, World War I, and (among civilians) World War II. Epidemic typhus fever dramatically affected the course of military operations. In 1632 typhus fever and scurvy killed 18,000 soldiers of two armies prepared to fight before the city of Nuremberg. Both sides withdrew to escape the disease. This situation was repeated in 1643, when Charles I, prepared to march on London, abandoned his plan in the wake of an epidemic of typhus fever. Prague was surrendered to the French army in 1741 because 30,000 of the opposing Austrians died of typhus fever. Epidemic typhus fever was particularly devastating to members of the medical profession, claiming more of their lives than any other disease. In the 1741 conflict all the French medical staff died of the disease; in the 1915 epidemic in Serbia all 400 medical doctors became infected and of these, 126 died. Among 1,230 physicians, 550 died of typhus in a period of 25 years in Ireland.

Even in times of political and military peace, epidemic typhus fever continued to be a major cause of distress to populations. In the Irish epidemic of 1816–19, 700,000 cases occurred among 6 million inhabitants. The typhus epidemic that ravaged Serbia in 1915 accounted for over 150,000 deaths in less than six months. Between 1918 and 1922 estimates place the number of typhus fever cases in Russia as high as 30 million and deaths as many as 3 million. The foregoing accounts are only representative of the enormous toll of human life and havoc attributable to typhus fever epidemics.

Almost 300 years elapsed after Fracastoro's historic treatise until another significant contribution was added to the meager scientific knowledge of epidemic typhus fever. In 1837 the American physician W. W. Gerhard established criteria for differentiating typhoid fever from typhus fever that helped dispel the persistent confusion in the diagnosis of the two diseases. Not until the early part of the twentieth century was the role of insect vectors in the transmission of rickettsial diseases discovered, the etiological agents of the major rickettsioses identified, the methodology developed to advance our understanding of the complex nature of rickettsial infections. The outstanding investigations of the brilliant American scientist Howard Taylor Ricketts on Rocky Mountain spotted fever in the first decade of the 1900's not only resulted in the first description of a rickettsial agent and a definitive study of the major aspects of the disease but also signaled the beginning of modern experimental studies on rickettsial infections. His techniques, protocols, and methodology for cultivating the infectious agent in laboratory animals showed researchers the means by which systematic investigations on rickettsial diseases could be pursued. In the same decade Charles Nicolle solved the enigma of how epidemic typhus fever is transmitted to man. Nicolle proved that epidemic typhus fever is passed from man to man by the body louse. In the light of past history of typhus fever epidemics, this discovery was a significant achievement. It was now possible to alter the course or even control outbreaks of typhus fever by the simple measure of attacking the louse vector. Ricketts and others shortly thereafter confirmed Nicolle's findings and demonstrated the rickettsial etiology of epidemic typhus fever. In 1916 the Brazilian scientist H. da Rocha-Lima confirmed and clarified the etiology of epidemic typhus fever and suggested, in honor of Ricketts, the name *Rickettsia* to designate the new group of infectious microorganisms. The name was later extended to include not only newly discovered pathogenic rickettsiae but nonpathogenic microorganisms of similar character that inhabit various species of arthropods.

With rickettsiae established as a new group of microorganisms capable of inducing disease in man, a wide variety of typhus-like fevers and spotted fever infections, known under different names, were soon recognized and described in several parts of the world. The ultimate clarification of the relations among these newly described rickettsial infections involved extensive laboratory, clinical, and epidemiological investigations that sometimes spanned a decade or more. A particularly perplexing problem, for example, was the relation among such rickettsioses as Brill's disease, epidemic typhus fever, and murine typhus fever that existed concomitantly in the United States and in neighboring southern countries. Through studies of the biological properties of the isolated agents and of the role of arthropod vectors, and through astute epidemiological deductions substantiated by laboratory and field data, the interrelations existing among these infections were eventually defined. A similar situation existed in various localities in many parts of southeast Asia and adjacent islands. Tsutsugamushi disease (scrub typhus), disguised under a variety of names, existed simultaneously with murine typhus fever. The Weil-Felix reaction, a diagnostic serological test in which *Proteus* strains are agglutinated by rickettsial antiserum, aided immeasurably in differentiating the forms of typhus-like fever prevalent in those areas. It is of interest to note that whereas filtration was instrumental in establishing the etiology of virus infections, this procedure did not attain a position of similar prominence in rickettsial studies. Results of filtration experiments were often conflicting and were far less informative than the more reliable microscopic examination of stained preparations of rickettsiae.

Many of the early research activities on rickettsial infections had a practical orientation in that they were concerned with the isolation and cultivation of the infectious microorganisms, tests for serological diagnosis, and attempts to produce, in particular, prophylactic vaccines against epidemic typhus fever. The success of these endeavors was in many instances limited owing to the difficulty of cultivating rickettsiae in abundant quantities. Live vaccines were produced that conferred protection, but they were not without risk. Killed vaccines were prepared from rodent lungs, ticks, tissue culture, suspensions of microorganisms from the peritoneal cavity of the rat, and the intestines of infected lice. The latter type of vaccine has historical interest because it was one of the first killed vaccines that conferred good protection against epidemic typhus fever. When it was found that infected lice harbor a considerable concentration of epidemic typhus rickettsiae, R. Weigl in 1920 devised a method for inoculating the louse intrarectally with suspensions of living rickettsiae. His phenol-killed vaccine was produced on a comparatively large scale for human use. An effective vaccine for Rocky Mountain spotted fever was produced in ticks, but its manufacture, too, was a laborious, expensive process that was not without considerable hazard to personnel engaged in its production.

The cultivation of rickettsiae in the yolk sac of the developing chick embryo, demonstrated by Herald R. Cox in 1938, was an invaluable and timely discovery of both practical and fundamental significance for researchers. This procedure practically superseded all other methods for growing rickettsiae, and it contributed directly to the subsequent development of highly specific complement-fixing antigens and to the detection of rickettsial soluble antigens and toxins. These developments added new dimensions to the serological diagnosis of rickettsial infections. In addition, Cox's technique was a significant breakthrough for the production of rickettsial vaccines. Formalin-killed vaccines were prepared from infective chick embryo tissues for Rocky Mountain spotted fever, murine typhus fever, and Q fever. A vaccine for epidemic typhus fever produced by this technique, modified by incorporating Craigie's procedure for the separation of rickettsiae from yolk sac suspensions by the ethyl-ether-water interface effect and the inclusion of soluble antigen, proved effective in helping to lower the incidence of typhus fever during World War II. The total number of epidemic typhus fever cases that occurred in immunized American troops for the 1942 to 1945 period was only 104, with no deaths.

In the light of past wartime experiences with rickettsial diseases, these infections became the focus of increasing attention and intensive investigation at the beginning of World War II. In the search for insecticide powders to combat the insect vectors of the rickettsioses, a compound first synthesized in 1874 by a German student, Othmar Zeidler, was brought to the attention of American authorities in 1942 by the Swiss firm J. R. Geigy. The compound, dichlorodiphenyltrichloroethane, to become known in abbreviated form as DDT, displayed distinct insecticidal value. Tests conducted by a group of entomologists at Orlando, Florida, indicated that DDT was highly effective in killing lice. Confirmation of the efficacy of DDT in controlling an epidemic of typhus fever was obtained at Naples in 1943–44 in a typhus fever epidemic that was raging among the civilian population. The conditions that existed in the heavily bombed, overcrowded city were conducive to a typhus outbreak. Although immunization helped to safeguard personnel engaged in disease control measures, it was the vigorous application of delousing procedures employing DDT that checked the spread and terminated the epidemic. The significance of the events that transpired in the Naples outbreak was that they represented a milestone in the field of public health and preventive medicine. It was the first time in the history of epidemic typhus fever that a major epidemic of the disease was actually brought under control.

While it was anticipated at the onset of the war that epidemic typhus fever might become a hazard to American troops, totally unexpected was the encounter with the mite-borne rickettsial disease known as scrub typhus (tsutsugamushi disease) by American personnel engaged in military operations in the southwest Pacific and China-Burma-India areas. The disease had not been considered of great military importance, and consequently medical personnel were unfamiliar with its diagnosis, clinical course, therapy, or the preventive measures to be employed. Explosive outbreaks of the disease accounted for approximately 16,000 cases among Allied soldiers and sailors. The experience and information attained from encounters with the disease were bought at a great cost in human suffering, but they advanced our general knowledge of the typhus-like fever and the measures necessary for its future control.

Q fever was still another rickettsial disease of little-recognized importance to man at the beginning of World War II. It was first described in 1937 by E. H. Derrick in Australia, and almost at the same time in the western United States; it was believed to be indigenous to these areas. During 1944–45 more than 1,000 cases of the disease occurred among Allied troops stationed in the Mediterranean area. The case incidence was second only to scrub typhus. The studies and observations that were made during the war and the years immediately following, established the extensive geographical distribution of Q fever; it is now recognized as an important world health problem. From this brief outline it is evident that military medical authorities were justified in their concern over the role of rickettsial diseases during the war.

One of the outstanding achievements during the World War II years, resulting from laboratory investigations directed toward specific chemotherapy of rickettsial infections, was the discovery of the rickettsiostatic activity of para-aminobenzoic acid (PABA). In experimental animals and in clinical trials the compound—generally regarded as a vitamin—shortened the duration, lessened the severity, and reduced the mortality of certain rickettsial infections. A fundamentally significant aspect of the initial studies on PABA was the recognition of metabolite interference as the guiding principle in the chemotherapy of rickettsial diseases. The management of the rickettsioses with PABA was supplanted by the postwar development of broad-spectrum antibiotics, e.g., Chloromycetin, Aureomycin, Terramycin. PABA, however, still maintains a useful role in basic physiologic and metabolic studies on pathogenic rickettsiae. The spectacular success of antibiotics in the treatment of rickettsial infections is exemplified by the subjugation of scrub typhus. This accomplishment was aptly summarized in the 1951 Jubilee Volume of the Institute for Medical Research in Malaya: "Overnight as it were, a once severe and often mortal disease, centuries old, much feared by planter and serving soldier alike, had become trivial."

In the past decade and a half, basic studies on rickettsial infections have added much new information to advance our understanding of the parasitic nature of the infectious agents, while applied studies have supplemented our armamentarium for diagnosis, treatment, and control of these diseases. Investigations on the internal structure, metabolic activities, and chemical constituents of the rickettsiae have emphasized the striking resemblances between these microorganisms and bacteria. Epidemiological surveys have revealed the worldwide prevalence of certain rickettsial infections, while studies of ecologic cycles and patterns have indicated the extensive variability of relations among the infectious agents, vectors, and animal population. In some instances this has resulted in a re-evaluation of ideas on vector-control measures. With improved techniques to facilitate the growth and maintenance of cell cultures, tissue culture systems have been used to propagate rickettsiae; to define the conditions optimal for their penetration, replication, and stability; and to reveal the close relation between rickettsial metabolic activity and pathogenicity. The *in vitro* hemolysis of erythrocytes by rickettsiae and the specific sensitization of these cells by a serologically active substance (ESS) from rickettsiae are novel serological phenomena that have value as research aids as well as applicability in serological diagnosis of infections. The rapid diagnosis of rickettsial infections has been shown to be feasible by the fluorescent antibody technique. Efforts to improve the efficacy of rickettsial vaccines have led to the discovery of phase variation—the reversible adaptation of rickettsial strains. This phenomenon has been directly related to the protective potency of vaccines. The use of attenuated rickettsial strains in vaccines continues to show promise. Immunization of small groups of volunteers with a living avirulent strain of *Rickettsia prowazeki* (Strain E) has proven effective in producing durable immunity against subsequent challenge with the virulent rickettsia of epidemic typhus fever. The recent cultivation of the rickettsia of trench fever in cell-free medium adds impetus to studies concerned with the *in vitro* growth of other rickettsiae.

In the preceding paragraphs a brief account has been given of the development of our present comprehension of the nature of the pathogenic rickettsiae and the manifold diseases they produce in man. The significant discoveries and pertinent phases of research are considered in greater detail in the prefaces and papers in this collection. The decline in recent years in the incidence of the major rickettsial infections is a reflection of the development and application of our knowledge of preventive and control measures against these diseases. Even with this apparent conquest of the rickettsioses, new problems continue to arise to challenge our existing knowledge. Constant vigilance and continual investigative studies are required if effective containment of rickettsial infections is to be achieved and maintained. Hans Zinsser's admonition of three decades ago on epidemic typhus fever is relevant to rickettsial infections in general and appropriate in our present time: "Typhus is not dead. It will live on for centuries, and it will continue to break into the open whenever human stupidity and brutality give it a chance, as most likely they occasionally will. But its freedom of action is being restricted, and more and more it will be confined, like other savage creatures, in the zoological gardens of controlled diseases."*

* From *Rats, Lice and History* by Hans Zinsser. Copyright, 1934, 1935, by Hans Zinsser. Reprinted by permission of Atlantic–Little, Brown and Company, Publishers.

The Fever Called Lenticulae or Puncticulae

Our recognition of the diseases caused by a distinct genus of microorganisms, the *Rickettsiae*, began with epidemic typhus fever. For centuries this ancient disease was a world scourge. History vividly records mankind's disastrous confrontations with the pestilence. The decisive role of epidemic typhus fever in decimating powerful armies, in depopulating cities, and in altering the course of world events is ominous evidence of its devastating power. An appalling toll of human life was exacted by the grievous visitations of the disease during those periods of history marked by chaotic existence brought on by wars, famine, plague, and natural disaster.

That the disease has been intimately associated with widespread human suffering is reflected in some descriptive synonyms for epidemic typhus fever, e.g., war fever, camp fever, famine fever, jail fever, hospital fever. The word *typhus*, derived from the Greek *typhos*, meaning smoky or hazy, had been used by Hippocrates to describe a "confused state of intellect accompanied by stupor," but the term was not related to typhus fever. *Typhus* was applied to the confused mental condition of individuals infected with the contagion beginning about 1760, and thereafter the term gradually came to denote the disease.

Although there are accounts of epidemics occurring before the sixteenth century that bear marked resemblances to typhus fever, the earliest lucid record of the disease is found in the classic dissertation by Girolamo Fracastoro (Latin form, Hieronymus Fracastorius), *De contagione et contagiosis morbis et eorum curatione* (Contagion, Contagious Diseases, and Their Treatment), 1546. This distinguished Italian physician and epidemiological writer is best known to medical historians for his precocious theories on the dissemination of infectious diseases and for coining the word *syphilis* in the poem *Syphilis sive Morbus gallicus* (1530).

Fracastoro's knowledge of typhus fever, related in his prose treatise of 1546, was based on his experiences with the Italian epidemic of 1528. The portion of the work reprinted here provided the first clinical description of typhus fever that established the disease as a distinct entity. He called the disease *lenticulae* or *puncticulae* fever because patients suffering from typhus fever exhibited red spots on their bodies that resembled lentils or flea bites. Although Fracastoro's publication was antedated by a contemporary physician, Gerolamo Cardano, in his work of 1536, *De malo recentiorum medicorum mendendi usu* (The Bad Practice of Healing among Modern Doctors), the latter's description of typhus fever had not the authority, clarity, or accuracy of Fracastoro's account.

There are also other fevers, which, in a manner of speaking, come midway between the truly pestilent and the nonpestilent, for though many die of them, many recover. They are contagious, and hence partake of the nature of pestilent fevers, but they are regularly called malignant rather than pestilent. Of this sort were those fevers which in 1505 and 1528 appeared for the first time in Italy, and had not been previously known there in our time. They are however familiar in certain parts of the world, for instance in Cyprus and the neighboring islands, and were also known to our ancestors. They are vulgarly called lenticulae (small lentils), or puncticulae (small pricks) because they produce spots which look like lentils or flea-bites. Others spell the name differently, and call them peticulae. We must study them carefully, because nowadays, too, they are frequently observed, not only as affecting many at once, but also as special cases, in individuals. Instances have been observed of persons who went from Italy to other countries where no fever of this sort existed, and died of it there, as though they had carried the infection with them. This happened to that very celebrated and learned man Andrea Navagero, ambassador from the illustrious Republic of Venice to the King of France, some years ago. For he died of this disease in a province where that sort of malady was not known, even by name. He was a man of such learning and genius that no greater loss to letters has been incurred for many a year.

This fever, then, is contagious, but it does not infect quickly, or by means of fomes, or at a distance, but only from the actual handling of the sick. Though in the early stages all pestilent fevers are gentle and mild, this sort invades so very gently that the sick are hardly willing to call in a doctor. Hence many doctors have been deceived at first; they expected a resolution of the malady in a little while, and so provided no remedy against it; soon, however, the symptoms of malignant fever began to show themselves. For though, according to the nature of fevers of this sort, a moderate temperature was felt, nevertheless a sort of internal disturbance became obvious, then prostration of the whole body, and a lassitude such as follows overexertion; the patient could only lie flat on his back, the head became heavy, the senses dulled, and in the majority of cases, after the fourth or seventh day, the mind would wander; the eyes became red, and the patient was garrulous; the urine was usually observed to be at first pale, but consistent, but presently red and clouded, or like pomegranate wine; the pulse was small and slow, such as I have described above, the excrement corrupt and offensive in smell. About the fourth or seventh day, red, or often purplish-red spots broke out on the arms, back and chest, looking like flea-bites (punctiform), though they were often larger and in the shape of lentils, whence arose the name of the fever. The patient felt little or no thirst; but the tongue became foul. Some were sleepy, others wakeful, while sometimes both conditions were experienced, in turn, by the same patient. The disease remained stationary in some cases till the seventh day, in others till the fourteenth, in others still longer. In some patients there was retention of the urine, and this was the very worst sign. Few women died of this fever, very few old men, almost no Jews, but many young people and children, and they were of the best families. This is the contrary of what happens in true pestilent fevers, which chiefly attack the common people, whereas these fevers seemed to strike at the nobility especially.

Special symptoms preceded death and likewise recovery. The following symptoms were bad: if the patient suddenly felt that all his strength had failed him; if the administration of a mild purgative had been followed by an abnormally large evacuation; if, after a crisis had occurred, there was no consequent relief; for I have often seen cases where three pounds of blood burst from the nostrils, yet the patients died soon after. Again, it was a bad symptom if the urine was held back; if the lentil-shaped spots remained suppressed, or, on the other hand, broke out with difficulty or were livid and very purple; and if all or several of these symptoms occurred, death was very certain to follow; on the other hand, recovery was certain, if all or several of the opposite symptoms appeared.

W. W. Gerhard

On the Typhus Fever, Which Occurred at Philadelphia in the Spring and Summer of 1836; Illustrated by Clinical Observations at the Philadelphia Hospital; Showing the Distinction between this Form of Disease and Dothinenteritis, or the Typhoid Fever, with Alteration of the Follicles of the Small Intestine

Several descriptive accounts of typhus fever epidemics appeared in the centuries after the disease was first recognized as a distinct clinical entity. One of the earliest medical contributions from the New World on typhus fever, or tabardillo, was published in Mexico by Francisco Bravo in the work *Opera medicinalia* (1570). In 1606 Tobias Cober gave vivid descriptions of typhus fever, which he called the Hungarian disease, in his treatise *Observationum medicarum castrensium Hungaricarum decades tres* (Three Decades of Medical Observations in Hungarian Camps). He commented on the abundance of lice in infected army camps but failed to correlate their prevalence with the dissemination of the disease. Although better known for his discovery of the true nature of scurvy, James Lind also wrote about typhus. In his *Essay on the Means of Preserving the Health of Seamen* (1774), he recommended the destruction of clothing and bedding of patients suffering from typhus, or jail fever. He cited several incidents to prove the contention that typhus fever was transmitted by fomites. In general, the meager information that existed on the nature of the disease was not supplemented significantly before the nineteenth century.

For many years the confusion among physicians in differentiating typhus fever from typhoid fever not only led to inaccurate diagnoses of the two diseases but compounded existing misconceptions about the nature of typhus fever. That typhoid fever was frequently referred to as *typhus abdominalis* attests, in part, to the perplexing state of affairs. This muddle was immeasurably clarified by the studies of the distinguished American physician William Wood Gerhard. His observations, published in 1837, lucidly depict the clinical and pathological distinctions between typhus and typhoid fevers. Although the two diseases had some analogous but distinctive symptoms, Gerhard noted that they differed radically in their pathological manifestations. The characteristic lesions of the glands of Peyer, mesenteric glands, and spleen prevalent in typhoid fever cases were not to be found in cases of epidemic typhus fever. Gerhard's classic study was an important contribution to medical science, providing criteria that are referred to, even today, for differential diagnosis of the two diseases.

During a residence of two or three years at Paris, I had studied with great care the pathology and treatment of the disease usually termed, in the French hospitals, typhoid fever or typhoid affection. There is another designation for it, founded on its anatomical characters, and therefore more directly in accordance with modern medical nomenclature; it is dothinenteritis. This variety of fever, which is identical with the disease termed typhus mitior or nervous fever, is frequent at Paris, and is almost the only fever which can be said to be endemic there. Intermittent and remittent fevers are rarely seen, except amongst those individuals who had already contracted some form of these diseases in the malarious districts of France. Some slight fevers, attended with a whitish or yellow tongue and gastric symptoms, occasionally occur; they scarcely assume the form of a fixed disease, and usually disappear under a very simple treatment.

These fevers were the only ones known at Paris for some years past; but in 1813–14, there occurred a severe epidemic fever, characterized by extreme prostration and strongly marked cerebral symptoms. This epidemic was first noticed amongst the troops who returned from Napoleon's unsuccessful campaigns in Germany and the east of France; it afterwards spread amongst the inhabitants of Paris and other large cities, and was everywhere extremely fatal. No accurate description of this fever is on record, although it was witnessed by several of the most distinguished French physicians. Some of these, more especially Louis and Chomel, are inclined to consider it as identical with the prevailing dothinenteritis, but their opinion is probably erroneous, and the disease, as far as we know, should be classed amongst the forms of continued fever, distinguished by the terms typhus, typhus gravior, petechial or spotted fever, etc.

There are, however, complete histories of the typhoid fever, or typhoid affection, or dothinenteritis (all names belonging to one disease). It is one of the most frequent and the most severe acute affections observed at Paris, and has been studied with extreme accuracy, more especially by Louis and Chomel, who have both published admirable descriptions of it. The work of Dr. Louis is especially interesting, and is a model in its kind; he has analyzed the symptoms and pathological phenomena of the fever so accurately and fully, as to surpass any other description of individual diseases. The typhoid fever was placed by this work of Dr. Louis in the same relation to other fevers that pneumonia holds in reference to the affections of the chest. They are both so well studied, and their symptoms are so well known, that they serve as types with which other less thoroughly understood affections may be compared.

It affords us, then, great advantages in the investigation of the history of fevers, to begin with the typhoid, as the best known of these affections. Assuming this disease as the basis of our investigations, one great point is gained, and much greater certainty can be given to our ulterior researches, if we compare the symptoms of any fever which is little known and imperfectly described, with those of the typhoid fever, or dothinenteritis, as it is now frequently called from its anatomical lesion.

This inquiry was in accordance with a desire which I had long cherished of investigating the most common fevers in the middle states of America, where, from our geographical position, we witness the fevers observed at the northern, and occasionally those of the southern states. The commercial relations of Philadelphia are so frequent with the whole southern coast of the United States, and the passage to the north so rapid in the summer and autumnal months, that we receive into our hospitals a considerable number of patients taken ill on the coast of North Carolina, Virginia, and even Alabama and Louisiana. There are, therefore, few places where such a study could be pursued to more advantage than at Philadelphia. During the last three years of a constant connection with our largest hospitals, either as resident or attending physician, I have not lost sight of this object of study, and I have already published in the American Journal for the year 1835, some cases of the dothinenteritis as well as of the remittent and intermittent fevers.

Dothinenteritis is by no means a rare disease at Philadelphia, although less common than at Paris. In the essay alluded to, I established the identity of the anatomical characters and of the symptoms of the fever occurring at Philadelphia with that observed at Paris. I also showed that the patients were chiefly those who had resided but a short time at Philadelphia, and that they were taken ill on shipboard, or under some other circumstances causing an abrupt change of food and habits of life. They were also young persons, but few having passed the age of twenty-five years. Both these conditions of age and change of habit are observed to be essential to the development of typhoid fever at Paris.

Having once established the complete identity of a fever which is so common at Paris and so well described, with a similar affection, not infrequently met with at Philadelphia, I examined the pathological phenomena of our remittent and intermittent fevers of the severe malignant character so frequently observed along the southern coast, and sometimes occurring in those malarious parts of the country which are situated within a short distance of Philadelphia. In all these fevers, the glands of Peyer as well as the other intestinal follicles were found perfectly healthy; the large intestine was occasionally but not constantly diseased, while the stomach, and to a still greater degree the liver and spleen were invariably found in a morbid condition. If the fever proved fatal in the course of the first fortnight, the liver and spleen were softened as well as enlarged; but if the disease assumed a more chronic form, the viscera were hardened as well as hypertrophied. The latter state was the first stage of these chronic lesions which are formed in the livers of patients long affected with remittents or intermittents, and which continue throughout the course of the ascites, which is so common a consequence of these diseases. I made numerous examinations of the bodies of patients who died of the same variety of malignant remittent and intermittent during the summer of 1835, and still more frequently in the epidemic of 1836, a year in which these diesases have been unusually fatal throughout the southern states. The results of these late examinations have confirmed those already obtained, and showed that the follicles of the small intestine are free from lesions, and that the anatomical character of the disease is to be looked for in the spleen, liver, and stomach.

The bilious and yellow fevers are probably referable to the same class as the malignant remittents, but in yellow fever the disorganization seems to be most extensive in the stomach, whence arises the black vomit, which forms a characteristic symptom of the disease. Bilious fever, or, in other words, the remittent fever attended with unusual alteration of the liver and a disordered secretion of bile, is common with us. Yellow fever is rare, and occurs in an epidemic form at such long intervals, that I have seen but few cases of it.

The typhus fever, which is so common throughout the British dominions, especially in Ireland, is not attended with ulceration or other lesion of the glands of Peyer.* From the account of the lesions presented by most of the writers upon the subject, it would seem that there is no constant anatomical lesion, but that the lungs present traces

* I mean that this lesion, when it occurs, is merely accidental or a complication not occurring in the ordinary course of the disease.

of disease more frequently than any other organ. My own observation of this variety of fever was limited to the examination of the fever patients under the care of the late Dr. Gregory of the Edinburgh infirmary. This observation was not sufficiently long or accurate to enable me to do more than refer to those physicians who have enjoyed extended facilities for the study of this affection. The lesion of the glands of Peyer is now well known to the British physicians, but an error frequently committed by them is that they regard this affection (dothinenteritis) as a mere complication of their ordinary typhus, or a modified form of it. At least I do not at this moment recollect any one who has clearly stated that the two diseases are always distinct, before the publication of a note in the Dublin Journal, by Dr. Lombard of Geneva (September 1836).

It is not possible to set this matter at rest unless a series of accurate histories of typhus with detailed symptoms and pathological lesions should be published by British physicians. With the aid of a statement of this kind, such a comparison might be made as to set the points of difference between the ordinary British or Irish typhus and the dothinenteritis of France in their true light. From the information we possess, we should conjecture that the two diseases are widely and entirely different in symptoms, anatomical characters, treatment, and mode of transmission. But the British typhus seems to us to be identical with the disease which forms the subject of the present memoir, and is apparently the same affection which is variously designated typhus gravior, ship fever, jail fever, camp fever, sometimes petechial or spotted fever. The term typhus mitior of the older writers seems nearly synonymous with that of typhoid fever, or dothinenteritis, of the French physicians.

In America there have occurred several epidemics of fever more or less similar in their nature to the British typhus. Some of these were confined to the New England States, where they were often known under the name of spotted fever, and are described by North, Hale, and others. Other epidemic diseases of a similar type extended to a larger district of country and overran a considerable portion of the Middle States, causing extensive ravages both in town and country. It was of epidemics of this kind that many distinguished physicians of Philadelphia perished in different years, amongst them the professors of the University, Rush, Wistar, and Dorsey. No distinct history of the typhus fevers which prevailed at Philadelphia at different periods between the years 1812 and 1820 is on record. I mean such an account of the disease as makes its diagnosis so clear that there can be no danger of confounding it with other analogous affections. The fever was well studied by the physicians who practiced at that time, but the habit of analyzing symptoms had not been introduced, and their experience, however valuable to themselves, was in a great degree lost for their successors. These remarks are so true, that although an eminent physician of Philadelphia pronounced the epidemic of 1836 to be the same as that of 1812 and succeeding years, another distinguished medical gentleman who was not familiar by his own experience with the former disease, considered them as distinct affections, and that the one which first occurred was a low grade of pulmonary inflammation.

That the fevers were really identical was proven by the opinion of Dr. Parrish, one of the most experienced physicians of Philadelphia, who practiced very extensively amongst all classes of inhabitants in the winter of 1812–13, and was remarkably successful in his treatment of the prevailing fever. He saw some of the cases at the Philadelphia Hospital in 1836, before the disease had extended to the wealthier classes, and immediately recognized its true character.

For a period of at least ten years there has been no epidemic of this nature at Philadelphia. In the year 1827, a large number of Irish immigrants were ill of a typhoid fever, with ulceration of the small intestines, which was probably dothinenteritis, and during several successive years there were more or less extensive epidemics of remittent and intermittent fevers, occurring in the neighborhood of the city, but not often extending into the central parts of the town. Occasionally, sporadic cases of fever of a comatose or typhoid character would occur, but these cases were nearly always either some form of malignant remittent, or else they occurred during the winter months, and were complicated with pneumonia. The inflammation of the lungs then appeared as the first stage in the disease, which afterwards assumed those cerebral symptoms of stupor and feebleness which have procured for it the designation of pneumonia typhoides. These cases I often witnessed while resident physician of the Alms-house infirmary during the years 1823–30.

At Boston, in the year 1833, there was an epidemic dothinenteritis of extreme gravity and unusually fatal. This fever was well studied by the late James Jackson, Jr., and other physicians, and was proven by them to be identical in symptoms and pathological lesions with the typhoid fever of Paris. Some of the physicians of that city are inclined to regard their former epidemics as of this nature, but this opinion seems to us more than doubtful. Since the epidemic, the typhoid fever is there a common sporadic disease, rather more frequent apparently than at Philadelphia.

In the winter of 1835–36, there was an unusual number of cases of gangrene of the lungs at the Philadelphia Hospital, and but few of decided pneumonia. Several cases of dothinenteritis occurred in the autumn, but there were few afterwards. During the winter, a form of fever not commonly met with at the hospitals was observed from time to time. It was characterized by pungent burning heat of the skin, dusky aspect of the countenance, subsultus, delirium, with great stupor and prostration; but there was no diarrhea, and but few other symptoms referable to the alimentary canal. It was the disease which afterwards appeared as an epidemic. At first it was not well understood by us, was sometimes confounded with bronchitis or pneumonia typhoides, from the complication of pulmonary disease with the symptoms of the fever. These cases recovered under the use of a mild stimulating and supporting treatment, with one exception, in which death ensued from sloughing of the sacrum and gangrene of the lungs.

In the early part of the month of March, the admissions for the fever were more numerous. They attracted the greater attention from their occurring in groups of several from the same house, and almost all coming from a particular neighborhood. Amongst the very first admitted were seven Negroes, the entire population of a cellar in the lower part of the city. The symptoms varied but little in the seven cases, and upon an examination of two of the number who died, no lesion of sufficient importance to account for the symptoms could be detected.

As soon as these patients were admitted, I resolved to note with care the pathological lesions presented by the bodies of most of those who should die of the fever, examine its symptoms and ascertain the influence of therapeutic agents upon it. This research was commenced with a view to obtain more precise notions as to the character of an epidemic which has probably more than once appeared in America, and seems to be endemic in Great Britain and Ireland. It was especially desirable to ascertain if there was a real fundamental difference between the form of disease which prevailed this year and the dothin-enteritis which is always to be met with in America as a sporadic affection. My friend and colleague Dr. Pennock had charge of one half the medical wards of the Philadelphia Hospital; his observations were conducted at the same time with my own, but the autopsies and the examination of doubtful cases were always made in the presence of both of us. Dr. Pennock noted a large number of cases, and has given me the privilege of adding his collections to my own. They are the more valuable from the familiar knowledge which he obtained of the dothinenteritis in the wards of La Pitié at Paris. Our inquiries were conducted so much in concert, and our opinions as to the symptoms and treatment of the fever were so often compared together, that this memoir is in most respects the expression of the results obtained by our joint labors.

A portion of the cases were treated by Dr. Pancoast; of these I have no notes excepting such as were obtained from the registers of the wards; they were chiefly admitted towards the close of the epidemic season, when we had already procured a large mass of materials.†

Many of the observations are deficient in the history of the early symptoms, as the patients at their entrance into the hospital often did not retain intelligence enough to recollect the previous symptoms of their disease. The autopsies were always made with great care, more particularly the examination of the small intestines; but the weight of occupation and the ennui of recording results which varied so little among themselves caused us to neglect committing some of them to paper. We have, however, noted in detail a very large number, showing the nature of the lesions; and we always took great care to remark the diseased or healthy state of the organs. We are quite sure that nothing of importance escaped us, and, above all, that the condition of the follicles of the small intestine was carefully ascertained. Our mass of facts is so considerable, that many important questions will be solved by them in relation to the history of this form of continued fever. They will clear up many questions relative to the disease; for although few cases are as complete as we could have desired, the information which is wanting in one case may be gathered from others; none are deficient in all the particulars, or fail to give a tolerably exact statement of the symptoms at one period or other of the disease.

In our investigations, we availed ourselves of the opportunities we possessed to inquire into the pathological anatomy, the symptoms, the mode of communication, and the treatment of this fever, which had not

† These inquiries were greatly promoted by the zeal and industry of the resident physicians of the hospital, who were all much interested in the examination of the disease, and untiring in their efforts to relieve the suffering of patients, who always required much more than ordinary care. In the rotation of service the most arduous duty fell to the lot of Drs. Bush, Stillé, Patterson, Elmer, Frisby, and Johnson, of whom the two last mentioned were themselves attacked with fever.

been witnessed at Philadelphia for some years, even if it were the same disease as that of former epidemics. At each step of this progress, I shall compare the facts before us with those relating to the history of the typhoid fever, or dothinenteritis, and when the symptoms differ, it will be easy to draw the line of distinction between two diseases, differing in their treatment, symptoms, duration, and pathological lesions.

There is some confusion in the designations of these fevers, but it is not my intention to enter upon the discussion of their nomenclature. It is sufficient to state that in using the terms typhus, typhus fever, typhus gravior, spotted or petechial fever, I mean that disease which forms the subject of this memoir, and that by the terms typhus mitior, typhoid fever, or dothinenteritis, I mean the disease described by Louis, Chomel, etc., and attended with a lesion of the glands of Peyer.

The number of cases admitted with typhus was 214. Of this number there were 120 men and 94 women. A few cases who were at the same time in the wards, and already under treatment for other diseases, are not included, although they were afterwards affected with the prevailing epidemic, but their names on the register present only the disease for which they had been admitted. The whole number of cases is, therefore, from 230 to 250. A large majority of the 214 patients were Negroes or mulattoes; there were 147 people of color and 67 whites. The disease first appeared in the former class of patients, and always prevailed more extensively amongst them than the whites who were living in the same part of the town and exposed nearly to the same causes of disease.

The patients were taken with the fever in various parts of the city and neighboring districts, but by much the greatest number came from that part of the town which extends from Lombard street to a little below Shippen, and from Fifth to Eighth streets; this small but crowded district became almost an infected suburb. Within these limits the poorest and most intemperate of the inhabitants of Philadelphia reside. It is the St. Giles or the Faubourg Saint Marcel of Philadelphia. The filthiest and most crowded alleys offered the greatest proportion of patients. Thus, Small street and St. Mary's street, with the numerous courts and alleys running from them, contained many more sick than other streets inhabited by a population nearly as poor and intemperate, but less crowded. The different streets were not infected at the same time, thus the earliest patients were taken ill in Shippen and in Small streets, while St. Mary's street, which furnished an immense number of patients, was comparatively free from infection until a month afterwards. The disease appeared very soon in the prison (now taken down) in Arch street, but as the inmates of the prison came in great part from the infected district, it is possible that the disease may have been introduced by those who were admitted while laboring under it. Towards the close of the epidemic, patients were admitted in considerable numbers from some of the streets in the Northern Liberties, and throughout its whole course there were scattering cases from different parts of the city, and a few from the country, where there were no others ill in the house from which the patient had come. But few cases, however, occurred in the central parts of the town, where the inhabitants are generally in easy circumstances, and comfortably fed and lodged.

Classes of Persons Affected.   The first patients were almost exclusively from the poorest and most intemperate class of people, chiefly day-laborers. Such was the case with most of the blacks, especially the men, who were almost without exception in the habit of drinking freely of ardent spirits. The women were without fixed occupations, or were servants out of place. As the disease extended to the different parts of the city, people of various occupations were affected, amongst them one respectable physician, who died of the fever. The extension of the disease to those in easy circumstances was shown in the practice of several eminent physicians of Philadelphia; they had not seen a case until the fever had prevailed some months at the hospital, although they afterwards met with it in their private practice.

Mode of Propagation of the Disease.   The origin of the disease is as unknown as that of most epidemics; according to the general rule, it attacked those who were sunk in poverty and intemperance, and huddled together in confined apartments. It also appeared at different and remote points, some miles distant from the focus of infection, without the possibility of tracing any direct communication between those already attacked. There was, thus, a general cause, which extended its influence throughout the vicinity of Philadelphia. But, besides the epidemic cause, from which the greater number of cases seemed to arise, the fever was evidently propagated in a considerable proportion of patients by direct contagion. Those who entered at an early period of the epidemic came in groups together, some from the prison, whole families from the same room or the same house. About that time, I made a careful inspection of the district as one of a committee of the Board of Health, and in some instances we found houses completely vacated, the tenants being either dead or at the hospitals. In other cases, the whole or a large proportion of the inhabitants of a room were ill.

It was rare to meet with a severe case without seeing others in the same house.

The evidence of contagion at the Philadelphia hospital was more direct and conclusive. Three of the principal nurses, and about a dozen assistant nurses, besides a number of patients ill with various diseases were taken with the fever. The three principal nurses belonged, two to the wards for blacks, where there were the greatest number of fever patients, and the third to a ward for whites, where there were several cases. There was only one nurse of a ward in which many of the patients were collected, who escaped, but several of his assistants and patients were taken ill. Two of the resident physicians in attendance upon the same ward, where the patients were most numerous, were also severely ill with the fever. On the other hand, no nurse from the part of the hospital where there were but few or no typhus cases, suffered, and the number of patients taken ill in the surgical or lunatic wards was very small, not exceeding six in number. The wards in which fever patients were placed did not contain more than a third or a fourth of the population of the hospital, yet the number of cases originating in them after the first introduction of the disease was at least four times as great as in all the other parts of the building. The Alms-house and house of employment, which are separated from the hospital by a space of at least forty feet at the nearest points, furnished five or six cases, probably not more than the same number of poor in any other part of the neighborhood would have done.

The proportion of attendants upon the sick who suffered was in exact relation to the number of fever patients in the ward; thus in the wards for blacks (both men and women) and in the men's medical, No. 1, scarcely an assistant escaped. In the other medical wards a few were taken ill, and in the surgical and lunatic wards all the nurses escaped. The matter of the contagion, be it what it may, was generally mingled with the air, but sometimes seemed to be combined with the pungent hot sweat of the patients. In some cases the contagion was evidently direct from body to body. This was established by the evidence of a nurse and an assistant, both persons of intelligence, and, from their familiarity with the disease, quite free from fear. The nurse was shaving a man who died in a few hours after his entrance, he inhaled his breath, which had a nauseous taste, and in an hour afterwards was taken with nausea, cephalalgia, and ringing of the ears. From that *moment* the attack of fever began, and assumed a severe character. The assistant was supporting another patient who died soon afterwards, he felt the pungent sweat upon his skin, and was taken immediately with the symptoms of typhus.‡ The wards in which the fever patients were placed were large and well ventilated. We were at first disinclined to believe that the disease would prove contagious, but as soon as the fact was clearly proven, measures were taken to remove the patients not yet affected from most of these wards, and, if it had continued for a longer period, an efficient local quarantine would have been adopted. Dead bodies either did not communicate the contagion or its influence was easily counteracted by favorable circumstances. Both Dr. Pennock and myself, and several of the resident physicians, were engaged nearly every day during the most intense prevalence of the disease in making long and laborious anatomical investigations, without suffering from the fever.

It is very clearly proven that the typhoid fever, or dothinenteritis, is not contagious. Dr. Louis informed me that, in the course of his long experience of the disease, he had never seen a single case originating in a hospital. I have seen but one. The contrast between the fevers, in this respect, is obvious.

Age of the Patients. After childhood, the age seemed to exercise but little influence upon the susceptibility to the disease. But children were rarely attacked by it. None of the children in the Asylum attached to the hospital, where there were about two hundred, were taken ill. Nor in the inspection which I made as a member of the Board of Health, of the houses in the infected district, did I discover many children who seemed to be laboring under the fever. After childhood, the age of patients seemed nearly without influence. Thus, of sixty-six whites, there were thirty-five below the age of 35 years, and thirty-one beyond that age, and, on adding the number of nurses and patients taken ill in the wards, we shall increase the number of persons older than 35 years, or past the middle of life. The blacks give a greater proportion of young persons, although there were patients amongst them who were far advanced in years. But their comparative youth is easily to be accounted for by the large number of blacks engaged as laborers and inhabiting the infected part of the town; very few of them are old or middle-aged men. Another reason is the habit of the blacks to state themselves younger than they really are, partly from ignorance of the value of numbers and of the precise year of their birth. It would,

‡ Two other cases of assistant nurses also originated from similar contact, but as they were persons of less intelligence, I have refrained from relating their cases as they offer less undoubted testimony.

therefore, give incorrect results to include them in our estimate. The age of these patients differs much from that of those affected with the typhoid fever, or dothinenteritis, who are all younger, the disease almost never occurring above the age of 35 years; the average for Paris and Philadelphia is 22½ and 22 years. (See Louis on Typhoid Fever and American Journal, 1835.)

Sex and Residence. The *sex* seems to exert little influence on the liability to the disease. The numbers were 120 men and 94 women, which is about the relative proportion of our ordinary patients. This result differs but little from that observed in typhoid fever, where, *caeteris paribus*, men are perhaps a little more subject to it than women.

The *change of life and habits* from country to town was of no importance. Our patients were nearly all resident for some years at Philadelphia, and some had been paupers for many years; their food and mode of living remaining unchanged during that period. The disease was not, as dothinenteritis, nearly confined to those persons who had recently removed from one place to another.

Use of Ardent Spirits. The most perfect temperance did not prove a safeguard when exposed to the contagion, as was shown by the cases of two of the resident physicians and of many others. Still, as a large majority of our patients were known to be intemperate, it would at first sight appear that intemperance was a powerful predisposing cause. But the habits of the day-laborers are such that but few of them abstain from using spirits more or less freely, so that the number of typhus patients who were intemperate does not greatly differ from that of those affected with other acute diseases. Most of the women were not given to intoxication.

Season of the Year. The epidemic began in March, and continued until August. There were a few scattering cases afterwards. The summer was unusually cool, and the spring and winter cold. It was remarked, that as the summer advanced, and an epidemic dysentery appeared, the fever was changed in character, and frequently offered a new symptom, that is diarrhea, which was wanting in the earlier months.

Occupation, etc. Our tables do not give us all the necessary information on this subject, nor would it be quite correct to receive their statements. The number of patients admitted with acute disease from the better classes of mechanics was extremely small, unless the subjects of it had been reduced to poverty by previous intemperance. Most of the blacks, like others of their race, were employed as mere day-laborers, chiefly masons' laborers, and stevedores. The poorest classes, whatever might be their occupation, were evidently more exposed to the disease than those who were richer, chiefly, perhaps, from their crowded and ill-ventilated rooms, as few of them had actually suffered from want of a sufficient supply of food.

Color. The proportion of deaths amongst the black men was much greater than amongst the whites: thus, of the whites, one died in $4\frac{2}{3}$; amongst the blacks, one in $2\frac{19}{28}$. Amongst the women the reverse was true: thus, one white woman died in $4\frac{3}{5}$; but only one colored woman in $6\frac{1}{5}$ nearly. These two results would, therefore, appear contradictory, unless explained by other causes.

Age. Twenty-two patients, eleven male and eleven female, both white and colored, were admitted under the age of twenty (from ten to twenty years); of these not one died. Youth, then, was almost a safeguard against the danger of the fever, and this charmed age (from ten to twenty) was as free from the danger of petechial fever as from most other causes of death. From the age of twenty to thirty, of women there died one in $5\frac{1}{5}$, and of men nearly one in 4. It should be recollected that the largest proportion of deaths amongst the men of the age above-mentioned occurred in blacks, who notoriously underrate their ages, especially the men who were employed in occupations and under circumstances which rendered it difficult for them to fix their dates as accurately as the women, many of whom were domestic servants. Amongst the whites the mortality of the men between the ages of twenty and thirty was only a twelfth, but amongst the women it was as high as a fourth. Therefore, after making allowance for the causes of errors alluded to, we shall have but a small difference in favor of women under the age of thirty. The deaths amongst the women above the age of thirty were one in five nearly. The influence of treatment upon the mortality will be afterwards noticed.

Pathological Anatomy. Dr. Pennock and myself examined a very large number of the bodies of those patients who died of the fever. Indeed, during nearly the whole epidemic scarcely a single examination was omitted, excepting in cases where it was impracticable from the removal of the body by the friends, immediately after death, or where putrefaction supervened, as it sometimes did almost immediately after dissolution. In this large number of autopsies, amounting to about fifty, there was but in one case, and that doubtful in its diagnosis, the slightest deviation from the natural appearance of the glands of

Peyer. In the case alluded to, in which there had been some diarrhea, the agglomerated glands of the small intestine were reddened and a little thickened; but there was no ulceration and no thickening or deposit of yellow puriform matter in the submucous tissue. The disease of the glands resembled that sometimes met with in smallpox, scarlet fever or measles, rather than the specific lesion of dothinenteritis. In all other cases, the glands of Peyer were remarkably healthy in this disease, as was the surrounding mucous membrane, which was much more free from vascular injection than it is in cases of various diseases not originally affecting the small intestine.

The mesenteric glands were always found of the normal size, varying, as in health, from the size of a small grain of maize to three or four times these dimensions. With the exception of a slightly livid tint, common to them and the rest of the tissues, they offered nothing peculiar either in consistence or color.

The spleen was of the normal aspect in one half the cases, in the other half it was softened, but not enlarged, and in one case out of five or six, enlarged and softened.

Thus, the triple lesion of the glands of Peyer, mesenteric glands and spleen, constituting the anatomical characteristic of the dothinenteritis, or typhoid fever, although sought for with the greatest care, evidently did not exist in the epidemic typhus. Indeed, it was a subject of remark, that in the typhus fever the intestines were more free from lesion than in any other disease accompanied by a febrile movement. This exemption extended to the large intestine until the summer heats began, when a few scattering cases offered some symptoms of diarrhea, during the prevalence of an epidemic dysentery; and, where they terminated fatally, softening and others signs of inflammation of the mucous coat of the colon were observed.

The fact that the morbid changes pathognomonic of dothinenteritis are not met with in the typhus fever would of itself seem conclusive that the two diseases are no more identical than pneumonia and pleurisy. Although, in some respects, the two affections are analogous, and even similar, the radical difference of anatomical lesions is at least as well marked as the distinction between the symptoms. It is, indeed, singular that there should of late be a strong tendency to confound two fevers, which were regarded as entirely distinct by some of the older physicians. The prominent symptoms and difference of treatment were particularly well pointed out by Huxham.

We will now give a series of dissections in the different stages of the disease. Some of the cases are detailed at length, the notes of others are not published, excepting that portion which relates to the pathological phenomena.

Case III

Precursory symptoms five days. Disease commenced with cephalalgia, muscular and erratic pains. Fever remittent, petechiae, vibices, great prostration. Death on the fourteenth day. Autopsy. Lungs friable, patches of Peyer healthy, black blood in arterial system.

Susan C——, aged 21, intemperate, entered the hospital March 27th. She was discharged from prison last winter, and has suffered from intense cold and privations of every description. Health generally good, with the exception of a syphilitic affection manifested a year since. She had been sick sixteen days, and although she was much prostrated, her memory was sufficiently accurate to fix the date of the occurrence of the different symptoms of the present disease. On the 16th, after experiencing lassitude, loss of appetite, and want of sleep during five days, she was seized with sharp pains in the calves of the legs, extending to the knees, thighs, and intestines. On the 19th, soreness of throat, great thirst, but no difficulty in deglutition. On the 20th, intense pain in the temples and eyeballs, with vertigo. On the 23d, acute pain was felt in the lumbar region. Constipation had existed two weeks previous to the 22d, when several copious, fetid, dark alvine discharges took place. The soreness of the throat disappeared spontaneously in two days, but the dizziness of the head and the local pains have continued, with but slight alteration, until the present time.

Present state, March 27th. Large frame, embonpoint considerable; dark blue eyes, chestnut hair, decubitus on either side; expression of the countenance anxious; skin of natural heat and dry; capillary circulation of the face, which is of a violet hue, languid, color disappearing upon pressure and returning slowly. Intelligence slightly obscured; tinnitus aurium, but no pain in the head; tongue dry, thick dark coating in the center, red on the edges; teeth covered with sordes; thirst very great, desires cold drinks. No soreness of throat, deglutition easy; abdomen distended, resonant on percussion over colon and stomach; pressure causes pain in left lumbar region; bowels opened; urine scanty, of high color, voided without pain or heat. Pulse 150 per minute, regular, of moderate volume, bounding, gaseous and extinguished on slight pressure. Carotids and vessels of the neck visibly pulsating, especially those on the right side. Heart yields no impulse, but its sounds are distinct over the praecordial region, with bruit-de-soufflet over the valves.

Thorax: Percussion anteriorly, resonant under both clavicles; obscure on the right side below the second rib. Respiration on the right, blowing, with sibilant ronchi; on the left side, in the clavicular region, strongly sibilant, occasionally sub-crepitant; over the praecordial region it is feeble, with mucous ronchus. Percussion posteriorly yields a dull sound in the entire extent of the chest, especially in the middle third. Respiration is extremely feeble, except at the root of the lung, where it is rude; the voice is there remarkably clear (argentine). Respiration 30, more abdominal than costal; sputa aerated somewhat viscid; slight cough, no soreness on pressure of larynx.

The body is covered with two varieties of spots; one of a brownish-red, varying in size from a pin's head to that of a ten-cent piece, do not disappear on pressure, and covered with slight scales, are the result of a syphilitic eruption; these, the patient says, had entirely disappeared previous to present illness. The other spots, which are of a lilac color, vary from a line to a quarter of an inch in diameter; they disappear on long continued pressure, reappear slowly, are not elevated or covered by scales, and are numerous, especially on the breast. Treatment: Tr. cinchona compos. ʒj. q. b. h. Solution of quinine, grs. ij. every hour. Effervescing mixture. Blisters to the thighs until redness is produced. Sulph. morph. grs. $\frac{1}{8}$ every hour until sleep takes place. Diet, essence of beef.

28th. Had disturbed sleep last night, after taking $\frac{2}{8}$ gr. of morphia; first sleep, the patient says, since the 21st. No delirium during the night; two slimy alvine dejections since yesterday, of a yellow color, without odor. Exacerbation of fever at three o'clock this morning, subsided at eight, and was followed by some moisture of the skin, but no decided perspiration. 11 o'clock, A.M., skin warm, soft; countenance flushed, capillary circulation of cheeks active, redness reappears immediately after pressure; eyes watery, conjunctiva congested; dimness of vision, which is increased by rising in bed; hearing very dull; no pain in the head, but noise in the ears, compared by the patient to blacksmiths hammering in the head; tongue less furred, edges cleaner than yesterday, violet color. Pulse still vibratory, but firmer, 138 per minute. Respiration 20, costo-abdominal; some cough, expectoration as yesterday. Continue treatment; dry cups to the chest, blister 4 by 6 to the back of the neck.

29th. Fever yesterday commenced at 12 M., continued four hours; skin was exceedingly hot, thirst intense, desiring ice; mind excited but not delirious, no perspiration was observable after subsidence. Fever recurred at 11 P.M., but less violent than in the afternoon. Delirium throughout the night; blister drew well. This morning the skin is warm, soft, but without moisture; spots on the body and extremities are more numerous; arms and hands present a mottled appearance of white and deep rose color, which disappears on pressure and reappears slowly. Spots are not elevated; they vary in size from a pin's head to half an inch in diameter. Hearing very obtuse; eyes congested, pupils small, contracted, insensible to light; countenance flushed, capillary circulation rapid; tongue moist, violet color, some yellowish fur in the centre; no swelling of the tonsils; tickling in the throat, no pain in swallowing. Pulse 142, gaseous; respiration 30. Treatment: Solution of acetate of ammonia, ℥ss. q. h.; dress blistered surface with quinine; blister calves of legs to redness. Discontinue the quinine while the skin is hot. Diet, essence of beef, with eggs and wine

30th. Some fever yesterday afternoon, slight fever through the night, no sleep, constant moaning, but no marked delirium; had two alvine evacuations of a yellow color, good consistence, no odor. This morning, at 10:30 A.M., skin of nearly natural temperature, capillary circulation extremely languid. The spots which were yesterday of a lilac are now dark violet; do not disappear on pressure. Tongue is dry, coated with brown fur; deafness more marked. Intelligence languid; answers questions slowly, but correctly. Pulse 120, regular, small volume, extremely feeble. Respiration 15; carotid strongly vibratory. Treatment: Rub the limbs with a liniment of equal parts of turpentine and tinct. of cantharides; turpentine emulsion; small portions of brandy toddy. Diet as before. Death took place at 5 P.M.

Autopsy. Eighteen hours after death. No emaciation, great cadaveric rigidity; abdomen much distended, resonant on percussion. Body and extremities covered with petechiae and vibices as in life; those of the upper extremities and legs are of a deep purple color, especially those on the lower extremities, where they are numerous, and of half an inch in diameter.

Brain: A small quantity of black blood is found in the vessels of the dura mater; falx filled with soft coagulum, of yellowish-green color; no thickening or opacity of the tunica arachnoides; pia mater transparent, its vessels congested with black blood; no effusion of serum between arachnoid and pia mater. Cortical substance pale, medullary of usual consistence, of violet color; each ventricle contains about a dram of serum. Cerebellum normal.

Thorax: Adeps considerable over the thorax and abdomen.

Larynx: Lining membrane reddened, transparent, its consistence natural. Mucous membrane of the fauces tumid, of violet color; amygdala contain numerous cicatrices filled with calcareous deposit. *Left lung:* Contracted, not crepitant upon pressure, extremely friable. *Right lung:* Congested, especially in the middle lobe, infiltrated with bloody serum, its structure not granulated, friable upon pressure, mucous membrane of the bronchi red but normal in consistence; each thoracic cavity contains about four ounces of red serum. No adhesion of lungs to pleura costalis.

Heart: Small, parietes of usual thickness and muscular, consistence good, valves healthy; coagula in the right ventricles thin and easily broken; a few drops of black blood in the left ventricle. Aorta contains black blood with some coagula.

Abdomen: The omentum charged with fat. Stomach and small intestines distended by gas; the mucous coat of the stomach in its large curvature stellated with red points of blood; its consistence, however, is normal throughout, excepting in the great cul-de-sac, where it is softer than natural. Small intestines contain some green feces; mucous coat normal, yields by traction strips from six to eight lines in length. *Peyer's glands* healthy. *Brunner's follicles* not developed. *Caecum* and *colon* healthy. *Liver* natural size, structure normal. *Bile* thick, ropy, and of very dark color. *Spleen* twice the natural size, by six four inches, structure much softened (diffiuent). *Kidneys* natural in consistence and size. *Bladder* not distended, contains a small portion of light-colored mucus. *Pancreas* usual size, violet hue. *Uterus* natural.

Remarks: The fever in this, as in the case of Walters, was remittent; the presence of black blood in the arterial system was also observed; the lungs were much more friable and more impermeable to air. The brain exhibited a state of passive congestion of some of its larger vessels; meninges unchanged in structure.

Case IV

Precursory symptoms, anorexia, lassitude, constipation. Disease commenced with nausea, vomiting, frontal cephalalgia, sore throat. Delirium, extreme prostration, petechia on the gums and lips. Death on twenty-ninth day. Lungs friable, black blood in the arterial system. Patches of Peyer healthy.

Bush, Negress, washerwoman, aged 20, entered March 6th, 1836.

During the last winter, she, with four Negroes, occupied a small, damp, confined cellar in south Water street, near the Delaware, and suffered greatly from want of food and intense cold. Has been sick three weeks; at the commencement experienced lassitude, general debility, loss of appetite, followed on the succeeding day by nausea and vomiting. On the morning of the third day, whilst washing, was suddenly seized by violent pain in the forehead; in the evening the throat became sore, and continued so, with difficult deglutition, three or four days, when it disappeared spontaneously. Cephalalgia with tinnitus aurium, some deafness, and much thirst had been constantly present. Patient says she has slept very little, and that constipation has been constant. Ordered stimulating enema of ol. terebinth. sulph. morph. grs. $\frac{1}{8}$, every hour until sleep takes place. Bowels were opened by the enema, and patient slept after the exhibition of $\frac{3}{8}$ gr. of morphia.

Present state, March 7th. Decubitus dorsal; skin warm and dry; dark spots, not elevated, from two to four lines in diameter, cover the breast and abdomen; expression of the countenance anxious; intelligence confused, answers slowly but correctly, when her attention has been strongly directed to the question; constant moaning; conjunctiva injected; pupil contracted to a point and uninfluenced by light; pain in eyeballs; feeling of soreness rather than of pain in frontal region; no tinnitus aurium; deafness in the left ear; tongue moist, covered with light fur, edges red, papillae much enlarged; gums of a rose red color, mottled with dark purple spots which do not disappear upon pressure; teeth covered with sordes; great thirst; some soreness of the throat; amygdala not enlarged; deglutition not easy; anorexia; abdomen hard, slightly tumid, resonant on percussion over the coecum; some epigastric tenderness; liver (tested by percussion) not enlarged. Pulse 150, weak, jerking, thread-like, extinguished by the slightest pressure, constant spasmodic twitching of fingers, and subsultus of tendons of the arms. Respiration costal, short, contracted, irregular, 66 per minute (counted after interrogating the patient). Percussion of the chest, anteriorly; under both clavicles, normal; slightly obscure in the lower two-thirds of the right side, where the respiration is vesicular, but extremely feeble; on the left, respiration is expansive, with sonorous ronchus. On the back, percussion yields a dull sound, especially on the left side. Respiration very feeble, with occasional sibilant ronchi on the left. Voice transmitted near the root of the lung remarkably clear, not resonant (argentine). Soreness on pressure of left breast prevented percussion of praecordial region. The heart gives no impulse; second sound predominates; bruit-de-soufflet over the valves. *Treatment:* Dry cups to the anterior parietes of the chest; blister 4 × 6 between the shoulders; evaporating lotions to the head. Pulv. camph. grs. v. ol. terebinth. gtts. xv., in emulsion, every hour. Diet, essence of beef and wine whey. Sulph. of morphia, to be given at night, and quinine grs. ij. every hour, should the skin become cool.

8th. Took grs. xx. of quinine yesterday. Camphor and opium suspended in the afternoon. Blister to the back partly vesicated. Disturbed sleep, with delirium, hiccup and jactitation through the night. This morning (10 o'clock) expression of countenance wild and anxious; moaning, but no marked delirium. Hearing very obtuse; constant movement of head from side to side; cannot protrude the tongue beyond the teeth; tongue moist, rose colored at the point, coated posteriorly, dark incrustation, papillae enlarged; skin dry, temperature natural; pulse 144, less jerking, subsultus diminished; respiration 30, costal, no dilation of nostrils upon inspiration; urine scanty, high red color, resembling blood. Last evening had one alvine evacuation of natural color and consistence. ℞. Sulph. quinine grs. ij. every hour. Camphor julap and turpentine every third hour. Enema of essence of beef; wine. Diet, essence of beef; morphia at night. In the afternoon vomiting frequently took place, but was checked by exhibition of kreosote ♏ ⅛ q. h.

9th. Slept well last night after ten o'clock, without either delirium or moaning. (Took ⅜ gr. sulph. morph.) 9:30 o'clock, A.M., decubitus dorsal with legs drawn up on the thighs; abandoned; deafness increased; constant moving of head from side to side; twitching of lips; eyes much congested, half closed, balls constantly rolling in the orbit; speechless, cannot articulate; tongue cannot be seen, as the teeth are firmly closed and covered with sordes; lips are dry, covered with dark fur externally, internal membrane mottled. Pulse 132, thread-like, regular, extinguished by slight pressure. Respiration 36, more costal than abdominal; on the right side, anteriorly, rude; pure on the left. Posteriorly rude in the interscapular space. Subsultus diminished. Both arms swollen, slightest movement causing pain. ℞. Dress blister between the shoulders with quinine. Enema of essence of beef, with camphor, grs. x. Other treatment continued. Patient became gradually weaker, and was insensible to external impressions at 8 o'clock, P.M. Convulsions took place, and, at 10 o'clock, death.

Autopsy thirty-six hours after death. No emaciation; no infiltration of serum. Body covered with vibices varying in size from two lines to half an inch in diameter, particularly on the abdomen and thighs. Percussion of thorax same as during life.

Brain. The vessels of dura mater contain globules of black blood, separated by air, the falx contains dark dissolved blood, with some soft yellow green coagula. A large portion of bone was found in the anterior portion of the brain between the dura and pia mater. The large vessels of the pia mater are congested with black blood, the smaller are empty: no effusion of serum between the pia mater and arachnoid. Arachnoid transparent, the membranes do not adhere to the cortical substance, which is of a pale ash color, and of natural consistence. The medullary substance of usual consistence, and of a very slight violet tinge; its horizontal sections present numerous black points at the orifice of the vessels; ventricles each contain a dram of limpid serum; corpora striata and thalami, normal, cerebellum and central portions of the brain also normal; tunica arachnoidea somewhat opaque at the base of the brain.

Thorax: No adhesion of lungs to the ribs; on each side the pleura contains a small portion (one ounce) of bloody fluid (resembling blood). *The right side.* Lung compressed, permeable in the upper lobe, impermeable in the lower lobes, excepting the middle anterior portions; lower lobe is friable, not hepatized, contains some bloody serum; the bronchial tubes are of a red color, their lining membrane transparent and of good consistence; the *left lung* is condensed in its inferior portions, which are impermeable to air, friable, but not hepatized; upper lobe natural anteriorly; posteriorly, impermeable, congested and friable. On the surface of the lungs beneath the pleura are seen eight or ten ecchymosed spots of blood.

Heart: Enlarged, twice its usual size; no adhesions between the heart and pericardium, which contains one ounce of effused blood; the muscular parietes of the heart are of the usual thickness but softened; the valves natural: soft coagula in both cavities, those in the left ventricle surrounded by black blood; black blood, with coagula, is found in the aorta; the blood in the vena cava ascendens is thick, black, and oleaginous.

Abdomen: Stomach and intestines distended by gas; mucous coat of the stomach presents a dark slate color, with the exception of a space an inch square in the cardiac (cul-de-sac) extremity, in which the mucous coat is somewhat softened; this membrane is mammillonated and thickened near the pyloric orifice, and yields strips of eighteen lines in length. *Small intestines* natural throughout the whole extent except the middle portion, where are presented numerous purple spots from the blood effused into the cellular coat at the capillary extremities of the blood-vessels; mucous coat throughout natural. *Glands of Peyer* and *Brunner* healthy. *Spleen* natural size and normal. *Liver* not enlarged, fawn colored externally, softened.

I have prepared for publication a case of dothinenteritis, and one of malignant remittent, or as it is called in the southern states, congestive fever. These cases occurred during the past summer when the epidemic of typhus still continued. The appearances observed on dissection did not differ from those already described in this Journal, in the report of cases which I published in the year 1834. In the dothinenteritis there were inflammation, and ulceration of the glands of Peyer, with a diseased condition of the mesenteric glands, and of the spleen. In the case of remittent fever the lesions were limited to softening and enlargement of the spleen and liver, and inflammation of the mucous coat of the stomach.

As their publication would extend the length of this memoir beyond the limits of a Journal, I refer the reader to the cases reported in 1834. The fevers differed in their symptoms, as well as in their anatomical lesions. The symptoms of these different affections will be compared in the concluding part of this memoir, at present, and I shall consider the anatomical lesions only, which were as different in each form of fever as the pustules of smallpox are unlike the eruption of measles. The anatomical characters of these varieties of fevers are peculiar to themselves, and it is as impossible to substitute the lesion of the follicles of the small intestine observed in the typhoid fever for the pathological phenomena of typhus, as it is by treatment or other means to transform the eruption of measles into the pustules of smallpox.

We shall hereafter inquire if the symptoms are equally distinct and characteristic in these fevers, which, from an abuse of names, are so often confounded with each other.

H. T. Ricketts

Further Experiments with the Wood Tick in Relation to Rocky Mountain Spotted Fever

A milestone in the field of infectious disease is the group of classic studies carried out on the natural history of Rocky Mountain spotted fever from 1906 to 1909 by the brilliant American pathologist Howard Taylor Ricketts. His work—imaginative, direct, and comprehensive—provided the fundamental approach and methodology for modern experimental investigations on rickettsial diseases.

In preliminary studies he quickly and conclusively showed, by infecting monkeys and guinea pigs with the blood from a spotted fever patient, that the infectious agent was present in the blood and that the disease was systemic (1). This was the first successful infection of laboratory animals with a rickettsial microorganism. By direct inoculation of infective material from one animal to another, he demonstrated that cultures of the agent could be maintained indefinitely. Laboratory investigations on the disease could now proceed independent of the limited seasonal appearance of the disease.

Testing the theory of transmission of the infectious disease by the wood tick (*Dermacentor occidentalis*), proposed on epidemiological evidence by Wilson and Chowning (2), Ricketts proved that both male and female ticks fed previously on infected guinea pigs could transmit the disease by their bite to healthy animals (3). Quasi-independently, Dr. W. W. King reported similar results using the same experimental approach (4). These findings confirmed the important epidemiological principle—the transmission of infectious disease by arthropods—advanced a few years earlier by Smith and Kilbourne, based on their studies on Texas fever (5). In subsequent studies Ricketts explained the sharp limitation of the disease to spring months from a study of the life history of the wood tick and showed further that the infection in ticks passed through all three stages of its life cycle but that only the adult tick was dangerous for man. The existence of a local animal reservoir for the disease and the detection of infected ticks in nature, combined with other evidence, further substantiated the tick theory of transmission (6).

The paper reprinted here, representative of Ricketts' pioneer studies, established the hereditary transmission of Rocky Mountain spotted fever from infected ticks to their offspring through eggs; this demonstration, together with the existence of an animal reservoir, helped explain the permanent maintenance of the disease in nature. From earlier experiments which indicated that an attack of the disease in animals conferred strong immunity to subsequent infection (7), Ricketts made additional valuable observations concerning immunity to the disease, e.g., serum therapy, sero-vaccination (8). He was the first to employ serological tests with rickettsiae and to prepare a successful killed vaccine.

Ricketts is credited with describing the first rickettsial microorganism, the etiological agent of Rocky Mountain spotted fever (9). He demonstrated the rickettsiae of Rocky Mountain spotted fever in the blood and serum of infected guinea pigs, and in infected ticks and their eggs, and showed their causal relation to the disease by positive agglutination tests. Unknowingly he had not only discovered a species but a whole new genus of infectious microorganisms. Further studies by Ricketts on the etiological agent revealed some paradoxical and disturbing observations. Rickettsiae were found in the tissues of ticks that were morphologically and serologically identical with the rickettsiae of spotted fever but were without virulence. He was able to explain this enigma by surmising correctly that the rickettsiae became avirulent as a consequence of long residence in the tissues of the tick. Later, Spencer and Parker (10) demonstrated that avirulent organisms in ticks may regain virulence after the tick has ingested fresh blood. This important phenomenon, called reactivation was later duplicated biochemically *in vitro* (see paper by Gilford and Price, 1955), and it helped resolve some of the puzzling aspects of tick transmission of the disease.

Experiments which I previously reported show that the adult male and female and the nymph of the Rocky Mountain wood tick (*Dermacentor occidentalis*) are able to acquire and transmit spotted fever.

In this paper experiments will be reported which show: 1) that the larva may acquire the disease and remain infective during the nymphal stage; 2) that the virus may be transmitted from an infected female to her young through the eggs; 3) that the virus exists in both the gut and the salivary glands of the infected tick.

I. Infection of the Larva

In these experiments the possibility of the larvae having acquired the disease from the female parent through the egg was excluded by testing the females on healthy guinea pigs before they deposited their eggs, and it is to be understood that all the larvae used in these experiments came from females which had been tested in this way and found uninfected.

When from one-third to three-quarters of the eggs of one or more females had hatched, the bottle which contained them was placed in a tick-proof cage with a guinea pig. As the eggs hatched, the living larvae were removed from the bottle and placed on the guinea pig, where they were left to feed or to drop off until ready to feed. Within a few days the guinea pig was inoculated with spotted fever and the course of the fever and the condition of the animal were observed daily. When the larvae had fed sufficiently they fell from the animal and crawled up on the canvas which covered the cage. From this location they were removed and placed in boxes to await moulting and the nymphal stage, and when a sufficient number had reached this stage they were placed in a fresh cage with a healthy guinea pig on which they were allowed to feed.

It was considered preferable to carry on the experiments in this way, i.e., to infect as larvae and to test as nymphs, rather than to attempt both steps during the larval stage. The latter course would have involved serious difficulties, and, moreover, the results have a more practical bearing when it is shown that the tick, having acquired the disease as a larva, remains infective after reaching the nymphal stage.

Larval infection 2. On July 8 several thousand normal larvae were placed with an infected guinea pig (670). A large number fed, dropped off, and were isolated, and when they began to moult were placed with a normal guinea pig (717). After a period of six days the temperature of the latter rose to 105.7°F., and on subsequent days it registered 105, 106, 105.4, and 105°F. The animal was found dead on July 20, after six days of fever and twelve days after it was placed with the ticks.

The condition at autopsy was typical for spotted fever in the guinea pig. The spleen was enormously enlarged, fairly firm, cyanotic, and granular. The inguinal, axillary, and mesenteric lymph glands were deeply congested or hemorrhagic, and the surrounding areolar tissue was congested. The kidneys and suprarenal glands were enlarged and congested. The liver was somewhat enlarged. The heart and lungs appeared normal. No hemorrhages had occurred in the external genital organs. The guinea pig was a female, and hemorrhages are less constant in the vulva than in the scrotum. Cultures on agar slants made from the heart, spleen, and kidney remained free from growth. Twelve enlarged nymphs were removed from the pig and cage, and this may be taken as a fair index of the number which had fed.

Guinea pig 732 likewise was infected with the remaining nymphs, the animal making an eventual recovery.

Of the several thousand larvae placed with the infected guinea pig (670) only a small proportion fed during the course of the fever. Under the title of larval infection 7 the remaining larvae were exposed to infection on guinea pig 637, which was inoculated on the fourth day after being placed with the larvae. This animal had been used previously in testing ticks found in nature, but had not been infected, a fact which was shown by the typical course of fever which followed inoculation.

The larvae which fed on guinea pig 637 were collected and after they had reached the nymphal stage were placed with a normal guinea pig (725). The temperature of the latter rose to 104.7°F. on the sixth day and death occurred three days later. Although this is a rapid course for spotted fever, the anatomic changes were characteristic. There were enlarged and intensely congested lymph glands; enlarged, cyanotic, and rather firm spleen, and incipient scrotal hemorrhages. No gross changes were discoverable in the other organs, and inoculations of agar slants from the liver, spleen, and heart's blood showed no growth. At least seven nymphs had bitten the guinea pig. In order to corroborate this result further, a monkey was inoculated from an emulsion of the liver, spleen, kidney, and suprarenal gland. The temperature of this animal on the second day rose to 104°F., and on subsequent days registered 105.8, 104.7, 105.4, 104.1°F., and death occurred on the seventh day after inoculation. The following were the essential changes seen at autopsy: beginning hemorrhages in the skin of the eyebrows and cheeks; the whole perineum was cyanotic and showed a roseolar eruption; the lymph glands everywhere were enlarged and congested but were not hemorrhagic; the spleen was greatly enlarged, rather firm and cyanotic. No changes could be noted in other organs. The virus was again passed through another guinea pig which reacted typically and the strain was then dropped.

Still another test was made with the nymphs which remained. After an incubation period of five days the guinea pig (739) showed a temperature of 105.3°F. and died six days later with characteristic anatomic changes. No ordinary microbes could be cultivated from the tissues. At least six nymphs had fed on the guinea pig.

Larval infection 4. On July 10 about 2,000 normal larvae were placed with guinea pig 659 and a few days later the animal was infected by inoculation. The guinea pig died on July 21 and was replaced by another (688) which was infected similarly and died on August 2. A third guinea pig (714) was introduced on this date, was inoculated on August 5, and died August 14. All three animals presented the course and anatomic changes of spotted fever.

The larvae which had fed were collected and, after hatching as nymphs, 360 were placed with a normal guinea pig (726), the nymphs being added as they moulted. None of the nymphs became attached for seven to ten days, and about ten days after feeding was discovered a course of fever began in the guinea pig and the latter died in six days, showing the characteristic anatomic changes of spotted fever.

In a similar manner the nymphs of larval infection 6 killed two guinea pigs successively (731 and 751), and the combined nymphs of experiments 2 and 7 produced spotted fever in guinea pig 674, which eventually recovered.

II. Transmission of the Virus from the Infected Female to Her Young, through the Egg

On hypothetical grounds these so-called heredity experiments were performed in two groups: First, certain females were exposed to infection before they were impregnated, by permitting them to feed on guinea pigs which had been inoculated with spotted fever. This was done in experiments 3 and 5. Second, the ticks of experiments 4 and 6 had been impregnated before their infection was attempted. This course was pursued, since it has been suggested in the literature that failure in hereditary transmission may depend on the time of infection with relation to the impregnation of the female. After impregnation many of the ova begin to enlarge, and, if the female is provided with food, they become surrounded by a denser pellicle. Presumably a microbe could penetrate such eggs less readily than the more minute and more delicate, immature ova or germ cells of the unimpregnated female.

In this instance, however, the point just discussed is not an essential one, since the most satisfactory results which I obtained involved females which were impregnated before their infection was attempted. Casual observation of the manner in which the eggs mature makes it clear why the conception mentioned is to a certain extent irrelevant in so far as the probability of infection of the eggs is concerned. If one exposes the viscera of a fully developed female which is on the point of laying its eggs it is seen that only a small proportion of the ova have matured, i.e., have reached the limit of size and the appearance which they habitually obtain before extrusion. Hundreds of smaller and still smaller ova are seen in the sac as one follows it back, a fact which makes it apparent that the eggs are matured *seriatim*, the food which is found in the greatly distended alimentary sac being gradually consumed in the meantime. Hence, even in the thoroughly ripened female one finds many minute and delicate ova which apparently would be susceptible to penetration.

None of the females used in these experiments was infected in the first instance. They were among ticks which had been collected from animals and from the woods during the search for infected ticks in nature, and each had fed on a normal guinea pig for a period much longer than that required for the transmission of the disease.

If the female failed to enlarge after prolonged feeding and after the passage of abundant feces the result was considered as proof that she had not been impregnated.

It is not my intention to analyze all the experiments in detail at this time. In addition to reporting two positive transmissions through the egg, I may mention the fact that short courses of fever were produced by the larvae in several instances, without the development of cutaneous phenomena. Immunity tests are still to be made with such animals, in order to determine whether these occurrences represented mild attacks of spotted fever.

The technic was similar to that used in the experiments termed larval infections, i.e., the larvae, as soon as hatched, were placed with normal guinea pigs in tick-proof cages.

Both experiments concern heredity experiment 4, in which infection of the ticks took place subsequent to their impregnation; that is to say, the ticks were not allowed to feed on infected guinea pigs until the character of their enlargement after feeding on normal guinea pigs indicated that they had been impregnated. The rather scant supply of guinea pigs rendered it impossible to prove the infectivity of all females before the eggs were laid. This was done in several instances, however, and all which were so tested proved to be infected. Concerning the two experiments to be reported, the infectivity of the larvae is ample proof that the females had been previously infected.

The precaution was taken to perform the experiments in entirely new cages, so that the larvae had no opportunity to come in contact with spotted fever virus other than that contained in the female parent.

Females 7 and 9 of heredity experiment 4 fed on four infected guinea pigs from May 22 until June 14, and at this time they were ready for oviposition.

Experiment with female 7.   This female was removed from an infected guinea pig June 14; it began laying eggs June 27; hatching began on or about July 27. It was estimated that about 2,000 eggs were laid.

Beginning on July 30, the larvae, as they hatched, were placed with a normal guinea pig (707). Inasmuch as they do not feed for some days after hatching, immediate results could not be anticipated.

On August 22 or 23 the temperature of the guinea pig rose to 104.5°F., the following day to 105.5°F., in the vicinity of which point it remained until the animal died August 28. The following notes were made at autopsy: The lymph glands are deeply congested and considerably enlarged and the surrounding areolar tissue is congested. The spleen is about twice its normal size, is fairly cyanotic and moderately firm, resembling the spleen of spotted fever when death occurs at an early stage. The kidneys are congested and degenerated, and the suprarenals are congested and enlarged. The appendages of the testicles show a good deal of congestion. There is no enlargement of the scrotum and no hemorrhages have occurred into it. (I have stated hitherto that these scrotal changes are sometimes missed when death occurs early.) Other organs appear to be unchanged.

Agar slants inoculated from the heart's blood, from the liver and the spleen, remained free from discoverable growth.

Two hundred and eleven enlarged larvae were removed from the cage, hence this number at least had bitten the guinea pig.

In order to verify the suspicion that this animal had died of spotted fever, an emulsion of its spleen and liver was injected into guinea pig 746. The temperature of this animal was recorded as follows on successive days: 103.7, 102.7, 104.1, 105.5, 105.6, 105.4, 105.8, 105.3, 104.8, 104, and 102.2°F. Death occurred on the fourteenth day following inoculation.

Autopsy Notes: Lymph glands are enlarged and deeply congested or hemorrhagic; spleen is greatly enlarged, cyanotic, and fairly firm; kidneys are swollen and congested; the scrotum is greatly enlarged and intensely hemorrhagic, and the tunica vaginalis is deeply congested. No gross changes are seen in other organs. The diagnosis of spotted fever was made positively.

Experiment with female 9.   This female was removed from an infected guinea pig June 14; it began laying eggs June 28; hatching began about July 28. Several hundred eggs were laid.

Beginning on July 31 the larvae were placed with a normal guinea pig (710) as rapidly as they hatched. Ticks were first seen attached after thirteen days and the first enlarged larvae were removed on the fifteenth day. Ten or eleven days later the temperature of this animal rose and continued within the limits of 104.3 and 105.3°F. for seven or eight days. Following this the fever subsided and the animal recovered. Slight enlargement of the scrotum after several days of fever was the only condition, aside from the temperature, which suggested spotted fever.

Inasmuch as in some other animals in these experiments the disease had run a similar course, with eventual recovery, it was suspected that the condition represented a mild attack of spotted fever. In order to decide this point if possible, 3 c.c. of blood were drawn from the heart of guinea pig 710 during the height of fever and injected into a normal guinea pig (749). The following course of the temperature in this animal was observed on successive days: 102.4, 103.4, 103.4, 105.6, 104.8, 106.7, 106.4, 106, 104.6, 105.4, 104.4, 104, 104.2, and 103.5°F. The guinea pig recovered. On the fourth day the scrotum began to swell, and on the tenth day the swelling was extreme and extensive hemorrhages had appeared. With recovery the hemorrhagic areas in the scrotum became gangrenous, and following separation of the sloughs a deformed and cicatricial scrotum remained.

A positive diagnosis of spotted fever in this animal was made, and the diagnosis was confirmed later by a severe immunity test, in which no reaction occurred.

Approximately two hundred larvae had bitten guinea pig 710.

The results of these two experiments prove, without question, that the virus of spotted fever may pass from an infected female to her young through the egg. The practical importance of this fact will, to a certain extent, depend on the viability of the virus in larvae which have been infected in this manner; this is to say, will such ticks be infective in their subsequent nymphal and adult stages? Although one probably should not try to forecast results, the positive results which I have obtained in infecting normal larvae and nymphs suggest that larvae which have acquired their disease through the egg will also prove infective when they have reached the adult stage. This suspicion is particularly well founded since the process of moulting does not destroy the infection in either the larva or the nymph.

III. The Infectivity of the Salivary Glands and the Alimentary Sac of the Diseased Tick

I wish to report a single experiment in which the salivary glands and the alimentary sac of an infected male tick (15) were dissected out and injected separately into normal guinea pigs. Male tick 15 had been infected by feeding on a diseased guinea pig and its infectivity was proved on normal guinea pig 677.

One cannot well remove the alimentary sac without contaminating all other viscera with its contents. On the other hand, one can grasp a salivary gland with forceps near the excretory orifice and, after a little careful dissection, remove the entire gland without rupturing it.

Hence in this experiment the salivary glands were removed first and without rupturing the alimentary sac, after which the latter was removed without regard to remaining structures. The glands and the sac were then triturated separately in sterile salt solution and injected, the salivary glands being inoculated into guinea pig 683 and the alimentary sac into 694.

From the date of inoculation, July 15, the following record of the temperature of guinea pig 683 was made on successive days: 104, 102.4, 102.3, 105.7, 105.7, 105.8, 105.9, 105.1, 105.4, 105.4, 104.1, 103.2, 102.1, 102.6, 102.7°F., etc. There was eventual recovery. Four days after inoculation the scrotum began to swell and on the seventh day it was extremely hemorrhagic and enlarged. On recovery the hemorrhagic areas sloughed. The course of fever and scrotal changes in guinea pig 684 were similar, though not so extreme.

On August 8 both animals were given immunity tests with three cubic centimeters of infected blood, a quantity which contained from thirty to sixty minimum pathogenic doses. Neither animal showed any reaction to the second inoculation.

In a repetition of this experiment two ticks should be used, the salivary glands being taken from one and the alimentary sac from the other.

It seems probable that the virus passes from the alimentary sac of the tick to the salivary glands; possibly this can be determined experimentally. Indeed, since the oviducts and the eggs of the female are invaded, at least in certain instances, it is not unlikely that spotted fever exists as a generalized infection in the tick for a greater or less period. Whether it eventually becomes localized in certain organs is a question for future investigation. However this may be, the disease is often, if not always, a comparatively harmless incident for the tick.

Summary

I have established the following points concerning the relationship of the Rocky Mountain wood tick to the spotted fever of western Montana:

1. Infected ticks exist in the so-called infected districts in nature.

2. Both the adult male and the adult female may acquire the disease by feeding on an infected animal, and may transmit it to a normal susceptible animal for a period of several weeks thereafter.

3. During either of its intermediate active stages, larval or nymphal, the tick may acquire the disease in the same manner, retain it during moulting, and prove infective when it reaches the subsequent active stage.

4. The infected female may transfer the disease to her young through the egg. It is possible that this does not happen in all instances, and it is quite certain that the brood of an infected female may include many uninfected larvae. This seems to have been proved in three of my experiments in which the infectivity of the females had been proved before oviposition; the larvae in these experiments failed to infect normal guinea pigs.

5. The virus exists in both the salivary glands and the gut of infected ticks at a certain time, and since it also invades the generative organs of the female the condition is probably one of a generalized infection, at least for a period. The disease is not highly destructive for the tick.

At least two important steps may now be taken in an aggressive fight against the disease: first, a thorough dissemination of the knowledge that the tick is the agent of infection; second, a massive reduction of the number of ticks in infected districts by means now used in the destruction of the cattle tick of the southern states. Extermination of the tick in the mountains will not be possible so long as native wild animals inhabit the soil and roam the hills. On the other hand, it is known locally that the number of ticks in the Bitter Root Valley has increased enormously as greater numbers of domesticated animals have been introduced, and the latter now seem to be the chief hosts for the tick.

Acknowledgments

This work has been supported by an appropriation made by the legislative assembly of the State of Montana, at the solicitation of the Montana State Board of Health, and aid has also been rendered by the University of Chicago, and by the Memorial Institute for Infectious Diseases, Chicago.

Charles Nicolle, C. Comte, and E. Conseil

Experimental Transmission of Exanthematic Typhus through Body Lice

Charles Nicolle, novelist, philosopher, scientist, and Nobel laureate in Medicine (1928), made numerous significant contributions in the fields of immunology and microbiology. For instance, he used immune serum as a prophylaxis against infectious disease (measles); demonstrated that leishmaniasis is transmitted by the dog flea; and years before it was established, proposed a viral etiology for influenza. His foremost contribution came, however, from his investigations on typhus fever.

Although the role of lice and fleas in the transmission of typhus fever was referred to and hinted at as long ago as 1876 by C. Murchison, in 1903 by Cortezo at the International Sanitary Congress in Paris and in 1907 by Matthew Hay (1) there was no experimental evidence available to substantiate these hypotheses. The work of Mackie (2) and of Sergent and Foley (3) on the relation of *Pediculi* to relapsing fever led Nicolle to suspect the louse as the transmitter of typhus fever.

In 1909 Nicolle supplied the experimental proof that solved the ancient mystery surrounding the transmission of epidemic typhus fever. In a preliminary study he found that typhus fever could be transmitted to a chimpanzee by the injection of a small quantity of blood from a patient in the acute stages of the disease (4). This was the first experimental infection of an animal with typhus fever. Shortly thereafter, in the historic report presented here, he demonstrated that monkeys could be infected by injection with blood from a chimpanzee ill with typhus fever, and most important, that the infection could be transmitted from animal to animal by the bite of infected body lice. This latter finding was confirmed by Ricketts and Wilder (5) and Anderson and Goldberger (6). With the knowledge that the human body louse is the most important agent in the spread of epidemic typhus fever, the simple measure of attacking the vector provided for the first time a sound defense and control measure against epidemics of this ancient disease.

The study of recent epidemics of exanthematic typhus which have harried Tunisia, especially Tunis and Metlaoui and Redeyef (phosphate mining installations at Gafsa and Kerkennah islands), had led us to consider that the probable agent of transmission of the malady was an insect.

In Africa Minor (Carthage area) typhus is a consequence of overcrowding and need; it harries the poorest populations and those which are the least careful in regard to hygiene; it is not contagious in a clean house or in a well-appointed hospital. In those conditions only parasite insects of the lodgings, of the clothing, and of the body—lice, fleas, bedbugs—could be suspected. The period at which typhus epidemics appeared (spring) made it unthinkable that mosquitoes, ticks, or stomoxes had any role in them.

Several observed facts led us to limit out hypothesis to the louse. At the native hospital in Tunis the incoming patients are washed and clad with clean clothes; no case of internal contagion was observed there, notably during the epidemics of 1902 and 1906, in spite of the absence of isolation and of the presence of numerous bedbugs in the rooms. The only contagion cases that were observed had occurred on the personnel whose duty it was to collect and disinfect the belongings of the incomers. In the Kerkennah islands, which are an endemic hotbed of typhus, bedbugs are rare. In Djerid, where the disease shows itself as elsewhere, fleas are absent. These insects, however, swarm all over the galleries of phosphate mines; there they attack without discrimination both the Europeans and the natives, and yet the latter alone are afflicted with typhus. Finally, we are acquainted with two cases where, after the ordinary incubation period, typhus has obviously followed the bite of a louse.

Those observations were present in our minds when one of us succeeded in inoculating typhus to a chimpanzee (1) and after it had passed through the latter, to a Chinese macaca (*Macacus sinicus*). Thus, from the very outset of our research, we have attempted to achieve the transmission of the malady from monkey to monkey by means of a body louse.

Our experiments were done as follows:

On Chinese macaca I, which had been infected with the blood of a chimpanzee, we placed 29 lice on the 16th day of the inoculation, in the hours that followed the appearance of the eruption. The lice had been collected that very morning on a person and had been kept without food for eight hours.

On the next day and the days that followed, we transferred the lice onto Chinese macacas A and B. Monkey A was bitten for six consecutive days by 15, then by 12, 13, 8, 6, and 3 lice, and monkey B on 12 days by 14, then by 15, 13, 9, 5, 5, 6, 5, 5, 4, 2, and 1 lice. Each day after the bite, the lice were mixed and put at a temperature of 16 to 20°C.

The two monkeys A and B had previously served in experiments on Kala Azar. Both were cured at the time of their inoculation, and—an important fact—their temperature, which had been taken twice daily for the past five months (monkey A) and one year (monkey B), had never shown any thermic rise.

Monkey A. (See Fig. 1.) Nothing to note until the 22d day of the inoculation. At that date there was a rise of temperature to 39 and 39.9°C.; then the temperature fell on the 23d and 24th days. The temperature rose on the 25th day to reach or surpass 40°C. on the 26th, 27th, and 29th days. Slow defervescence on the 30th to 34th days. On the 39th day the temperature rose again; relapse of five days of duration with a classic thermic curve (maximum of 40.5°C. on the 41st day). Dead on 44th day in the morning.

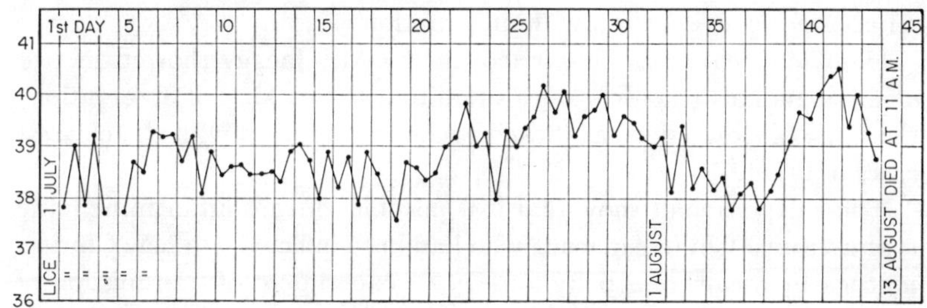

Fig. 1.

General state rather good until the 30th day; at that date there was weakness, the animal ate less, was easier to catch. No eruption. Extreme agitation during the second fever period. Violet coloration of the lips on the last two days. Autopsy showed no lesion except an ulceration at the cecum with an irregular surface covered with a diphtheroid exudate. Spleen, 8 g. The weight of this monkey went down from 1,500 g. to 1,300 g.

Monkey B. (See Fig. 2.) Nothing until the 40th day of the inoculation. On the 41st day, rise of temperature coinciding with the second fever push of monkey A. On the 44th day the temperature was 40°C.; defervescence starting on the 46th day, and on that same day, eruption. The only symptoms observed were a little weakness and a little less appetite; almost immediate return to health.

With the blood of those two monkeys we inoculated several Chinese macacas. But as we already have noted in all our past experiments, the virulence had rapidly descended. Out of four Chinese macacas

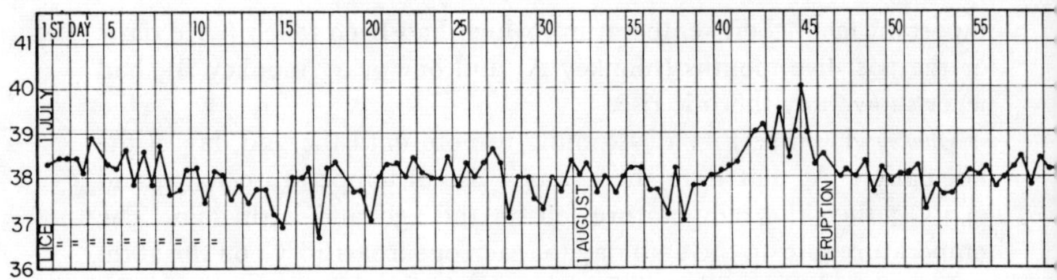

Fig. 2.

inoculated with monkey A, three (including one previously vaccinated with a virus inoculation) had an eruption; two had an aborted rise in temperature. Two Chinese macacas inoculated with monkey B showed an aborted fever reaction without eruption.

Hematological research carried out by Mr. Jaeggy showed in two of those animals (the only ones submitted to this kind of observation) the same bloody lesions as those in monkeys afflicted with the clearest cases of typhus.

These experiments show that it is possible to transmit exanthematic typhus from a Chinese macaca who had been infected to a new Chinese macaca by means of a body louse. (An experiment of transmission of typhus to *Macacus cynomolgus* with body lice collected on a patient afflicted with typhus had yielded a negative result when we tried it.) The application of this finding to the etiology and the prophylaxis of the malady in man should be made. The measures against the ravages of typhus must aim at the destruction of the parasites, especially those on the body, the body garments, the clothes, and the bedding of the patients.

H. T. Ricketts and Russell M. Wilder

The Etiology of the Typhus Fever (Tabardillo) of Mexico City

Tabardillo is the Mexican name for typhus, derived from the Spanish *tabardo*. The latter referrred to a gaily colored coat or cloak; it was a fitting but dreaded description for the rash that resembled a "red cloak or mantle" seen on patients infected with typhus fever.

Ricketts had been impressed for some time with the superficial resemblance between Rocky Mountain spotted fever and typhus fever. The epidemic of tabardillo occurring in Mexico City in 1909 provided him and his volunteer assistant, Russell M. Wilder, with an opportunity to investigate the disease at first hand. Within a short time after initiating their research they not only confirmed the transmission of typhus fever by the body louse, demonstrated earlier by Nicolle, but where the latter had obtained negative results, they were able to infect monkeys directly by inoculation with blood from a human patient (1). Subsequently, from a comparison of clinical evidence and by cross-immunity tests, they showed that spotted fever and typhus fever, although similar in certain aspects, were distinct entities. Fleas and bedbugs, often suspected as vectors of typhus fever, were shown to be unimportant in the transmission of the disease (2).

The most singular finding of their research on typhus fever in Mexico was the description of the etiological agent, reported in the paper reprinted here. Their experimental studies and observations clearly demonstrated and accurately characterized a bacillus-like organism found in the blood of typhus patients and in the intestines of infected lice as the causal agent. The promising research of these investigators was abruptly halted when, ten days after the announcement of their discovery, on April 23, 1910, Ricketts died of typhus fever at the age of 39 years.

The dedication, integrity, and sacrifice of Howard Taylor Ricketts is an outstanding model of the spirit of scientific research in the highest tradition. His investigations on Rocky Mountain spotted fever and on typhus fever marked the beginning of the modern era of experimental research on rickettsial diseases and contributed directly to the subsequent rapid progress on these infectious disorders. In the succeeding 50 years more knowledge was amassed to elucidate the nature of rickettsiae and the diseases they produce than in all the preceding centuries.

Some months ago we reported an experiment in which the virus of typhus, as it exists in the diluted serum of the patient, failed to pass through a Berkefeld filter. The monkey which received the unfiltered serum exhibited a severe course of fever after an incubation period of five days, whereas the animal which received the filtered serum developed no fever and remained perfectly well.

The immunity test, which has not been reported heretofore, confirmed the conclusion that the virus did not pass through the filter. This test, which was given about one month following the "filtration experiment," consisted of the intraperitoneal injection of 7 c.c. of diluted defibrinated blood drawn from a human patient on the tenth or eleventh day of his fever. No. 3, which had tolerated the filtered serum without visible disturbance, showed a course of high fever lasting eleven days, and preceded by an incubation period of seven days, as the result of the immunity test. The animal which had received the unfiltered serum died as a consequence, and of course no immunity test could be given.

This experiment has been repeated with a similar result. No. 19, which received filtered serum, showed no signs of infection, whereas No. 18, which was given unfiltered serum, passed through the customary incubation period followed by a severe course of fever.

Anderson and Goldberger (1) obtained a similar result.

It seems, therefore, that the evidence is sufficiently strong that the virus of tabardillo does not pass through a filter of the type mentioned. This being the case, the result may be taken as offering a suggestion in regard to the probable or approximate size of the virus. It seems not unlikely in view of its nonfilterability that the microorganism is of such size that it should be susceptible to observation microscopically, provided its tinctorial affinities and density are favorable.

Prompted by this probability, we have been engaged in a careful search of the blood of patients for the presence of microorganisms, correlating our findings with the microbic content of the organs of the body louse, which has the power of carrying the disease. It will be apparent that the results do not prove that the organism to be described is the cause of typhus, but to our minds they have a suggestive value which is sufficient to render their preliminary presentation justifiable. They may be stated briefly as follows:

1. In the stained (Giemsa) preparation of the blood of patients, taken on from the seventh to the twelfth day of the disease, we invariably have found a short bacillus which has roughly the morphology of those which belong to the "hemorrhagic septicemia group." Usually it appears to stain solidly, but on minute examination an unstained or faintly stained bar is seen to extend across the middle. Occasionally two organisms are

seen end to end. Exact measurements have not been made, but when compared with the size of the erythrocyte, their length is estimated at hardly more than two micromillimeters, and their diameter at about one-third this figure. Certain other bodies, the identity of which is not so clear, may represent degeneration or involution forms of the above. They consist of two stained granules, connected by an "intermediate substance," which is stained faintly blue or not at all. Frequently one of these granules, or "poles," is larger than the other and stained a deep purple, whereas the smaller takes a faint blue color.

2. In moist preparations of the blood of patients, bacillary bodies, with a structure like that mentioned above, have been encountered in all cases. The differentiation of the forms into two halves, separated by a line or narrow zone of a substance of different refractive power, may be observed. They possess no active motility, but vibrate more or less rapidly.

3. The dejecta and various organs of a large series of lice have been stained in a similar way and examined for the presence of micro-organisms. Certain groups had been deliberately infected by permitting the lice to feed on patients, while others were supposedly normal, having been collected from healthy individuals. Streptococci, staphylococci, an oval bacillus occurring in clusters, and certain solid-staining bacilli are encountered irregularly and indifferently in the feces and intestinal contents of both "normal" and "infected" lice. Polar-staining organisms have been found occasionally in the feces, and intestinal contents of "normal" lice, whereas they are present almost constantly, and often in large numbers, in similar material from "infected" individuals.

Protozoa have not been recognized. Microorganisms are encountered occasionally in preparations of the salivary glands, ovary, eggs, and testes of the louse. Further study is needed to determine whether they are present in these tissues as a result of faulty technic, or not.

Technic

Probably no field of microscopic research is more exposed to errors and misinterpretation than the search of the blood for microorganisms of an unknown character. We shall not at this time consider the many sources of confusion which are inherent in the blood itself, and in methods of its preparation. Naturally, we have attempted to avoid being led astray by these conditions. Accidental contaminations from outside have been guarded against carefully. Slides and cover-glasses were cleaned in sulphuric acid and potassium bichromate, washed in freshly distilled water, and preserved in absolute alcohol. The latter was removed by freshly laundered linen just prior to making the preparations. Forceps previously flamed were used in manipulating the glass. The water employed in diluting the Giemsa stain was distilled, then filtered, autoclaved, and preserved in small flasks, which had been cleaned and rinsed repeatedly with filtered water. Preparations of the blood were covered at once to avoid contamination from the air. The blood was taken from the ear after the latter had been scrubbed with green soap and absolute alcohol by means of sterilized cotton.

Frequency of the Bacilli in the Blood

The organisms described have been found to be more numerous in the blood within three or four days prior to crisis than before this period. In comparison with the frequency with which the organism of malaria and trypanosomiasis are encountered in the blood of patients, the bacilli would be considered quite rare. It is rare to recognize a bacillus short of one trip across a three-fourths-inch cover-glass, and frequently it is necessary to cover this distance two or three times. This is true of both the stained and the fresh preparations. A rough, and naturally inaccurate, idea of their number may be obtained from the consideration that 0.01 c.c. of blood made from fourteen to twenty-four smears on the three-quarter-inch cover-glass, as determined in two observations. With the 2-millimeter apochromatic objective of Zeiss and with the No. 6 compensating ocular, and with the tube drawn out to 16 millimeters it is required to traverse the preparation from 80 to 90 times in order to observe the entire surface of one cover-glass. Hence one might expect, roughly, to find from 300 to 2,000 bacilli in 0.01 c.c. of blood.

In the intestinal contents of the "infected" louse, it is occasionally necessary to search for three or four minutes before bipolar organisms are found, but in most instances organisms of this type are much more numerous in the intestine of the "infected" louse, and fifteen or twenty may be found in a single field.

It has occurred to us that the segmented bacilli observed in the blood may be identical with the bipolar forms, which are found in the intestinal contents of the louse. The differences are not greater than those which are encountered in the known organisms of this type, such as the plague bacilli and that found in association with Rocky Mountain spotted fever.

The Typhus Fever of Mexico City

Theoretical Considerations

Considering that typhus is an insect-borne disease, the first thought in regard to its microbic etiology would naturally involve an organism of protozoan character, on the basis of analogies which are known to all. Yet our knowledge of the role of the flea in the transmission of the bacillus of plague, of the tick in South Africa in carrying the spirillum of tick fever, and of the same insect in carrying the bacilli which are associated with Rocky Mountain spotted fever, should leave us without prejudice regarding the etiology of some other insect-borne disease. It seems, therefore, that our minds should be open to conviction in relation to a bacterial cause for typhus as well as protozoan.

There are, in addition, at least two features of typhus which would suggest a bacterial rather than a protozoan cause.

The first consists of the fact that typhus is an acute self-limited disease, in so far as clinical evidence can show. This condition is more in harmony with a bacterial rather than a protozoan cause, inasmuch as the protozoan diseases, in so far as their etiology has been determined, are chronic in character, provided the animal survives the initial acute attack.

A second condition which suggests bacterial etiology consists of the fact that one attack of typhus, at least in the monkey, confers immunity to further inoculations. It is true that not all bacterial diseases confer such immunity, but it is equally true that immunity is not recognized as a distinctive feature of protozoan infections.

If we may be permitted to resort to another analogy, some ground may be found for the theory that typhus is caused by an organism of the "hemorrhagic septicemia group" of bacteria. This relates to the fact that typhus actually is a hemorrhagic septicemia from the clinical and experimental standpoints, and that it has certain points which are distinctly common to plague and Rocky Mountain spotted fever, both of which may be classed as hemorrhagic septicemias. We are inclined to consider, therefore, that the three diseases mentioned constitute a group of human "hemorrhagic septicemias."

We are aware that others have described organisms more or less similar to the one we have considered in relation to typhus, but in so far as we know they are organisms which are susceptible to cultivation by ordinary means. Gaviño and his assistants in Mexico City and Anderson and Goldberger have failed to cultivate an organism of any type from typhus, and this has been our experience also. We consequently conclude that the organism we described is not susceptible to cultivation under ordinary conditions. This is corroborated by the fact that two experiments failed to yield an organism of this type from the intestinal contents of the louse.

It is the purpose of this paper to present the observations and the theoretical considerations which have been mentioned solely because of their suggestive value. It is clear in our minds that the grounds are not sufficient for claiming an etiologic role on the part of the organism described, yet the conditions under which they are found, together with the theoretical argument presented above, appear to demand that they be taken somewhat seriously and subjected to further study in their relationship to typhus.

Acknowledgments

We desire to express our obligations to the Department of Public Instruction of Mexico, to Director Gaviño of the Bacteriologic Institute, to the authorities of the General Hospital, and particularly to Dr. Escalona, for their numerous courtesies.

1910

A. Conor and A. Bruch

An Eruptive Fever Observed in Tunisia

The following selection by Conor and Bruch (1910) is historically significant because it was the first clinical description of tick-borne typhus. The disease that they described and named Tunisian pimply fever was later renamed boutonneuse fever. The latter is more descriptive because a nodule characterized by a black spot, *tâche noire*, always develops at the site of infection. Boutonneuse fever was subsequently found to be representative of a wide range of tick-borne rickettsioses that occur in the Mediterranean coastal countries of three continents (Europe, Asia, and Africa) and throughout Africa, Australia, and possibly Russia (1).

Various forms of tick-borne typhus, e.g., Indian tick typhus, Nigerian typhus, tick typhus of Abyssinia, South African tick typhus, Kenya typhus, have been grouped together under the general category of spotted fevers. *Rickettsia conori* is believed to be common to all these varieties. Cross-immunity tests have revealed that a reciprocal relation exists between Rocky Mountain spotted fever and tick-borne typhus. Although the latter is a typhus-like, febrile disease, it is immunologically unrelated to epidemic (louse-borne) typhus.

We have had the chance to observe in Tunis and in the immediate neighborhood of Tunis an eruptive fever whose special characteristics seem to us to be worth relating.

Observation I. Madame C.P., 45 years old. Lives in Tunis on an avenue outside the center of the town. On July 30, 1910, she complained of stiffness in the back and limbs and of gastric trouble. Fever appeared on August 1st and lasted until August 14th—irregular and with morning let-ups. (See Fig. 1.) There was some constipation, some nausea and vomiting, pains in the joints of the limbs.

At the same time there appeared, without forewarning rash, first on the abdomen, then on the whole surface of the body, including the face, an eruption with the following characteristics: dermo-epidermic elements, which partly faded through pressure, which were pink or dark red, and which were the size of a lentil; they were nonconfluent, leaving between them a zone of normal skin. These lesions gave the impression of minute swellings which were not noticeable to the touch; they were neither pruriginous nor painful and appeared in successive waves. There was no edema around them. They are difficult to classify in the

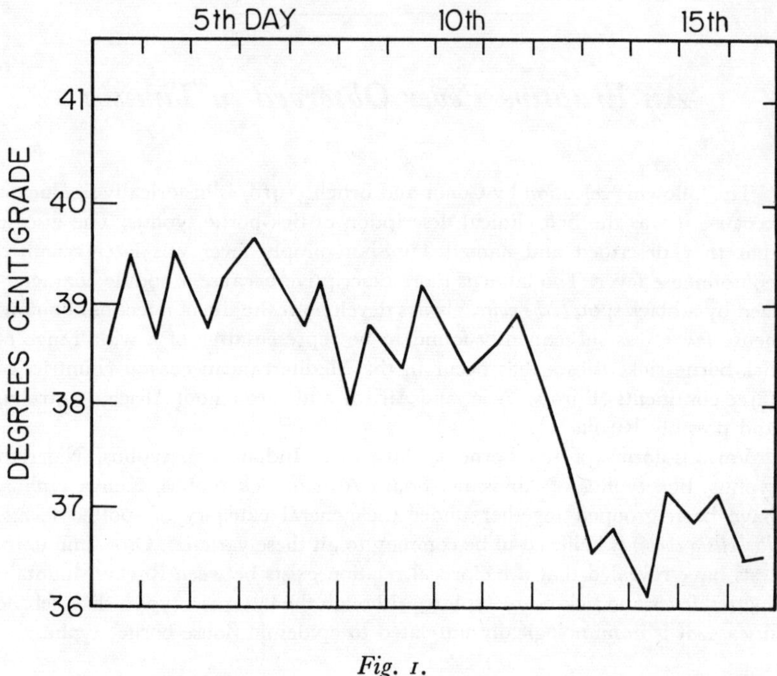

Fig. 1.

nosological framework of skin diseases. They were not spots or stains or pimples. The term which suits them best is pimply lesions, which may lack precision but seems to us to be the most exact. There was no enanthema. The leucocytary formula on the tenth day was: polyn. 52; large and medium monon. 13; lymphocytes 31; transition forms 3; eosinoph. 1; absence of hematozoaries. Negative sero-reaction with the typhus b. and *M. melitensis.*

During the fever period the general state remained very good. Slight stiffness, no headache, no albumin in the urine. During the course of a few days we noted a passing irregularity of pulse and the persistence of pains in the joints which had little intensity and did not present rheumatic characteristics.

The patient had fever until August 14th. Convalescence was short, but the eruption persisted for about a week after the fall of temperature.

Observation II. 26-month-old child, living in the Mornag plain (17 km. to the southeast of Tunis). Previous health was very good. On August 4, 1910, the child's parents noticed he was fussy, had fever, lack of appetite, constipation. On the next day an eruption appeared, with the same characteristics as the one described in observation I, first on the upper limbs, then on the whole body. A mosquito sting was noticed on the antitragus of the left ear. It was slightly infected. The general state of health remained good; no digestive troubles; the tongue was normal. The fever was irregular, reaching 39°C. in the evening. Soon the temporomaxillary area became painful, without swelling, but that pain did not last more than two or three days. At the same time the child complained of pains in the lower limbs.

On August 16th, after 13 days of illness, the child was cured. Nevertheless, for some time he remained tired and lacked appetite. Leucocytary formula on the fourth day: polyn. 42; large and medium monon. 15; lymphocytes 24; transition forms 11; eosinoph. 5.

Observation III. Miss T., 22 years old. Previous health very good. Lives during the summer on Cape Bon Peninsula, northeast of Tunis. On September 14, 1910, she dines with good appetite, but during the night she is suddenly seized with shivers and sweat. Next morning she gets up and feels better, but soon goes back to bed with shivers, fever, and vomiting. She feels stiffness, pains in the joints, especially on the left side. She dares not move, believing herself paralyzed. At the same time pimples appear on the arms, then over the whole body, including face. The fever reaches 38.8°C. in the evening. Neither constipation nor diarrhea. The appetite remains. At the beginning there is passing enanthema in the mouth and under the tongue.

We saw the patient on the 20th. The general state of her health was very good. The eruption was identical to that in the two cases already described; it was rather discreet (did not show too much), but existed on the palms and on the soles. The left eye was bloodshot. There was a slight pain in the left knee. The temperature did not go above 38°C. The patient remembered having been stung by very small mosquitoes some days before she felt ill. The description she gave made it possible to recognize the *Phlebotome*. At that time there had been a flight of those mosquitoes during a spell of wind from the East: in the area [where the patient had been] there are usually no mosquitoes. The convalescence of the patient was rather slow.

Observation IV. Mrs. C. Lives in Maxula-Rades, a small town on the seashore 10 km. east of Tunis.

On September 19, 1910, the patient is stung by a very small mosquito on the left pupil and on the right breast. The latter sting, a trace of which is still visible, was very painful. At Rades there are very few mosquitoes, and the doors and windows of dwellings are protected with iron nets.

On the 23d the patient feels tired and has fever. On the 24th the patient gets up, then goes back to bed quite soon. In the evening there is intense stiffness, shivering, sweat. On the 27th the eruption appears first on the limbs, then extends over the rest of the body and on the face. There is a slight constipation, some headache, some vomiting. The temperature, taken irregularly, oscillates between 38 and 39°C.

We saw the patient on October 1st. The eruption was very clear, generalized, nonconfluent, possessing all the characteristics described above; it extended to the palms and to the soles of the feet. The joints and the muscular masses were slightly painful, but the pains had been violent; the patient could not move without suffering and said she felt as if she were paralyzed. On October 3d there was a passing enanthema on the mouth mucous.

The general state of health was good. Nothing wrong with the heart. The patient had appetite. Leucocytary formula on the eighth day: polyn. 50; large and medium monon. 12; lymphocytes 35; transition forms 4. Temperature fell on the 12th day.

Previous to these recent cases, which were observed within a period of two months, one of us had observed three other cases, whose observations we briefly condense here.

Observation V. Mrs. W. Lives in Chaouat, 30 km. northwest of Tunis. Suddenly fell ill in October 1902. Irregular fever, stiffness, pain in the joints. On the third day there is eruption, first on the abdomen, then a generalized eruption. The temperature varies between 38 and 39°C. On the 12th day fever ceases and the symptoms gradually disappear.

Observation VI. Mrs. J.P., 50 years old. Excellent previous health. In April 1909 she was seized with stiffness, fever, stomach trouble, slight constipation, pain in the joints, slightly irregular pulse. Then there appeared an eruption similar in every point to the one described in observation I. That eruption first appeared on the abdomen, then was generalized in successive waves.

The general state of health remained good: no headache, no albumin in the urine. After 12 days of irregular fever (see Fig. 2), fever disappeared suddenly. Short convalescence. The eruption persisted one week after the fall of temperature. This patient lives in the same house where case I occurred later.

Observation VII. Mr. G., 53 years old. Lives in Tunis. Sick in April 1910. Irregular fever, suburral tongue, constipation, moderate headache,

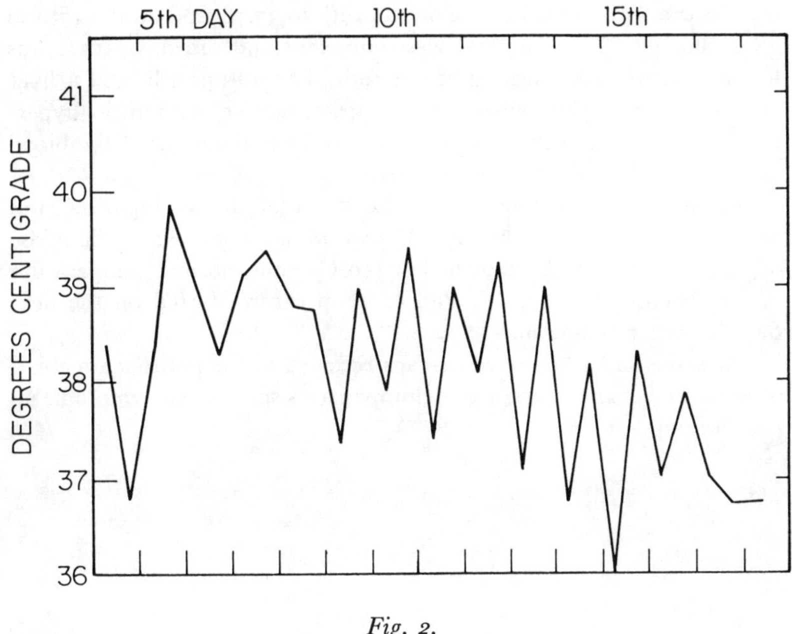

Fig. 2.

downcast, painful joints, no albumin in the urine. Same eruption as in the preceding cases, sores on the palms. The illness lasted 12 days. For two months some traces of the eruption persisted on the feet. The patient remembers having been stung by very small mosquitoes.

These observations are superposable. They do not show the characteristics of ordinary eruptive fevers, of polymorphous erythema, of knotty erythema, or of exanthematic typhus.

Without entering into the question of diagnosis, with which we shall deal later, we shall note that this malady approximates in certain aspects, but as notably differs in other aspects from, the eruptive ailments of the Mediterranean basin, such as dengue, Dalmatian phlebotome fever, phlebotome fever of India and Malta, as well as the Rocky Mountain spotted fever. We propose, for this fever, the name of Tunisian pimply fever.

We have carried out attempts of transmission to the monkeys. On August 8, 1910, we took by veinous tapping 1 c.c. of blood from the patient of observation I. We inoculated that blood under the skin of a chimpanzee that had recovered from an experimental typhus infection 45 days earlier. The temperature, which varied between 36.7 and 37°C., rose on the 15th to 37.6°, then on the 16th to 37.7°, and on the 17th to 38.6° and 38.9°. The animal was somnolent and did not eat. It was found dead on the morning of the 18th. The autopsy showed a liver afflicted with a generalized fatty degenerescence, and little hypertrophied spleen. No eruption. Cultures and examinations of the blood and of the spleen tissue were negative.

We took 2 c.c. of blood from the heart of this chimpanzee and inoculated it under the skin of a *Macacus rhesus*. There was a slight rise of temperature on the fourth day (40°C.), the normal temperature having been 39° and 39.5°. Fall of temperature started on the next day. No other symptom.

The same day a bonneted macaca received in the peritoneum 1 c.c. of emulsion of the pulp of the chimpanzee's spleen. No symptom, no rise in temperature.

1910
Nathan E. Brill

An Acute Infectious Disease of Unknown Origin: A Clinical Study Based on 221 Cases

Discerning clinical studies by American physicians contributed significantly to the early recognition and understanding of rickettsial infections. In 1898 Nathan Brill described a mild febrile disease resembling typhoid fever in which the Widal reaction was negative (1). His report, based on 17 cases, presented evidence to show that the atypical cases were not typhoid fever. In 1910 he published an account of his observations of 221 cases of the disease occurring sporadically in New York over a decade. He noted the similarity of this endemic infection to typhus fever, but he believed that it was a new clinical entity. Because the disease was not epidemic, lacked a high mortality rate, and was not associated with body lice, Brill was logically reluctant to consider it to be typhus fever. He preferred to call the disorder "an acute infectious disease of unknown origin," which later became known in the United States as "Brill's disease."

In 1912 Anderson and Goldberger demonstrated by cross-immunity tests that Brill's disease and Mexican typhus (tabardillo) were identical (2). From an article published by Brill in 1919 (3) it is apparent that he eventually became convinced of this identity. The epidemiological significance of Brill's classic clinical studies, and the relation of the disease he described to Old World (epidemic) typhus, were revealed almost 15 years later by Hans Zinsser (see Zinsser's paper, 1934).

For many years great confusion prevailed about the two diseases which are now known as typhus and typhoid fever, even after clinical knowledge of these diseases had separated them from the large group of "pestilential fevers" with which they had previously been confounded. This confusion was due to the fact that, irrespective of the lack of pathological investigation and the ignorance of the causative factors of these diseases, no well-systematized analysis of the clinical features of them had been carried on. At the end of the eighteenth and the beginning of the nineteenth centuries the first great work on the differentiation of typhus and typhoid fevers was begun. We owe to Prost (1), in France, the recognition of the intestinal lesions as the important distinctive lesion of typhoid fever. Even with the great contribution of Petit and Serres (2), who followed and elaborated on

Prost's work, showing that the lesion was limited especially to the lower part of the small intestine, and of Bretonneau (3), of Tours, that the lesion was always localized in the agminated and solitary glands of the ileum, the great acumen of Louis (4), who gave the name typhoid, and of Chomel (5), could not dissociate clinically typhus from typhoid fever. They all regarded the contagious fever of camps, of armies, and that of the English writers as identical with the disease whose lesion they so meritoriously discovered and analyzed.

Just as important as this was the work at differentiation being done in Great Britain by James Muir (6), Edmonstone (7), Hewett (8), of St. George's Hospital, Bright (9), Alison (10), Craigie (11), Cheyne (12), who were able to support the findings of the French authors, but only in a limited number of the immense number of cases at their disposal. Thus, it came about that the French pathologists rarely failed to find the intestinal lesions, for they were dealing with typhoid fever cases mainly, and the English investigators, who were dealing with much the greater number of typhus fever cases, rarely found the lesion. In 1835 Peebles (13) pointed out to Perry (14) of Glasgow, the rubeoloid eruption of typhus which he had learned to recognize in the typhus of Italy. Perry, thereupon, in the following year in a paper, correctly described many of the differences between typhus and typhoid, and showed the absence of the rubeoloid eruption in dothienenteritis, although Stewart who was present at the Glasgow hospital when Peebles demonstrated the rubeoloid eruption to Perry, insisted that Perry had maintained (even though Perry in his writings had not stated that dothienenteritis had an eruption of its own) the complete difference between the two eruptions. It was Lombard (15), of Geneva, in 1836, who was the first to state definitely that there were in Great Britain two distinct and separate fevers, one of them identical with contagious typhus, the other a sporadic disease, identical with typhoid fever, or dothienenteritis, of the French. In Germany, however, as early as 1810, Hildenbrand (16) distinguished between the contagious typhus and the noncontagious *Nervenfieber.*

To this country belongs the honor of definitely and firmly establishing the two diseases as distinct entities, owing to the epoch-making work and contributions of Gerhard and of Pennock (17), of Philadelphia. They had studied in Paris under the great Louis, had been shown typhoid there, and on their return had investigated the disease in Philadelphia, but more especially an epidemic of typhus in Philadelphia in the spring and summer of 1836. They recognized the distinction between the disease of this epidemic and the typhoid fever in Paris demonstrated to them by the master clinician Louis. These observations were published by Gerhard in 1837, in February and August, and constitute the final differentiation between the two diseases. There is no chapter in the history of medicine more interesting and fascinating than the evolution of the clinical entities of typhus and typhoid fevers.

I have utilized this brief description of the course of the differentiation between these affections because it indicates how many workers in a field are necessary to establish the entity of any disease, the difficulty encountered, and finally the doubt which arises in many minds before final adjudication removes it. Bearing this in mind, I hesitate to submit the following theme, which is based on an experience of 221 cases of an acute infectious disease which has probably for a long time been considered by others as typhoid fever, but which I hope to show by definite clinical symptoms can have no relation to typhoid fever per se, but that it has a distinct clinical entity, entirely separate from typhoid, from typhus, or from any other disease known to me. My object in presenting this study is to enlist the attention of others who may have recognized the essential attributes of this disease, in the hope that by discussion the truth of my observations may be substantiated, or what would be equally advantageous to all, the error of my deductions be indicated.

There can be no doubt that the remarkable discovery of agglutinins by the work of Pfeiffer (18), Durham (19), Brünbaum, and that of Widal (20) in establishing the practical basis upon which serum reactions can be made in typhoid fever, has made the diagnosis of typhoid fever, by their demonstration in the blood, much more easy than before the discovery. Equally important with this reaction in simplifying the diagnosis was the establishment of the fact that typhoid fever is a bacteremia and is characterized by the presence of the Eberth bacillus in the blood, more or less constant, at all times of the disease. The practical application of cultural methods to recover the organism from the blood in this disease, demonstrating its presence in over 90 per cent of all early cases of typhoid fever, has been also of inestimable service in establishing the identity of typhoid and separating it from other bacteremias. Hence it is fair to assume that the recovery of the typhoid organism from the blood has much facilitated the diagnosis of the disease.

Everyone who has had considerable experience with typhoid fever and who has studied the voluminous literature of this disease has learned that the disease is so protean and complex in its clinical picture that at times a diagnosis can only be established with difficulty. Fortunately, deviations from the usual clinical picture are not common. There is a general congener of symptoms, however, whose existence establishes the presence of the disease clinically. While no one symptom may be said to be characteristic of the disease, there are two signs whose presence establishes the disease peradventure. Fortunately these two signs are the most constant, in fact, the only constant factors of the disease: (1) the presence of agglutinins which occur in over 95 per cent of all typhoid fever cases; (2) the typhoid bacteremia, or the presence of the Eberth bacillus in the blood of patients suffering with this disease, which is constant in over 90 per cent of cases.

It would seem to me that a clinician would be stepping on very thin ice were he to make a diagnosis of typhoid fever in the absence of the roseola, of the enlarged spleen, of the Widal reaction, of the typhoid bacilli from the blood, from the stools, and the urine, of the symptoms of intestinal ulceration, especially if the fever of the infection ran but a ten to fourteen day course. He certainly would find it well nigh impossible to prove his position. If this proposition be true, its corollary may also be assumed to be true, viz., that given a disease of definite duration, twelve to fourteen days, having a most extensive nonroseolar eruption, giving no clinical signs of intestinal ulceration, with the Widal reaction invariably absent at all times of the disease, with no organisms in the blood at any time during its course, and with a fever that falls by crisis, such a disease is most likely not typhoid fever.

It may be noticed in this argument that I have made no reference to a pathological basis of the disease I am about to describe, or to that of morbid anatomy. I wish I could, because knowledge from those sources might establish the truth, as occurred with typhus and typhoid fevers in England and France just one century ago. But in my study of the disease which forms the subject of this communication, I have not met with a single fatal case and therefore can offer no contribution to its pathology and morbid anatomy.

HISTORY.   The theme, as may be inferred from these preliminary remarks, is based on a careful clinical study of 221 patients suffering from an acute infectious disease, and was begun late in 1896 and carried on since then. At that time, with a fairly large typhoid fever service at Mount Sinai Hospital, I noticed a type of disease occurring mainly in the summer and fall months, somewhat similar, but characterized by many features irreconcilable to the picture of typhoid fever, such as the course (being twelve to fourteen days), the temperature descent, which was mostly by crisis, the eruption, which was maculopapular and did not disappear on pressure, and the absence of the Widal reaction in this group.

Widal had just published the agglutination test which is now known by his name, and we began our investigations with it. What struck me forcibly was the positive results we got with the typhoid fever cases and the invariably negative results with this group which we had separated clinically from these cases. Our investigation was further carried on during 1897. We attempted to recover, if possible, either a typhoid bacillus or some other pathogenic organism from the feces, the urine, and, even at that date, from the blood of the spleen obtained by aspiration puncture, but with negative results. The results of this clinical work were published by me in an article entitled "A Study of Seventeen Cases of a Disease Clinically Resembling Typhoid Fever, but without the Widal Reaction, together with a short Review of the Present Status of the Serodiagnosis of Typhoid Fever" (21).

With the limited material of this type of disease at my disposal at that time, my judgment as to the eruption was not as matured as it is now. I spoke of the eruption being roseola and disappearing on pressure. This was a mistake which I have long corrected, and was occasioned by the fact that there may be found here and there among the spots of the characteristic type of eruption, a few which may disappear on pressure. Since that time I have constantly and persistently watched for similar cases, and have collected up to December 1, 1909, from my service and my colleague's at Mount Sinai Hospital, 221 patients with the following type of disease. The most of these I have seen personally.

DEFINITION. An acute infectious disease of unknown origin and unknown pathology, characterized by a short incubation period (four to five days), a period of continuous fever, accompanied by intense headache, apathy, and prostration, a profuse and extensive erythematous maculopapular eruption, all of about two weeks' duration, whereupon the fever abruptly ceases either by crisis within a few hours or by rapid lysis within three days, when all symptoms disappear.

GENERAL DESCRIPTION. After a period of three or four days, during which the patient suffers from malaise, loss of appetite, nausea, and slight headache, the disease begins rather abruptly, many times with a chill or chilly sensation. This is followed occasionally by vomiting, by general body pains or pain in the back; epistaxis sometimes occurs. The headache now becomes intense and apathy and prostration supervene with the rapidly rising temperature. The fever reaches its height in two to three days, when it remains constant thereafter, the temperature showing but slight diurnal remissions. During the fastigium of the fever the patient lies very quietly, sometimes moaning or groaning, with facial expressions of pain shown by the contracted and furrowed brow. His eyes are dull and suffused, his conjunctivae congested, and his face, especially over the malar prominences, flushed. He is rather drowsy, his sensorium dulled, and he resents being disturbed by more marked expressions of pain; any attempt to move him increases his headache. The tongue is usually coated and moist, only occasionally is it dry and furred. The skin of the body feels hot and dry. The headache remains intense without diminishing in severity, and about the sixth day a rash appears. The eruption is found over the abdomen and back, and quickly spreads to the thorax and to the arms and thighs and occasionally to the neck, forearms, hands, legs, and feet. I have seen the whole body, even including the palms and soles, excepting the face, covered by the eruption. The rash is dull red in color, very slightly raised, and when subjected to pressure does not disappear. The individual spots on pressure fade slightly in color, and only very rarely can they be obliterated, but return to their florid efflorescence as soon as pressure is removed. The bowels are obstinately constipated, as a rule, and in many cases can only be moved by laxative agents. The pulse is full, rather slow, not nearly as rapid as might be expected with the pyrexia. It is soft and of low tension and often dicrotic. These symptoms remain in full development until about the twelfth day, when the fever abruptly disappears, the patient's temperature suddenly dropping in a few hours to normal, the rash fades, the headache leaves, the apathy and prostration vanish, and the patient feels perfectly well, taking an interest in his surroundings. A rapid convalescence follows. During the progress of the disease slight emaciation may develop, but rarely very marked. The urine is scanty, high colored, and at times contains albumin. Delirium is only exceptionally noticed, and then only at night in the patients with hyperpyrexia. A few patients show rigidity of the neck, and the presence in them of the Kernig sign may be elicited.

Etiology and Analysis of Symptoms. I have selected the histories of the last 50 cases of my series, chiefly because these histories were readily accessible and because I have had the symptoms tabulated for the purpose of comparative study. These 50 cases have come under my observation since June, 1906, and extend to December 1, 1909.

Sex. Males show a greater tendency to be affected than females. There were 34 males and 16 females.

An Infectious Disease of Unknown Origin

Nativity. Inasmuch as the largest number of patients at Mount Sinai Hospital are Russians, Russia leads the list of cases with 30; Austria, 12; United States, 2; Ireland, 2; Germany, 1; not noted, 1.

Month. By far the largest number of cases occur in the summer months. Of this group there were 1 in January, 3 in February, 3 in March, none in April, 3 in May, 8 in June, 8 in July, 2 in August, 6 in September, 11 in October, 3 in November, and 2 in December.

Age. The disease is most common between the twentieth and fortieth years of life. In this group 33 appeared in that period: First to second decade, 9 cases; second to third decade, 19 cases; third to fourth decade, 14 cases; fourth to fifth decade, 4 cases; fifth to sixth decade, 2 cases; sixth to seventh decade, 2 cases. The youngest patient of this group was aged seventeen years, the oldest was sixty-five years.

Contagion. I can find no evidence of the disease being directly communicable. In the 221 cases we have not had, so far as I can learn, two members * of the same family, nor two from the same household or same house. The patients are admitted into the general wards, and the disease has never been communicated to any other occupant of that ward; nor has the disease ever arisen among the patients in the hospital. One of the nurses of the Training School who, in December, 1896, went through a severe typhoid fever infection, was attacked six months later with this disease, though at that time there was no other case of this disease in the hospital or training school. She was the only person I have seen developing the disease within the hospital.

Food Poisoning. It might be asked whether the disease has any relation to the ingestion of certain foods or to the toxins contained in decomposing food. The prima facie evidence seems to be against this view, for, if such were the cause, the disease would necessarily be widespread in special districts and affect many in a single family; secondly, the infection is not confined to any race, even though some races eat certain articles of food proscribed by others. We have found the infections in Germans, Americans, Austrians, and in the Celtic race. There is no analogy between this affection and the group of meat-poisoning cases known as botulism, and which seem to be due to the special organism of the Gärtner group—*Bacillus enteritidis* group. This group has the quality of interagglutinating, and its bacilli are often agglutinated by typhoid serum. In our examinations no such agglutination

* Since this was written I have had the opportunity to see at Bellevue Hospital, through the courtesy of Dr. Warren Coleman, four members of one family who were attacked almost simultaneously with this disease.

could be obtained. It seems highly improbable that a constantly definite and distinct type of disease, with unvarying type of eruption, running a definite course, subsiding at a definite period, and showing the character of this disease, could be due to a chemical ptomaine rather than to an infectious organized agent.

Incubation. The period before the acute symptoms begin varies in duration from sudden onset without premonitory symptoms to fourteen days. In 15 of this group of 50 cases the incubation period could not be ascertained, in 35 it varied from a few hours to fourteen days. The average of this stage of the disease was four and eight-tenths days. During it the patient suffered with malaise, fatigue, anorexia, constipation, dull feeling in the head or a distinct headache. Sometimes he complains of nausea and indigestion and painful sensations over the body. After this stage the disease in its intensity may be said to begin.

Onset. This may be sudden, when it is marked by a distinct chill, or chilly sensation, with increased general body pains or pains in the back, by nausea, and sometimes by vomiting. Now the headache becomes intense. Or the onset may be gradual, when it cannot be separated from the incubation period. In the latter case only the development of the fever and the increasing headache permit one to define this stage of the disease. In 19 cases the onset was sudden; in 31 the disease began gradually.

Epistaxis. While it occasionally occurs, is not common. It was noted during the course of the disease in three cases.

Headache. This is one of the most pronounced features of the disease and is almost invariably present. It may start in with the incubation or it may not appear until the onset. It becomes intense and at times agonizing, and in severity is only equalled by the headache of a meningitis, of a cerebral tumor, or the head pains occasionally present with syphilis. It lasts, as a rule, in all of its intensity throughout the disease, and then only disappears with the crisis. In the latter respect it differs from the headache of typhoid fever, which, as is well known, diminishes in intensity in the second week of that disease and is then no longer the chief subject of the patient's complaints. In this disease the headache is much more severe, and it lasts throughout its course until convalescence begins. The headache is general and is not confined to any locality of the head, being as severe in the occiput as in the frontal and temporal regions. In the cases in which the headache is most intense rigidity of the neck is sometimes observed; when the latter is present, a distinct bilateral Kernig sign may be observed. Rigidity of the neck and Kernig's sign were noted in four patients of this group. Lumbar puncture was made in these four patients, and the cerebrospinal fluid was examined culturally and cytologically. The growth was sterile in all, and the proportion of lymphocytes was slightly increased. The headache was agonizing in 8, intense in 33, and moderate in 9. With rigidity of the neck, there may be contracted pupils and, rarely, muscular twitchings and active reflexes.

Facies.   The patients suffering with this disease look sick, much more so than a patient in the corresponding period of typhoid fever. The face is flushed, especially deeply over the malar prominences, the flush being, sometimes, not noted about the nose and mouth, which then may look unusually pale. The conjunctivae are congested, the eyes suffused and later may become dull in expression. The forehead is wrinkled and the brows drawn together giving the expression of headache with which they suffer. The attitude in bed is generally relaxed, the patient being inordinately quiet. He does not toss about, as motion increases the headache. He resents being disturbed, and responds with reluctance to questions. He utters moans and groans and points to his head when asked where he suffers. It would seem to me that the physical relaxation and the indifference shown to the examiner represent an apathy which is only disturbed by an attempt to move him. This apathy is marked in most of the cases. In 6 of our group it was extreme, it was marked in 17, and absent in 12. In 15 the condition was not recorded.

Prostration.   There can be no doubt, after one has seen a few of these patients, that this symptom is a striking one. It is marked by the general muscular relaxation, the posture of the patient in the bed, the indifference of the patient to his surroundings, and his lessened ability to move. It usually corresponds in intensity with the intensity of the infection, and is more marked with patients showing a hyperpyrexia than in the milder cases of the disease.

Skin.   During the course of the disease the skin is hot and dry. Between the fifth and seventh day of the disease a maculopapular eruption appears, first on the back and abdomen and then over the trunk. The rash may spread rapidly, and in a great number of cases the arms and thighs may be covered. In a few cases the eruption involves, in addition, the neck, forearms, hands, legs, and feet, even exceptionally the palms and soles. At times the eruption is more profuse on the extremities than on the trunk. The eruption does not appear in crops, as in typhoid, but the spots appear synchronously over the area of the body which they invade. Each spot lasts throughout the rest of the course of the disease. It is noticeable that the rash is the most profuse when the attack is most severe. The spots are distinctly maculopapular, are only slightly raised and may be designated as an erythema. They are dull red in color. They vary in size from two to four millimeters, and uneven in contour, and are irregularly round or oval, their periphery being commonly diffuse and indistinct. If subjected to pressure they do not disappear, but fade slightly. This is best tested by pressing them with and under a glass microscopic slide, when all gradations of pressure effects may be observed. The eruption is more nearly morbiliform or rubeoloid than roseolar. In three of this group the eruption in places was distinctly petechial, suggesting a typhus fever eruption more than any other eruption.

From this description it may be seen that the eruption in no respect resembles that of typhoid fever, the eruption of which is characteristically papular, circumscribed and lenticular, appears in crops, very rarely involves the extremities, is never more profuse on the extremities than on the trunk, has never to my knowledge been observed to attack the palms and soles, and almost always disappears completely on pressure excepting in hemorrhagic typhoid fever. The eruption of typhoid fever consists of hyperemic spots; in this disease it is distinctly erythematous, some of the capillary contents escaping into the surrounding tissues, leaving a more or less permanent zone which pressure cannot remove. I have looked for the subcuticular mottling of typhus, but have never observed it in these cases.

The eruption does not begin to fade until the crisis, then it rapidly becomes paler, and in two days thereafter only dirty yellowish-brown stains mark the site of the former spots. When petechiae are present, the punctate hemorrhages disappear much more slowly. The rash is not nearly as discrete as it is in typhoid, for two or more spots frequently coalesce, a condition which is commonly seen. I have never observed the eruption on the face, but have seen it occasionally extend up the sides of the neck, involving the skin over the mastoids and even the back of the ear. Contrary to the typhoid eruption, which, as a rule, is not abundant, but occurs in varying crops of ten to twenty in number, this is, as a rule, an abundant eruption. In our series the following was the distribution of the eruption: abdomen, chest, and back, 13 cases; abdomen, chest, back, arms, and thighs, 22 cases; abdomen, chest, back, arms, thighs, forearms, and legs, 9 cases. Distribution not noted, 6 cases.

Of those with profuse rash involving the forearms and legs—9 in number—the eruption was observed on the palms and soles in 4, and on the neck in 3 cases.

Herpes.   Labial herpes was noted as an accompaniment in 3 out of the 50 cases.

Pulse.   The pulse rate, considering the fever, is not very high; it averages between 86 and 100 beats per minute. It is full, soft, and of low tension. Dicrotism is not infrequently observed.

Temperature.   The course of the fever is rather distinctive. The patients' temperature begins to rise at the onset, usually three or four days after the stage of incubation, and then with rapid strides, so that on the second or third day from the onset it may have reached its fastigium. It then averages between 103.6 and 104.2°F. It is but slightly higher in the evenings, and continues high throughout the rest of the disease. The remissions between morning and evening seldom exceed 1°F. With the exception of these remissions the temperature remains constantly and uniformly high until the day before the critical fall, when a precritical rise may occur. In four of these 50 cases a precritical rise between 105 and 106°F. was observed. The precritical rise, however, is not the rule and only occasionally occurs. On the twelfth to the fourteenth day the temperature begins to drop. The fall is quick and abrupt, and in some of our cases within ten hours from 105°F. to normal. The critical fall occurs in a large number of the cases. In also a fair proportion of the group the temperature falls by rapid lysis (Figs. 1, 2, and 3). In this connection we have assumed as a standard by which judgment may be expressed the following: a crisis to be a fall in temperature to normal within twenty-four hours; rapid lysis to be a fall to normal in forty-eight hours; and lysis to be a fall to the normal within seventy-two hours. As a rule, after the fall, whether by crisis, rapid lysis, or lysis, the temperature does not rise again. Exceptionally a short rise, lasting but a few hours or a day thereafter, was observed. The most remarkable feature of this disease is that with the fall in fever all the signs clear up, and the patient, who may have felt and looked very sick, becomes alert, interested in his surroundings, and says he is well; the headache is dispelled, as if by magic; the eruption rapidly fades, and convalescence is established. In this group there was a critical fall in 16 cases, a fall by rapid lysis (less than forty-eight hours) in 17 cases, a fall by lysis in 17 cases. I have not seen a single patient whose temperature took more than sixty hours to fall to the normal, excepting with a complication.

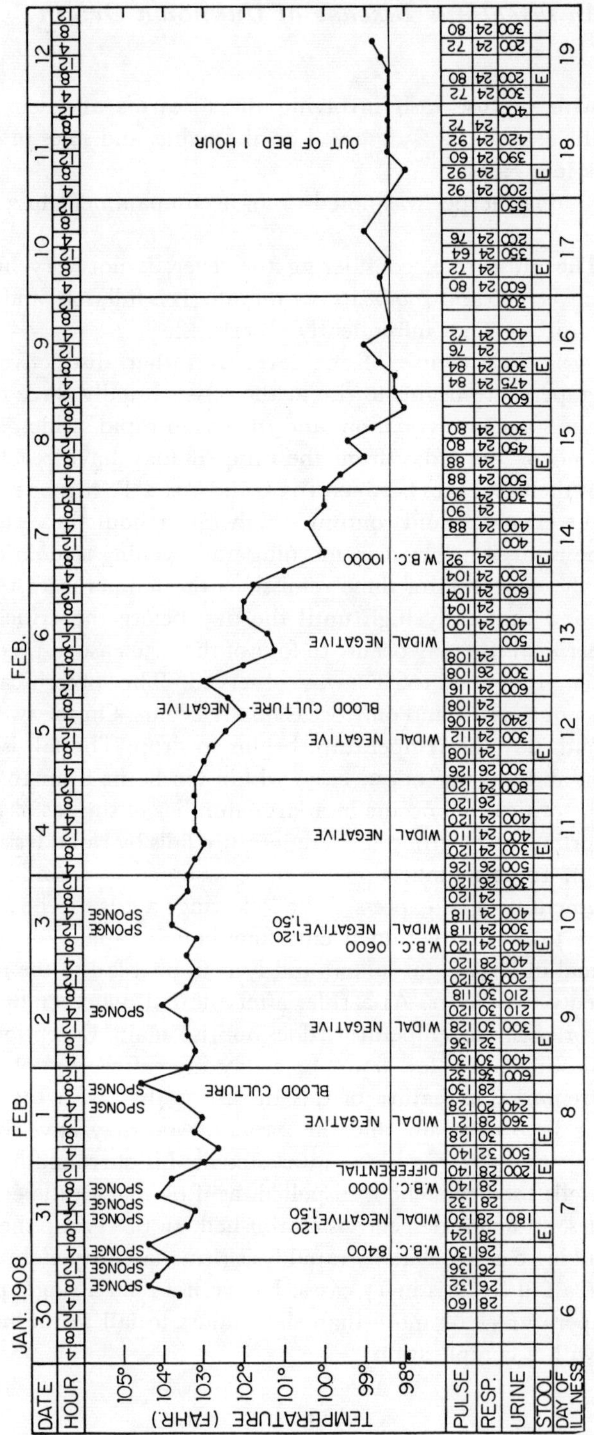

Fig. 1. The temperature record, showing a fall by lysis within sixty hours, beginning on the thirteenth day.

Eyes. In 28 cases the eyes were suffused and the conjunctivae congested; in 18 they were not affected; the condition was not noted in 4.

Tongue. The tongue is at first moist and coated with a white fur, the tip and sides remaining red. This condition may last throughout the disease, although in some of the cases with hyperpyrexia the tongue becomes dry and brown.

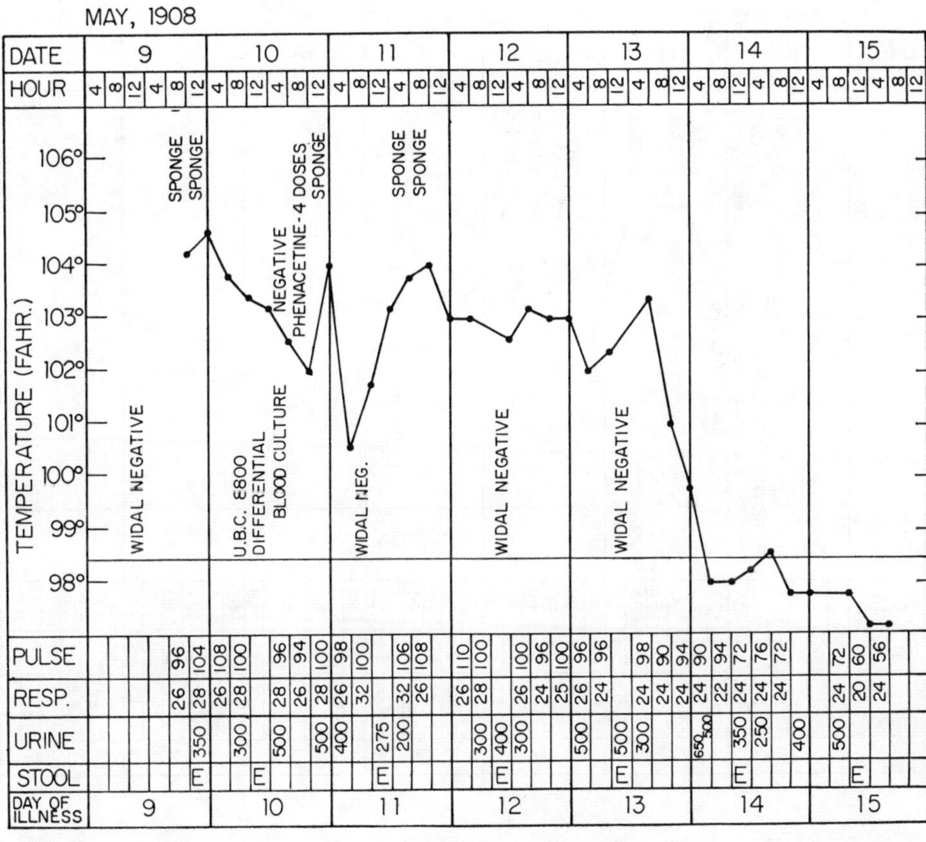

Fig. 2. *The temperature record, showing a critical decline (slight precritical rise) to normal within twelve hours, occurring on the thirteenth day.*

Constipation. This is a marked feature of the disease. It was present in 42; in 6 the bowels were regular, and in 2 there was a diarrhea following a previous constipation. Very frequently the bowels can only be moved by the use of cathartics. Blood has never been found in the fecal discharges, either macroscopic or microscopic. The guaiac and benzidin tests for occult bleeding have been negative.

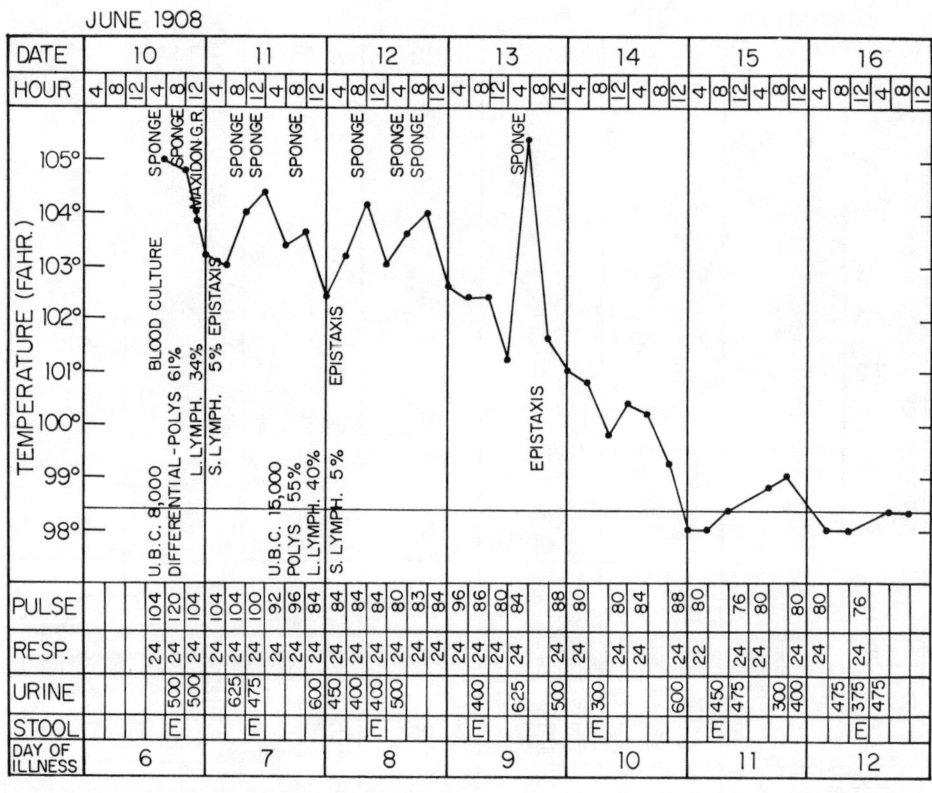

Fig. 3. The temperature record, showing the precritical rise to 105°F. and decline by rapid lysis within thirty hours, on the ninth day.

Tympanites. This is not a feature of this affection. In 9 cases a slight abdominal distension was observed.

Spleen. This organ is frequently enlarged to palpation. In 27 cases of the series it was distinctly palpable below the costal margin. At times the spleen extends for a considerable distance below the ribs, four centimeters below being the maximum. In 16 cases it was one centimeter below; in 7 cases, two centimeters; in 2 cases, three centimeters; and in 2 cases, four centimeters.

Mental Symptoms. The apathy and dulled sensorium have been mentioned in the general description. Delirium is only occasionally present, and it does not assume the active type so commonly seen in typhoid fever. It usually occurs in those running a high febrile course, and then only at night. It is muttering in character.

Blood. The average white blood cell count is higher than it is in typhoid fever; there is not the tendency to leukopenia which typhoid fever blood shows, the count being between 9,000 and 11,000. When bronchopneumonia exists as a complication the count is, of course, higher; our highest in such a case was 23,600. The average of the series—in only one case was no white blood count noted—was 9,394, the lowest being 4,200 and the highest 23,600, the last being in the patient with bronchopneumonia. The average count of polymorphonuclears was 69.4, and the lymphocytes, 30.6 per cent.

Urine. The urine is generally high-colored and clear. It contains a faint trace of albumin in many cases and occasionally granular casts. Albumin was noted in 19 of the cases. The diazo reaction is not infrequently obtained, but it is more frequently absent than present. It was demonstrable in 9 cases, and no reaction could be elicited in 30; in 11 cases it was not noted.

Agglutination Reactions. In the 221 cases there has not been a single positive reaction to the Widal test. The test has been carried on perhaps much more assiduously than would have been the case had positive results been obtained. The blood has been sent to the laboratory daily in most all of the cases, not only during the course of the disease, but during the period of convalescence until the patient left the hospital. No positive reactions have been obtained. Tests were made in dilutions of from 1 to 20, and in some cases up to 1 to 1000, because it has been shown that agglutinations with the typhoid bacillus in some cases of typhoid fever are demonstrated only in high dilutions. Agglutination tests were also made in some of the cases with various paratyphoid bacilli, with several colon strains, and in a few cases with the Gärtner bacillus. The results were all negative. I believe that the absence of positive results speaks very strongly against these cases being due to infection by the typhoid bacillus or members of the intermediate group.

BACTERIOLOGY. The evidence of infection by the recovery of the offending organism in this disease is entirely wanting. Since 1896 we have persistently tried to isolate a specific organism from these cases, but without success. Blood cultures have been made in a very large number of the cases. During the past three years cultures have been made from all of the cases that have come under observation. The cultures in these cases were made under the direction of Dr. Libman. The methods used in this work during the past three years are the same as those that were used in the studies of the bacteremia in typhoid fever made by Dr. Epstein (22). Dr. Epstein obtained positive results in nearly all of the cases of typhoid fever. This makes all the stronger the proof that in the set of cases which I am describing we are not dealing with typhoid fever or paratyphoid fever.

The clinical aspect of the disease is strongly in favor of its infectious nature, because it has a definite incubatory stage, one of onset, one of duration, and one of decline. We regard typhus fever, measles, scarlet fever, and the like as infections, and have no definite knowledge as to the nature of the infection, hence the absence of such knowledge as to this disease should not militate against considering it an infectious disease.

PREVIOUS TYPHOID. We carried on an inquiry based on immunity which typhoid fever gives to the one who suffered previously from typhoid, and found that in the group of 50 there were 10 who had had typhoid fever previously, 37 who had not suffered from typhoid fever, and 3 could give no information concerning previous illnesses.

If typhoid fever produces a short immunity, as has been shown, we would have a strong argument in favor of the cases here described not being typhoid, in the case of the nurse in the Training School, who had a severe typhoid infection in December, 1896, and who suffered with this infection in September, 1897.

RELAPSES. I have never seen a relapse in this disease. When the temperature once falls the disease ends. Unless there be a complication the fever does not rise again. This is so entirely different from the course of typhoid infections that in itself it would cast a serious doubt on the probability of this disease belonging to the typhoid fever group, with which some of my professional colleagues insist it belongs. They have stated in medical meetings that they see no reason why these cases should not be classified as atypical or abortive typhoid fever. I shall discuss this later in the section on diagnosis; for the present, however, I wish to call attention to the subject of relapses in abortive typhoid fever as presented by Dr. J. B. Briggs from Professor William Osler's clinic at Johns Hopkins Hospital. Dr. Osler (23) says: "J. B. Briggs has studied 44 of these mild cases from my clinic, in which the fever lasted fourteen days or less. Rose spots were present in 24, and the Widal reaction in 26. There were three relapses."

According to Murchison (24) and Curschmann (25), relapses are especially prone to occur in the abortive type of typhoid fever.

With such a weight of authority as to the occurrence of relapses in abortive typhoid and the entire absence of relapses in this affection, one should at least be guarded in making positive statements as to the identity of this disease with typhoid infection.

COMPLICATIONS. *Bronchitis* is a common accompaniment of the disease and is present to a greater or less degree in the majority of the patients. When it develops, it is seen early, sixth or seventh day. It lasts as a rule, throughout and disappears in convalescence.

Bronchopneumonia was observed in 3 of the group.

Meningismus. What clinicians call signs of "serous meningitis," such as rigidity of the neck, contracted pupils, the presence of bilateral Kernig phenomenon, stupor, etc., are sometimes present. These signs were noted in four of the 50 of this group.

Phlebitis cruris was observed once.

Otitis media occurred in one patient.

Cystitis was observed twice, but I think it was due to some error in the technique of catheterization, which was done on both these patients.

DURATION. The disease lasts about two weeks. In our series the average duration was thirteen and three-tenth days. In one case it lasted five days and in one, twenty-two days. The last case, however, was accompanied by a bronchopneumonia and it was difficult to determine when the original infection terminated. The detail of the series is as follows:

5 days	1 case	14 days	5 cases
6 days		15 days	5 cases
7 days	1 case	16 days	2 cases
8 days	1 case	17 days	3 cases
9 days	1 case	18 days	
10 days	2 cases	19 days	1 case
11 days	4 cases	20 days	
12 days	13 cases	21 days	
13 days	10 cases	22 days	1 case

It will be seen from this that almost half the cases terminated between the twelfth and thirteenth days. This has been our experience with the rest of the 221 cases. A prediction may almost be made that the disease will terminate on one of the two days just stated.

DIAGNOSIS. To one who has had the features of the disease pointed out to him, the diagnosis is relatively easy. For the past few years the members of my house staff recognize the disease and make the diagnosis before my visit to the wards. This is also the case with the members of the "Admitting Department Staff" in the hospital. It is only on rare occasions that their judgment is found to be incorrect. It seems to me, if it be possible on first examination to predict, as it has been almost invariably, in these cases, that a patient having an eruption of this type will not show at any time a positive Widal or give a positive blood culture, we are dealing with a disease *sui generis*. The positive factors of this disease which would suggest its presence when first seen by the examiner, are the facies, the headache, especially and definitely the eruption, the apathy, prostration, and the palpable spleen. It requires no great clinical acumen to differentiate the eruption, after its characters have been pointed out a few times. I have shown the eruption and alongside of it in a typhoid fever patient, a roseola eruption, and the differences were so striking that the members of the house staff quickly learned to detect the differences.

DIFFERENTIAL DIAGNOSIS. Inasmuch as these cases have been considered by almost all my colleagues in New York, in the past, as typhoid fever cases, it will be necessary to show the marks of differentiation. The parallel column offers itself for this purpose as most convincing:

Typhoid	*Unknown Infection*
Usually long incubation.	Short incubation, four to five days.
Onset not commonly abrupt.	Commonly with chill or chilly sensation.
Fever; gradually increasing ascent of temperature to fastigium—in all about ten days.	Fastigium reached in three days.
Remissions of temperature occasionally more than a degree.	Rarely more than one degree.
Fall usually by gradations to normal, taking commonly one week.	Fall commonly by *crisis*, not longer than sixty hours.
Eruption, circumscribed, lenticular, papular.	Maculopapular, periphery indistinct and irregular.

Distribution, chiefly, back, and abdomen, seldom appearing on upper and lower extremities; almost unknown on palms and soles.	Distribution in addition to trunk on upper and lower extremities not infrequent, on palms and soles occasionally.
Eruption appears in crops throughout the disease.	Does not appear in crops.
Spots rarely confluent, and then confluence of but two spots.	Confluence may occur with three or four spots forming a number of patches.
Roseola disappearing on pressure.	Erythema, not disappearing on pressure.
Petechial spots (hemorrhagic) very rare.	Petechiae occasionally.
Apathy and prostration late in development.	Apathy and prostration early.
Labial herpes rare.	Labial herpes in 6 per cent. of the group.
Diarrhea fairly common.	Constipation an almost invariable accompaniment.
Hemorrhages from the bowel often observed.	No intestinal hemorrhages or blood in feces.
Headache disappears in second week.	Is more intense and lasts throughout the disease.
Relapses observed by all observers.	Relapses have never occurred.
Widal reaction positive in over 95 per cent of the cases.	Widal reaction invariably absent.
Blood cultures positive in over 90 per cent of the cases.	Blood culture invariably negative.
Convalescence slow.	Convalescence speedy.

Typhus Fever. In the case of an epidemic of typhus fever, in my opinion, it would be simply impossible to say that these cases which I have described were not mild typhus fever. From the clinical aspects no lines of demarcation can be fixed. The onset, the eruption, though subcuticular mottling is absent, the critical decline, the absence of relapses, are almost identical in both. If one can believe that typhus fever has been so modified by modern conditions of hygiene as no longer to be communicable, but to exist at all times in a community, to have lost its notoriously epidemic character, and to have been deprived of the grave nervous symptoms and its toxemia so as to be a nonfatal disease, then one could say that these cases deal with a modern typhus fever, or rather with a peculiar typhus fever which has been evolved by modern improved hygiene and sanitation. The preference of the disease for developing in the summer months is against the probability of its being typhus. Clinically this disease resembles typhus fever more than it does any other disease, and I should have felt that I had offered nothing to our nosology if it had been proved that typhus fever had lost its virulence, that it was constantly present in a community, that it was not communicable, that when it was present epidemics of it did not occur, and that it was no longer a grave and fatal disease. But with typhus fever, as the great masters of medicine have taught, and as I have seen it, such a conception would be unjustifiable; therefore, I believe this disease not to be typhus fever.

Meningitis.   The occasional occurrence of signs of meningismus in this disease might suggest epidemic cerebrospinal fever (spotted fever). There would be no very great difficulty in determining the presence of that disease if spinal puncture were carried out and the cerebrospinal fluid examined culturally. Its cytology and bacteriology are definite, and the recovery of *Meningococcus intracellularis* would settle the diagnosis.

Influenza.   In epidemics of this disease some cases might appear which have a great similarity to our disease. Those of us who dealt with the type of influenza as it appeared here in 1890 will no doubt recall cases very similar. The protean forms that were then observed would very likely suggest that perhaps this disease might be one of the multi-varied or protean forms of influenza. Influenza appears pandemically, is very sudden in its onset, and prostration is the earliest symptom; it has no definite incubatory stage; it is accompanied by signs of cardiac weakness with rapid pulse and often with diarrhea. It is par excellence the disease of complications and sequels, and especially of slow convalescence.

PROGNOSIS.   Thus far it has been invariably good. No fatalities have ever occurred in my cases. Sick as the patients are and grave as the symptoms sometimes appear to be, one ought from this experience to be justified in predicting a favorable issue to the disease.

TREATMENT.   This for the present should be entirely symptomatic. Personally I have used no stereotyped plan. The usual remedies have been employed for the symptoms which required relief. The diet has been restricted to fluid and soft nourishment. For the present I deem it wise, especially in cases occurring in institutions to use the usual precautionary measures which are employed in typhoid fever cases to prevent infection; nurses are so instructed in handling these patients. Such precautions, however, would seem to be unnecessary; nevertheless in the indefinite state of knowledge concerning the causative factors of this disease no injury can be done in using preventive measures.

Epicritical.   More difficult than separating this group from typhoid fever, among which it has been in all these years included, is the difficulty of giving a name to this disease. To my mind there can be no doubt that the clinical picture is so definite, so marked that it cannot escape recognition. If this should be the view of others, the disease must represent a distinct clinical entity. I am convinced it does and is entitled to a place in medical nosology. There is no sign in the clinical picture which would characterize the disease. The critical fall is definite and I thought it might be wise to use that feature for a provisional name, calling the disease critical fever; but pneumonia and typhus fever are likewise critical fevers. On this account the name is not desirable. I should emphatically deprecate calling the disease pseudo-typhoid fever because the affection has nothing in common with typhoid, paratyphoid, and typhoid-colon, or intermediate group infections. Some years ago, before we had done reliable blood work on this group, I believed that it might represent paratyphoid infections, and so I wrote (26), but retracted that idea long ago, after I had convinced myself that the disease had nothing in common with paratyphoid. If it be typhus fever Health Boards should take cognizance of the fact that there exists in New York City at all periods of the year a nonfatal and noncontagious typhus fever which may possibly give rise at any time to an epidemic, though it has not done so in the last fourteen years. For the present, owing to ignorance of the pathology and etiology of the disease, I deem it wise not to give a name to the affection. I prefer to speak of it as an "acute infectious disease of unknown origin." My chief desire, in recalling to the attention of the profession this disease group, is to enlist its attention, in the hope that other observers may find similar or identical cases. Let us trust, if they do, that they can give us more definite and accurate knowledge than I have been able to offer. If this be the result of this contribution, or, if further inquiry shows that my attempt to establish a clinical entity has been based on poor observation and defective deductions, I should have almost as great satisfaction as would corroboration and additional proof bring to me, for it would have further and more forcibly taught me that while it is human to err, still truth will always prevail.

H. da Rocha-Lima

On the Etiology of Typhus Fever

The untimely death of Ricketts from typhus fever prevented the completion of his studies on the causal agent of that disease. His preliminary publication, however, attracted the attention and interest of other researchers, who confirmed his original findings (1, 2, 3). But there was no unanimity of opinion among investigators about the nature of the etiological agent despite the creditable experimental data that had been accumulated. Viruses, protozoa, and cultivable bacteria were variously considered to be the causative agents of epidemic typhus fever.

The confusion was resolved by the important investigations of da Rocha-Lima, who reaffirmed the etiological role of the microorganisms found in typhus-infected lice. His studies were published in 1916 in two reports, of which the first mentioned the observations made with von Prowazek before the death of the latter from typhus fever during the course of their investigations (4). Da Rocha-Lima also contracted the disease but recovered. The second paper, reprinted here, was a continuation of the work, and records the first experiments in which lice were sectioned to follow the development of the microorganism of typhus fever. His report describes in detail the agent of typhus fever in infected lice and demonstrates its intracellular location and proliferation in the epithelium of the louse's stomach. These findings proved useful for differentiating the pathogen from similar microorganisms later encountered in the alimentary tract of normal lice. Any doubts that existed as to the causative relation between the microorganism found in infected lice and epidemic typhus fever were eliminated by the similar results obtained by Wolbach, Todd, and Palfrey (5).

The work of Ricketts and von Prowazek was commemorated by da Rocha-Lima in naming the etiological agent of epidemic typhus fever: he designated the genus *Rickettsia* and the species *prowazeki*. Subsequently *Rickettsia* became established as the generic name for microorganisms possessing the characteristics of the group.

A portion of the results of experiments conducted by Prowazek and myself in the prison camp at Cottbus in the early months of the year 1915 on behalf of the War Ministry were made public by me, after new important factors for a better interpretation of the results had been obtained, in No. 2 of the 1916 *Archive für Schiffs- und Tropenhygiene* [Archives of the Institute for Maritime and Tropical Hygiene].

On the Etiology of Typhus Fever

Despite the fact that in about 95 per cent of the typhus fever lice which were examined, microorganisms uniform in appearance were found in unbelievable numbers, not only in the contents of the digestive tract, but also principally as parasites of the epithelial cells of the stomach and intestines, and that, on the other hand, in more than 100 lice from an area free of typhus fever (Hamburg) which were examined in the same manner a similar finding was not made once, I was still at that time unable to bring myself to express an opinion as to the importance of these microorganisms in the etiology of typhus fever. The fact that I am doing so now is due to the finding of new and important elements of proof during the most recent epidemic in Wloclawek. In the meantime, the results given here were the subject of an address which I gave before the German Pathological Society in Berlin on April 26. Until this date, there had been no reports of any checking on my numerous experiments in connection with the finding of the characteristic features and the importance of the *Rickettsia prowazeki*. The fact that similar small bodies occur in smear slides prepared from typhus fever lice was of course mentioned by Prowazek and other authors before me. Recently Töpfer also saw bodies near a spirochete in a smear slide which are said to be very similar morphologically to rickettsia.

In the course of the past year H. Sikora has with much patience and skill worked out the technique of experimentation with lice practically to perfection. As I was now given the opportunity to continue my typhus fever experiments in Wloclawek, I was able to let lice of various origins, and in any desired numbers, suck on typhus fever patients. It was then possible to observe them under various conditions and to answer the key question as to whether the microorganism found in typhus fever lice in Cottbus was perhaps an incidental finding, i.e., an epizoon which occurred in the Russian lice independently of typhus fever, or whether it is the typhus fever blood that causes the infection of the louse with this body.

If this were to be the case, then the lice experimentally infected in this manner must also yield the same results as those infected by natural means. And this was also found to the fullest degree. In healthy lice which had been allowed to suck on typhus fever patients, the microorganism in question was found to develop regularly as a parasite of the stomach and intestinal cells, whereas lice which were kept under like conditions but allowed to suck only on healthy persons or those who had recovered from typhus fever were not infected. This microorganism, which enters the louse only through drinking of typhus fever blood, settles in the cells of the intestinal walls and multiplies rapidly. It probably also reaches the salivary glands of the typhus fever transmitter. Furthermore, the characteristics of the typhus fever virus and of these parasites, insofar as they are known, are identical. And since the only shapes that can be found with the microscope in the blood of typhus fever patients have the same shape and size as our bodies, no other logical conclusion can be drawn from the results of my experiments than that the microorganisms with which we were occupied are none other than the long-sought causative agents of typhus fever.

The exterior form of this microorganism is suggestive of a bacterium, but the characteristic difficulty in staining, the resistance to culturing, and the tendency to gather together in sharply defined parts of the protoplasm of the affected cell much in the same manner as chlamydozoa suggest rather a strongyloplasm or chlamydozoa. Whether bacteria or strongyloplasm, the variations from known types are great enough to allow the assumption that it is a special species. As to the question of order, we do not yet have sufficient information. This remains an open question, and the required name for this microorganism, which has until now been referred to as *body*, might be most practical if a possibly prejudicial terminology were avoided. Therefore I should like, in honor of the great researchers who have fallen as victims of typhus fever—Prowazek and Ricketts, to suggest the name *R. prowazeki*.

The only identifying characteristic of *R. prowazeki* known at present is its ability to penetrate to the digestive tract cells of the louse and there to multiply rapidly. Organisms similar in appearance can therefore be identified with certainty as rickettsia only if in addition to morphological characteristics this activity is also demonstrated. This postulate of course applies to all investigations which are conducted in an effort to answer any basic question. The monotonous and trying examination of sectional slides of the respective lice is absolutely necessary. The mere determination of similar bodies in smear slides from typhus fever lice cannot be taken as a sure confirmation of our investigation, nor can the same finding in normal lice be considered as a reliable argument against them. For in my first publication I have already pointed out that similar shapes sometimes occur in smear slides of normal lice.

This is not to say that the examination of smear slides has no importance, but only that special care must be taken in the interpretation of findings. This caution is particularly important in the absence of sufficient experience in the observation of fine morphological details; for small round shapes which now and then are seen to lie in pairs can be found in just about any slide preparation, and actual microorganisms of spherical shape always seem to like to lie in pairs. The finding of small double bodies, or perhaps rods with pol-coloring, does not suffice to speak of *similar bodies* in the sense of an apparent identity.

The morphological characteristics of *R. prowazeki* can only be recognized clearly on heavily stained Giemsa preparations at about 1,500 times magnification. They are somewhat smaller than the smallest bacteria (*M. melitensis, M. prodigiosus*) and take on a red color and tone similar to chromatin red. The shape is not spherical but rather bluntly elliptical, olive-shaped. They often lie together in pairs, bound by a substance of much lighter color which surrounds them. Exceptionally short or long individuals occur now and then, but in spite of having given particular attention to finding other shapes which might indicate a kind of development and multiplication other than simple division, I have never been able to observe them.

Breeding of these microorganisms has as yet not succeeded, either under aerobic or anaerobic conditions, in spite of the addition of albumin-rich ascites, fresh blood, rabbit organs, and lice extracts to the culture. Further experiments are still in progress.

Isolated single individuals in tissue or blood smears are at present hardly recognizable with certainty, for they are easily confused with other shapes. Slides in which the organisms occur in very thin concentration are therefore to be looked upon with doubt. In the naturally, as well as in the experimentally, infected lice they are present in tremendous numbers and are therefore easy to recognize. The smear slides present the appearance of smears of bacteria cultures.

In the blood of sick persons, I have seen objects with the shape and color of *R. prowazeki* only within the leukocytes. Without wishing to identify these with certainty, I consider it not improbable that they represent the seeds of the disease slowly circulating in the blood stream. This agrees with the observations of Prowazek, the first to believe that he recognized the causative agent of typhus fever in the "Giemsa-carmine-red-colored, distinct, elongated or round bodies and double bodies with fragile bonds." In any case, the Prowazek bodies—and only in the strictest sense of their discoverer—are the only microorganisms of all those found in typhus fever which can be considered with (albeit an uncertain) probability to be identical with rickettsia in organs of the louse. The histological examination of the large amount of material which I preserved for this purpose will serve to indicate this.

My investigations have yielded the noteworthy fact that the temperature at which the lice are kept is of great importance. This finding might also explain the fact that the head louse does not play as great a role in the transmission of typhus fever as does the body louse, which exists usually only under more favorable conditions of warmth. When I kept the lice which were fed twice daily on persons sick with typhus fever at about 23°C., no rickettsiae developed, and these lice proved to be not infected in experiments with animals (guinea pigs). In lice which were fed on typhus fever cases in the same manner but kept at a temperature of 32°C., rickettsiae did develop and guinea pigs injected with them became sick almost without exception. Until the fourth day after the initial feeding of lice on patients the tests for rickettsiae, as well as the experiments with animals, gave negative results. After the fifth day both tests gave positive results.

Experiments dealing with the inheritance of the infection in the louse, which are partly still in progress, have already yielded positive results. Here the larvae from eggs laid on the sixth day of the female's infection have been shown to be infected also.

Experiments conducted to date concerning the possibility of the transmission of the infection via the excretions of the louse, which also contain the germs, have as yet yielded no single positive indication.

The methods which I used in these investigations enable me to explain the required amount of blood, the optimum time for extracting blood from patients for the infection of lice, and the time at which the typhus fever patient is most infectious. Later reports will discuss the as yet unfinished experiments dealing with the production of a vaccine from the intestine of an infected louse which is maintained in the form of a culture, and with obtaining a serum.

We see that there are still a number of important questions concerning the etiology of the causative agent of typhus fever that must be investigated. As shown by the progress of my experiments up to this time, work with lice will furnish the best possibility of success in this effort.

On Serological Diagnosis of Spotted Fever

In 1910 W. James Wilson of Ireland found in the feces of one case, and in the urine of two, a variant form of *B. coli communis* that was agglutinated by the serum of 17 cases of typhus fever but not by normal serum (1). A similar phenomenon was discovered during World War I and was developed into the Weil-Felix reaction, a unique serological test for the diagnoses of rickettsial infections.

During a study of epidemic typhus and typhoid fever cases, referred to in the paper presented here as spotted fever and abdominal typhus, respectively, Weil and Felix isolated a strain of *Proteus* bacillus that was agglutinated by the serum of a typhus patient in a dilution of 1:200. In the same study another strain of *Proteus* was isolated; the first was designated X-1 and the second, X-2. A third strain of *Proteus*, X-19, was later found that was agglutinated by typhus serum in titers much greater than that obtained with either the X-1 or X-2 strains (2).

In subsequent studies terms were introduced to designate the motility characteristics of the *Proteus* group: nonmotile "O" (*ohne Hauch*, "without film") and motile "H" (*Hauch*, "film"). By separating *Proteus* microorganisms into "O" and "H" types, Weil and Felix found that the agglutination of "O" *Proteus* by typhus serum was more specific than that of "H" *Proteus*. The classic strain employed in the reaction was thus designated *Proteus* OX-19. As commonly occurs in the course of a scientific investigation, the initial discovery had far greater significance and applicability than originally envisioned. In this instance the discovery of "O" and "H" antigens constituted a major serological breakthrough leading to the discovery of fundamental immunological relations and to analyses of bacterial microorganisms, e.g., the typhoid bacillus (3).

The Weil-Felix reaction is a nonspecific biological test in which there is no etiological relation between *Proteus* strains and rickettsiae. The phenomenon has been investigated extensively, and numerous hypotheses have been framed to explain it. Although the reaction is still not clearly understood, it is believed that strains of each microorganism possess cross-reacting antigens of accidental structural similarity. A common soluble specific factor, a carbohydrate antigen, has been demonstrated for *Proteus* OX-19 and *R. prowazeki* (4).

The importance of the Weil-Felix reaction in the diagnoses of rickettsial infections will be appreciated when one recalls that for years it was the only serological test of value in diagnosing rickettsioses. It was not until about 1940 that specific rickettsial antigens were prepared for use in complement fixation tests. On the basis of the reaction a scheme of classification for the rickettsiae was proposed (5). The Weil-Felix reaction has also proved useful in demonstrating the generic relation of some unknown diseases to the rickettsioses and in differentiating various forms of rickettsial infections, e.g., tropical typhus in Malay States (6).

In a small town (Rr.) in Eastern Galicia (Poland) at the end of September 1915 we had occasion to examine a number of spotted fever cases bacteriologically and serologically and also to observe some of them clinically. The patients were mainly civilians native to the town and its surroundings, and to some extent male and female nurses of the military hospital which was being utilized as an epidemic hospital. The investigation covered a period of two months during the first four weeks in the hospital itself and the second four weeks from a distance, after having been transferred.

In the first cases we were doubtful of the clinical diagnosis of spotted fever, which was based on the findings communicated by Weil and Spaet (1), in view of the simultaneously existing epidemic of abdominal typhus. However, we were struck by the fact that in the first nine cases observed, we were not successful in any of them in demonstrating *B. typhosus*, in spite of careful and repeated examination of blood, stool, and urine and although the Widal reaction was positive in some of them. These cases consisted exclusively of civilians not vaccinated against typhus.

However, we incubated from the urine of patient V (a Rumanian physician who admitted the first of these patients to the hospital and fell ill about two weeks later) a microorganism that was not agglutinized by typhus, paratyphus A and B, or dysentery sera but did agglutinize with autoserum in the dilution 1:200. Although in itself of little significance, this finding became of interest when the sera of nine spotted fever patients also showed agglutination with this strain. This induced us to examine the strain thoroughly in regard to:

1. Culture,
2. Serology,
3. The blood sera of spotted fever patients,
4. Control sera,
5. Other similar strains incubated simultaneously.

I. Cultural Characteristics

Appearance: Short, delicate, gram-negative rods similar to *Proteus*, slightly motile, forming pseudothreads.

On Serological Diagnosis of Spotted Fever

Drigalski-Conradi Medium: Blue colonies, even after weeks.

Endo's Medium: Colorless colonies after 24 hours which subsequently turn red.

Dextrose Agar: Fermentation after 18 hours.

Lactose Agar: Fermentation after 48 hours.

Milk: Peculiar coagulation after 40 hours.

Litmus Whey: After 24 hours, turns reddish more than typhus and less than paratyphus.

Gelatin: Liquefaction after 48 hours.

Plate Culture: Grows similar to *Proteus*.

These observations show that the germ is culturally sharply distinguished from typhus (fermentation of dextrose and lactose, liquefaction of gelatin), from paratyphus and dysentery (fermentation of lactose and liquefaction of gelatin), and from a slightly acid-forming colibacillus (liquefaction of gelatin). The reliability of our nutrient media was controlled through simultaneous vaccination with typhus, paratyphus, and colibacillus.

II. Serological Characteristics

Serological examination fully agreed with the cultural findings and showed the absolute difference from the types of bacteria mentioned above.

III. Specific Agglutination with Sera of Spotted Fever Patients

Thirty-three cases were observed in Rr. which had been diagnosed clinically as definite spotted fever. However, they showed some deviations from earlier findings both in serological and bacteriological characteristics. In five patients not vaccinated against typhus and with a negative reaction to *B. typhosus*, the Widal reaction could be demonstrated in dilutions above 1 : 75. Moreover, *B. typhosus* was demonstrated in five patients (four times in the blood, once in the urine). In one of these cases (B) spotted fever followed convalescence from typhus. Another case of this group died in the first days of the spotted fever, and autopsy findings were negative for abdominal typhus, although *B. typhosus* had been incubated from the blood. The third of these cases (L), with *B. typhosus* in the urine, was the brother of a female patient suffering at the same time from spotted fever with a high Widal reaction and negative to *B. typhosus*. The last two cases, as well as the other two cases with *B. typhosus* demonstrated in the blood, were believed by the attending physicians to be mixed infections of typhus and spotted fever.

Table 1

Agglutination with	Dilution			Reaction
Typhus antiserum	1:8000	1:200		Negative
Paratyphus A	1:1000	1:100	1:5000	Negative
	1:3500	1:100	1:1000	Negative
	1:2000			Negative
Gärtner serum	1:4000	1:100	1:1000	Negative
	1:2000			Negative
Dysentery Shiga Kruse	1:400	1:100		Negative
Dysentery Flexner	1:1000	1:100		Negative
Rabbit immune serum[a]	1:2000			Positive

[a] Obtained after injecting twice with 2 c.c. each of bacterial emulsion = 1 loop ["*Oese*"].

This is very probable because there was a severe epidemic of typhus at the same time. This raises the question of how to explain the positive Widal reaction in the five cases without *B. typhosus*. Three possibilities present themselves:

1. Simultaneous existence of abdominal typhus (as probably in the case of the female patient L);

2. A prior case of typhus and a nonspecific resurgence of the Widal reaction during the spotted fever (possible in view of the prevailing epidemic of abdominal typhus in this Eastern Galician district);

3. Coagglutination remains an open question, although the Castellani test with these sera would appear to eliminate coagglutination.

All of the 33 sera produced agglutination with the baccilus incubated by us as follows: 16 sera in the dilution 1:50; 5 sera in the dilution 1:100; 8 sera in the dilution 1:200; 3 sera in the dilution 1:500; and 1 serum in the dilution 1:25.

The specific agglutinins occurred in an early stage of the disease. At the time of manifestation of exanthema, they had already reached their maximum; they remained at the maximum during the fever period, lasting generally two weeks; and they rapidly disappeared after the patients were free of fever. About two months after the patients had been free of fever, the sera of the convalescents no longer produced agglutination in dilutions of 1:25.

The only case with an agglutination titer of 1:25 is explained by this manifestation because the serum was procured from the recovered patient three weeks after his discharge from the hospital. The greater number of the sera agglutinizing only at 1:50 originated either from the first start of the disease or from the period of convalescence. All of the cases with a higher titer had been examined during the acute stage.

Any kind of constant relation between this specific agglutination and the Widal typhus reaction could not be established. This is shown by the following consideration: all three sera with the highest specific agglutination titer (1:500) persistently showed a negative Widal reaction. Among eight sera with the specific titer 1:200, six also persistently produced a negative Widal reaction. This fact justifies us in the conclusion that the specific agglutination occurs completely independently of the typhus reaction.

These findings persuaded us to assume that we had found in the incubated germ an aid for the diagnosis of spotted fever. It merely remained to investigate whether the epidemic in Rr. concerned a particular disease similar to spotted fever, and what relation this affection had to cases of spotted fever of different provenance. We soon found an occasion for this.

In the town of Ra. (in Russia and more than 100 km. distant from Rr.) two cases of spotted fever were recorded, and repeated examination of the two sera produced the specific agglutination described in dilutions of 1:100 and/or 1:200. Both patients were Russian prisoners of war not vaccinated against typhus, and both sera persistently showed a negative Widal reaction to typhus and paratyphus.

For three members of a sick Russian family, exanthema in the wife led to a diagnosis of spotted fever. Serological examination was performed immediately (on the second day of appearance of the exanthema) and produced the specific agglutination at 1:100. Autopsy confirmed the diagnosis of spotted fever. In the other two patients (father and child), who had already begun to convalesce, the diagnosis of spotted fever could be made only subsequently from the result of the agglutination reaction, which was positive in the dilution 1:500 and/or 1:100.

From the many cases sent to the spotted fever hospital in P. (Russia) from a large army and rear-area sector, we were unfortunately able to obtain only 11 sera of patients and/or convalescents for investigation. The expected serological reaction fully agreed with the earlier results. Nine sera produced the specific agglutination, and in two cases the reaction remained negative. The latter were sera of convalescents who had been free of fever for more than six weeks. In the nine positive cases, the relation between the agglutination titer and the stage of the disease absolutely agreed with the circumstances described for the epidemic in Rr. The two acute cases (10th and/or 12th day of illness) showed the highest agglutination (1:200). The other seven sera showed a decreasing titer in relation to the increasing interval of convalescence (calculated from the day of return of normal temperature). Three of these cases with a titer of 1:100 had been free of fever 11, 8, and 2 days; three cases with a titer of 1:50 had been free of fever 47, 43, and 4 days; and one case with a titer of 1:25 had been free of fever for 55 days.

IV. Control Sera

We investigated 169 control sera for agglutination with the incubated strain. Our main attention was obviously directed to abdominal typhus, which is frequently indicated as differential diagnosis to spotted fever. We were able to investigate 95 sera of clinically confirmed typhus, in 11 cases of which we incubated *B. typhosus*. The agglutination test was performed each time in the dilutions of 1:25 and 1:50. It was positive in a dilution of 1:25 in ten cases, all of which concerned normal agglutination such as are known for any pathogenic microorganism. Two cases showed weak positive agglutination at 1:50. One of these had an extensive exanthema which became squamous during convalescence, and the second case (where any existing exanthema could not have been noted because of the strongly pigmented, dark-brown skin of the whole body) showed a critical return to normal temperature [*"kritische Entfieberung"*]. We are far from regarding these cases as spotted fever, because it is possible for the titer of standard agglutination to be somewhat higher in infrequent cases. However, this circumstance will hardly interfere with diagnosis, because the agglutination sets in generally more strongly and more quickly where spotted fever is concerned. In two cases with a strong clinical presumption of spotted fever where repeated specific agglutination tests remained negative even in a dilution of 1:25, a diagnosis of abdominal typhus was subsequently confirmed by the demonstration of *B. typhosus* and completely confirmed through the further progress of the disease.

We further investigated repeatedly 12 cases of bacteriologically determined relapse fever, with negative results in each case. From the further investigation of 62 sera of patients and/or convalescents with febrile enteritis, pneumonia, angina, bronchitis, pleuritis, erysipelas, etc., we obtained: 54 negative reactions; 8 positive reactions at 1:25.

Almost all these cases were military personnel vaccinated against typhus, and therefore had a positive Widal reaction.

Consequently, normal agglutinins were present in 12 per cent of 169 sera investigated. Differentiation between normal agglutination and specific agglutination does not cause any difficulty, however, because the normal is qualitatively distinguished from the specific by the loose flocculation and the much longer interval of several hours required for reaction. According to our present experience, specific agglutination occurs in 100 per cent of the cases investigated (47) at the height of the disease in a dilution of at least 1 : 50 within a short time (20–60 minutes) and as a rule reaches values of several multiples of this titer (see above).

V. Control Strains

During the investigation of this epidemic in Rr. we were successful only once in again incubating this germ during the acute stage of the disease from the urine of patient W. The identity of the two strains was confirmed by the absolute concordance of the cultural behavior and by the agglutination with patient sera and with an artificial rabbit immune serum.

During the epidemic we incubated from the urine and stool of spotted fever and other patients 28 different bacterial strains which became blue in the Drigalski medium, showed fermentation of dextrose in most cases, and were not paratyphus or typhus. Not one of these strains was agglutinized by our artificial immune serum and by patient sera with the highest titers. This indicates with absolute certainty that the two bacterial strains incubated by us were not any usual saprophytes of the human body. Although we had only few occasions to investigate cases in the acute stage and were not able to do so in the hospital itself, we still believe that the germ is extraordinarily difficult to find. The behavior of the blood serum already points to this. Since the agglutination titer reaches its maximum at the very beginning of the exanthema, the bacteria must have developed their activity in the organism for some time prior to this. We therefore feel justified in assuming that the bacteria have already disappeared at the moment where the clinical suspicion makes examination necessary and possible. The rapid decrease of the agglutinins, which can be explained only by the complete disappearance of the bacteria and their bodily substance, would also speak for this.

We do not feel justified in regarding this germ as the pathogen of the spotted fever. Clarification of its role in etiology would require experimentation which we are at present not able to carry out. However, it appears to us that this microorganism may be an aid for the diagnosis of spotted fever.

Addendum by Dr. O. Bail after proofreading: Through the courtesy of Dr. Weil, I recently received the bacterial strain described above, and by chance within the last few days had an opportunity to test it with serum from patients suspected of having spotted fever. All three cases were prisoners of war.

Case To.: Weil-Felix reaction at 1:25 doubtful, otherwise negative.

Case Ste.: Weil-Felix reaction completely negative.

Case Mi.: Within two hours at 37 per cent, Weil-Felix reaction at 1:25, 1:50, 1:75 complete; at 1:100 almost complete; at 1:150 and 1:200 pronounced agglutination. Repetition showed that positive agglutination still existed in a dilution of 1:400.

Concerning the negative cases, further investigation showed that To. did have a negative Widal reaction but that *B. typhosus* could be incubated from the blood clot with bile tubes. This was not successful for Ste., who had a slightly positive Widal reaction (1:75).

It is not permissible to draw any far-reaching conclusions from these few cases in which not even epicrisis is possible. However, your communication is justified on the one hand by the urgent necessity for facilitating the diagnosis of spotted fever and on the other hand because of its inherent epidemiological interest. Although the case Mi. very strongly showed the Weil-Felix reaction, it had most probably no relation to the Galician and Russian cases investigated by Weil and Felix.

1917

M. H. Neill

Experimental Typhus Fever in Guinea Pigs

The following paper by Neill, published in 1917, provided the first experimental evidence that there existed more than one form of typhus fever. He noted that 70 per cent of male guinea pigs inoculated intraperitoneally with strains of "Mexican" typhus exhibited an enlargement or swelling of the scrotal sac and adhesions of the testes. The reaction described by Neill was milder than the severe response that occurred in guinea pigs infected with Rocky Mountain spotted fever rickettsiae; it was also absent in animals inoculated with the microorganisms of Brill's disease and of epidemic typhus fever. Since the reaction had never been observed in the course of many years of study on typhus fever, it was difficult for typhus researchers to reconcile Neill's demonstration of a scrotal reaction induced by the agent of typhus fever with their own experiences.

Neill's findings were largely ignored until ten years later, when H. Mooser noted that over 90 per cent of male guinea pigs inoculated with strains of typhus fever rickettsiae isolated from patients in Mexico caused a pronounced swelling and reddening of the animal's scrotum (1). Mooser further demonstrated through careful pathological examination that the rickettsiae multiplied profusely in the tunic lining over the testes. Subsequently these cells packed with rickettsiae were called *celles de Mooser*, or Mooser cells, and the tunic reaction in guinea pigs was referred to as the Neill-Mooser reaction (2). This biological reaction, along with other epidemiological and laboratory evidence, helped affirm the existence of murine typhus fever.

The significance of Neill's and Mooser's findings is that they constituted evidence of a biological difference between "Mexican" typhus and the epidemic typhus fevers, including Brill's disease, and helped ultimately to clarify some of the confusion and seemingly contradictory reports on the identity of typhus fever forms in the Americas. Later it was established through a series of experimental and epidemiological investigations that the "Mexican" or "endemic" typhus was another form of typhus called murine typhus fever (see Maxcy's paper, 1929).

It is well known that the intraperitoneal inoculation of guinea pigs with 2 to 4 c.c. of blood containing the virus of typhus fever is followed by a rather characteristic elevation of temperature which will be observed about 10 days subsequently. Not many descriptions of pathological changes as a result of the above procedure have been reported. Bachr and his coworkers consider certain changes in the spleen, "which is enlarged and congested, with its malpighian bodies prominent" (1), as typical of typhus fever in the guinea pig. Aside from the above, most workers seem rather to have insisted on the absence of gross lesions due to the typhus virus in these experimental animals.

The striking similarity, in many respects, of typhus fever and Rocky Mountain spotted fever led to the examination of the scrotums of typhus-fever guinea pigs, since very definite lesions of the scrotal tissues are almost uniformly present in the former disease. These changes have been described by Ricketts (2) and other workers.

While the observations recorded in this paper have been in progress there has been ample opportunity for comparative study, as a strain of Rocky Mountain spotted fever has been carried on by transfer from guinea pig to guinea pig.

Lest there be any possibility of misunderstanding, it seems desirable to state that the nonidentity of the two diseases has apparently been thoroughly established by immunological studies.

The guinea pigs on which the observations were based were those inoculated with Mexican typhus directly from human cases or from other guinea pigs or monkeys in which the strains of Mexican typhus were being propagated. The observations were made during 1916 and 1917.

A series of guinea pigs infected with a strain of the so-called endemic typhus, or Brill's disease, which had been propagated in monkeys and guinea pigs for several years, was examined before attention was focused on the scrotal lesions. While it is possible that a mild type of the lesion may have been present, it certainly was not sufficiently conspicuous to attract attention.

In well-developed male guinea pigs, which had been intraperitoneally injected with the Mexican typhus virus, the following changes have been observed: from 9 to 15 days after inoculation, the temperature of the animal becomes elevated to from 40.5 to 41°C., and if the scrotum, with the testicles in place, be examined, a definite swelling is observed. If the skin be of a light color, some redness may be noted. These external changes subside in a few days. If the animal be killed when the fever and scrotal changes are at their height, dissection reveals the following gross findings: the skin of the scrotum looks apparently normal, but if it be carefully dissected from the tissues immediately beneath, definite hemorrhages appear in the cremasteric fascia, just external to the parietal laminae of the tunica vaginalis. If these structures be incised and the testicle and epididymis exposed, hemorrhages of a similar nature will be noted immediately beneath the visceral laminae of the tunica vaginalis. The extent of these hemorrhages varies, from a few minute petechiae to nearly complete envelopment of the testicles by hemorrhagic areas. If the animal be examined at the height of the process, i.e., one to two days after the swelling is first noted, the lesions above described are indistinguishable in their gross appearances from the lesions of Rocky Mountain spotted fever at the same stage of development of the disease, that is, one or two days after the swelling of the scrotum is first noted. In the spotted fever animals, in contradistinction to the typhus animals, the disease becomes progressively more severe. Hemorrhages into the skin of the scrotum take place, and in some cases typical necroses of the scrotum, paws, and ear tips are observed before the death of the animal, which usually follows. On the other hand, the lesions of typhus fever rapidly clear up and soon the animal is as well as ever.

Twenty-six out of 37 male guinea pigs killed at the height of the febrile reaction showed the lesions to be as described. These animals represent several strains of typhus received from El Paso, Texas, and Laredo, Texas, this year.

Lecount (3) and Wolbach (4) have emphasized the significance of vascular lesions in the pathology of Rocky Mountain spotted fever, both in human cases and in guinea pigs. These lesions consist of various grades of reaction to injury of the cells of the endothelium, i.e., endarteritis, and of rather peculiar and characteristic perivascular accumulations of cells.

E. Frankel (5), Aschoff (6), and Poindecker (7), and apparently several other workers whose publications are not now available, have described certain histological changes in typhus fever, especially as regards the exanthem. These writers all describe as characteristic, lesions of the smaller arteries consisting of necrosis of the intima and the perivascular accumulation of cells among which, as in spotted fever, the mononuclear elements predominate.

In the present study the writer reports that in guinea pigs infected with Rocky Mountain spotted fever and typhus fever, and killed at about the same stage of development of the lesions, sections of the testicles, epididymis, and their envelopes revealed similar changes. They were as follows:

A. Subperitoneal hemorrhages, presumably due to
B. Vascular lesions, characterized by degeneration of the intima, proliferation of the endothelium and connective tissue of the vessel walls.

Pronounced perivascular infiltration, as noted above, was found in both diseases. This consisted chiefly of cells of the lymphocyte series and of endothelial leukocytes. Polynuclear leukocytes were present, but distinctly in the minority. The changes were particularly abundant in the small vessels. Thromboses were occasionally observed in the early lesions.

The lesions in spotted fever showed more necrosis, exudation, and in older specimens, more proliferation in the vessel walls than occurred in the typhus fever animals.

Summary

1. Definite, gross, and minute pathological changes in the genitals of male guinea pigs reacting to Mexican typhus fever blood have been described. The gross lesions occurred in about 70 per cent of such animals examined.

2. These depend on lesions of the blood vessels.

3. The lesions are similar in process to, but milder in character than, those occurring in guinea pigs infected with Rocky Mountain spotted fever.

1929

Kenneth F. Maxcy

Typhus Fever in the United States

The first description of murine typhus fever is credited to J. E. Paullin, who in 1913 recognized a mild form of typhus fever occurring in Atlanta, Georgia (1). Before the disease was conclusively identified and established as an entity separate from epidemic typhus fever, it was the subject of intensive laboratory, ecological, and epidemiological studies which spanned a period of almost two decades.

During this time, research efforts on the disease were permeated with a certain amount of confusion and misunderstanding that may be attributable, almost directly, to the prevailing circumstances. On the Eastern Seaboard states, in addition to murine typhus there existed two other kinds of typhus-like diseases: Brill's disease and spotted fever. In Mexico, where much research on typhus originated, both epidemic and murine typhus existed concomitantly. An additional factor was unfamiliarity of the recently discovered genus of microorganisms, the rickettsiae, for whose investigation research techniques had not yet been fully developed. Furthermore, the terminology was woefully unclear: it was difficult to know what strain of typhus-like microorganisms or which disease an investigator was referring to when he used the names endemic typhus, sporadic typhus, Brill's disease, and Mexican typhus almost interchangeably to denote murine typhus fever.

An early indication that a biological difference existed among typhus-like diseases went unnoticed for a decade before Neill's critical observations were rescued from obscurity by Mooser (see preface to Neill's paper, 1917). Several views and observations were published in the 1920's by individuals in different parts of the world that hinted at the existence of a mild form of typhus fever differing epidemiologically from epidemic typhus fever (2, 3). The studies that directed research to the essence of the problem and led to the identification and confirmation of murine typhus fever as a distinct rickettsial entity came from a series of astute epidemiological deductions by Maxcy, based on a survey of a typhus-like disease in Montgomery, Alabama, and Savannah, Georgia (4). In the 1929 publication reprinted here, selected for its clarity and brevity, Maxcy postulated that apart from man a reservoir existed for endemic (murine) typhus of the southeastern United States and that rats or mice might serve as the reservoir. He further stated that the transmission of the infectious agent probably involved an insect vector such as fleas, mites, or ticks.

Maxcy's epidemiological hypothesis was corroborated when the etiological agent of murine typhus fever was isolated from fleas of rats trapped in typhus foci in Baltimore (5). A similar agent was obtained from the brains of rats

91

caught in the Belem Prison in Mexico City during an epidemic (6). The rickettsial agent was designated *Rickettsia mooseri* (7). Later, Dyer and his associates demonstrated experimentally the transmission of murine typhus from rat to rat by the flea *Xenopsylla cheopis*. Although the rat flea is the principal vector of the disease, Mooser and Castaneda showed that several species of fleas are equally capable of transmitting the infection (8). The first proof of antigenic differences between *R. mooseri* and *R. prowazeki* was demonstrated by Zinsser and Castaneda (9).

With definite knowledge of the basic epidemiology of the disease established, the name murine typhus fever was adopted to indicate its presence as a natural infection of rats (10). Because murine typhus may occur in epidemic and endemic forms, such synonyms as endemic typhus and sporadic typhus that still appear in texts are not descriptive of the disease. Once murine typhus fever was identified, its existence in most parts of the world was quickly established (11).

From time to time, when epidemics raged in Mexico, localized outbreaks of tabardillo have occurred in contiguous American territory, confined largely to the Mexican population living on this side of the border or brought into this country in labor gangs. The last epidemic was associated with the political upheaval and internal strife which racked that country from 1916 to 1918. Notoriously a disease of armies and refugee populations, tabardillo wrought havoc among the soldiers engaged in operations in the north of Mexico, states of Chihuahua, Coahuila, and Nuevo Leon, and came across the border with refugees to El Paso, Del Rio, and Laredo, Texas. Scattered outbreaks followed labor gangs into Arizona, Colorado, California, and central and eastern Texas.

In 1922 Armstrong investigated an epidemic of typhus among the Indians on the Navajo Reservation in New Mexico. There was no direct evidence but a strong presumption that the infection had been imported from Mexico.

There is a tradition that tabardillo is confined to the highlands of that country; that it rarely occurred and showed no tendency to spread in the low-lying land of the coast and the Rio Grande Valley. In 1925, however, an investigation (Sinclair and Maxcy) of some suspicious cases which had been reported in the vicinity of Rio Grande City and Fort Ringgold, Texas, led to the conclusion that a mild form of typhus was present and probably had been endemic for some years in the lower Rio Grande Valley and the nearby towns of southwestern Texas.

The importation of typhus into the eastern United States is apparently a much more recent affair. The disease was not clearly differentiated from typhoid until Gerhard's description of the fever which had prevailed in Philadelphia during the spring and summer of 1836. During the forties and fifties a considerable number of outbreaks were reported from eastern cities, associated with the arrival of immigrant ships, particularly from Ireland, where typhus was then epidemic. That the disease had gained no permanent foothold in this country is evidenced by the fact that during the Civil War it was of no consequence to either army. A few cases were reported among the Federal troops, but such an authority as Woodward (1863) questions the accuracy of the diagnosis in many of these.

The last outbreak of any considerable size on the Atlantic seaboard was that in New York City, 1892–93, when some 434 cases were removed to the reception hospital from the poorer tenements and lodging houses. Since that time, although occasional cases of typhus fever have come in on ships from European ports, there has been little, if any, secondary spread after arrival.

From 1893 to 1910 the United States was generally considered to be free from typhus fever except for the occasional case imported from Europe or Mexico. At this time Dr. Nathan Brill (1910) called attention to a disease occurring endemically in New York City which was clinically indistinguishable from typhus fever but presented certain epidemiological differences. The work of Anderson and Goldberger in the following two years indicated that in monkeys the virus of Brill's disease and that of tabardillo were identical and similar in all respects to the published accounts of virus of European and African typhus fever. Following these publications a considerable interest was aroused. Reports of cases similar to those described by Brill were made from several of the eastern cities. The impression still prevailed, however, that these cases were simply a mild form of Old World louse-borne typhus, attributable to imported infection, although their association with recently arrived immigrants could seldom be demonstrated.

Since 1915 there has been a growing appreciation of the fact that cases resembling typhus fever and corresponding to Brill's disease clinically were occurring on the soil of the United States under circumstances where the chances of recent importation of the virus seemed rather remote.

The discovery in 1923 that cases of this type were occurring in the native population of Montgomery, Alabama, led to a study of the situation in this city, which was later extended to other parts of that state and to the neighboring states by direction of the Surgeon General of the United States Public Health Service.

Clinical Observations

The clinical picture of this typhus-like disease in the southwestern United States was carefully observed and analyzed in a large series of cases. The syndrome is constant, clearcut, and easy to differentiate from other eruptive fevers. The uniformity with which the fever lasts just two weeks is remarkable, sometimes a day or two under, more often a day or two over, but always within this range. The eruption, too, is absolutely characteristic in the irregularity of the size, shape, degree of elevation, intensity of color, and amount of extravasation of individual spots. In a well-developed case the diagnosis may be made with maximum assurance on purely clinical grounds.

While the course is undoubtedly like that of typhus fever, when the physician consults his textbook on medicine he is puzzled because of the relative mildness of the symptoms, the rarity of complications, and the low fatality rate. The textbook descriptions are, however, based upon the severe and highly fatal typhus seen during epidemics.

It is not generally appreciated that the severity of typhus is exceedingly variable in different epidemics and in different localities and that between epidemics the disease is quite mild. In the Serbian epidemic of 1915 the mortality rate reached 60 per cent or more; in the Russian epidemic of 1919–22 it was in the neighborhood of 5 to 7 per cent. In the interepidemic periods it would be difficult or impossible to distinguish on clinical grounds alone the disease of the Old World from that seen in the southeastern United States. Here the disease is by no means always mild, though usually so. Especially when old people are attacked, it may run a virulent and rapidly fatal course, with death in the second week. It is difficult to determine the fatality rate with any degree of precision on account of unrecognized and unreported cases, but it is approximately 2 to 4 per cent.

Serological Confirmation

In 1916 Weil and Felix discovered that the serum of typhus fever patients would agglutinate certain proteus-like organisms which they cultivated from the urine of persons sick with this disease. The most sensitive of their strains was called *Proteux* X-19. They demonstrated that agglutinins for this proteus were ordinarily not present in the serum of normal persons except in low dilution. During an infection with typhus fever they appeared to increase toward the end of the first week, to reach maximum titer about the time of convalescence, and then gradually decline to their former level. In other words, the agglutination paralleled the course of the infection. Sera from patients sick with various febrile diseases did not show this phenomenon. Although an etiologic relationship for *Proteus* X-19 has never been demonstrated, the Weil-Felix reaction has been generally accepted to be peculiar to this disease.

Sera from several hundred cases of the endemic typhus of the southeastern United States have now been examined in various laboratories.* The Weil-Felix reaction has been found to be almost invariably positive in the disease where the blood was taken at the proper time or repeated specimens submitted. It has been of great assistance in establishing diagnosis in some cases where typhus was not considered by the attending physician.

Reaction of Experimental Animals

The susceptibility of the chimpanzee and, later, of the *Macacus rhesus* to the virus of typhus was established by the work of Nicolle and his coworkers in Tunis, 1909–12, and by Anderson and Goldberger, working with Mexican typhus, 1910–12. Most of the early researches were made upon the monkey. A little later Nicolle found that the guinea pig was also susceptible, and since that time most of the work in typhus has been done with this readily available species of experimental animal. Consequently the manifestations of typhus in the guinea pig have been thoroughly, even minutely, studied and described.

With the realization that a typhus-like disease was endemic and not uncommon in the southeastern United States, the question arose whether the causative virus was identical with Old World typhus.

Although the work of Anderson and Goldberger had been very convincing, it was thought worthwhile to repeat the observations on experimental animals, working with strains which were obtained from cases occurring in the southeastern United States where there is less chance of direct importation of infection from abroad.

Accordingly, during the past six years repeated attempts have been made to establish a strain from human cases of this endemic typhus in

* Particular interest has been taken in this investigation by Dr. L. C. Havens, director Alabama State Laboratories, Dr. T. F. Sellers, director Georgia State Laboratories; and Mr. Conrad Kinyoun, director Municipal Laboratory, Savannah, Georgia.

Alabama, Georgia, North Carolina, and Virginia. Many of these attempts were unsuccessful. In a few the result was apparently positive, but on account of failure, for one reason or another, to propagate the strain, the studies were not sufficiently complete to warrant conclusions. Finally, however, two strains have been carried through a long series of passages and carefully studied.

Briefly, it has been established that the virus of this endemic disease of the southern United States gives manifestations in experimental animals exactly like those of Mexican typhus or tabardillo. The reaction is similar to that of strains of typhus from Old World sources, but shows constant, though slight, differences in guinea pigs. With the endemic and Mexican strains, after intraperitoneal injection, guinea pigs show marked involvement of the scrotum, and it is very difficult to demonstrate the characteristic typhus nodes in sections from the brain, whereas in Old World typhus the involvement of the scrotum is much less marked and nodes can be constantly and easily demonstrated in sections of the brain after the fourth or fifth day of the fever. Notwithstanding these differences, all three strains immunize against each other. The study has enabled us to conclude, however, that our endemic typhus has common origin with Mexican typhus and is not dependent upon importation from Old World sources.

Incidental to these observations in the guinea pig, there have been found in preparations made from the surface of the tunica vaginalis at the onset of fever some very minute, pleomorphic, Gram negative, intracellular microorganisms which seem to correspond to the *Rickettsia prowazeki* of da Rocha-Lima, 1916. They were originally observed in the cells lining the gut wall of lice infected with typhus and much evidence has been accumulated to indicate that they bear an etiological relationship to the disease. The demonstration of these microorganisms constantly in the tissues of guinea pigs infected with typhus has added considerable weight to this evidence.

Epidemiological Observations

Having established, then, in experimental animals that the disease belonged to the typhus group, a good deal of concern was felt as to the possibilities of epidemic spread. It became necessary to examine the conditions under which this disease was able to maintain and propagate itself in this country. Earlier observations on its epidemiology have been confirmed by more extended experiences during the past six years.

Geographic Distribution.   The data which are available from morbidity reports, from the literature, and from field investigations give only a bare outline of the occurrence of typhus-like cases in the United States. So far as information is available, the disease is rather sharply limited to the Atlantic seaboard and the near-by piedmont sections as far north as Boston. It is present in nearly all of the seaports from New York southward and has attained widest distribution in Alabama, Georgia, and Florida. On the Gulf coast, while it is endemic in Tampa, Pensacola, Mobile, New Orleans, Galveston, and Houston, there is at present no information regarding its occurrence in Mississippi. The lower Rio Grande Valley from Laredo to Mercedes constitutes an important focus. On the Pacific coast only Los Angeles has reported a considerable number of cases. While an occasional case has been reported from the interior of the country, that section has been for the most part strikingly free.

Incidence. A study of the occurrence of cases emphasizes the fact that they are sporadic—scattered as to place and time. There is an entire absence of focal outbreaks.

In many places the occurrence of a case seems to be a chance happening which may not be repeated again for many years, if ever. For example, in 1928 there was a single case in the suburbs of Washington, D. C.; one in Laurel, Maryland; two, a mother and son, taken sick at the same time, at Alexandria, Virginia; one at Concord, North Carolina, in 1927; two at Rock Hill, South Carolina, etc. No other cases have been known to have occurred in these places previously or subsequently.

In certain towns in the southeastern states the disease occurs almost every year, but usually only one or two cases per year. In certain of the larger towns and cities many cases, scattered as to place and time, occur each year.

Seasonal Distribution. Undoubtedly typhus outbreaks can occur at all seasons of the year—modified by latitude, habits of living, and other factors—but it is generally accepted to be chiefly a disease of the cold months. The summer and fall maximum of the endemic typhus of the United States is in direct contrast with the high winter and spring incidences of typhus in the Old World.

Contact. Several interesting facts developed in the course of the study of the circumstances under which cases were occurring in Montgomery, Alabama, Savannah, Georgia, and Tampa, Florida.

In the first place, all attempts to trace the origin of one case to contact with a preceding case have been unfruitful. In the same way the disease when once introduced into a family, a boarding house, or a hospital has shown no tendency to spread. Occasionally multiple cases have occurred in the same household, but usually the persons attacked came down about the same time or within a few days of each other, suggesting a common source of infection rather than secondary attack. There have been no localized outbreaks in jails, asylums, or boarding houses. Many cases have been cared for in general hospitals each year without special precaution, and no instance of infection of physicians, nurses, attendants, or fellow patients has come to attention. *The disease does not seem to be communicated directly from man to man.*

Occupation. An occupational analysis indicated that persons engaged in "trade" (clerks, proprietors, managers, salesmen, dealers, etc.) had a significantly higher attack rate than those employed in manufacturing and mechanical industries. Furthermore, it appeared that one-third of the cases in Montgomery and in Savannah were engaged in handling foods, groceries, meats, produce, feed, and flour. If to this were added those patients who live in rooms which were adjacent to premises on which food stuffs were stored, the correlation is still more striking. This association has been evident in all the cities and towns in which the disease has been studied.

Social Status. It follows that the cases occurred among persons earning a reasonably good livelihood. It occurred among the average rank and file of the community. It did not select the poor and uncleanly; frequently leading citizens were attacked. The relative freedom of the Negro from the disease was a remarkable and unexplained fact.

Louse Infestation. In view of the evidence that the disease is typhus, and that typhus, as known in the Old World and in Mexico, is transmitted from man to man by the louse, as careful inquiry as possible was made in each case to detect lice or any evidence suggesting prior infestation with them. This inquiry consisted in asking the physician in attendance and the patient in all cases investigated whether louse infestation had been noticed, or, indeed, whether the patient had noticed insect bites of any kind. In all cases personally investigated by the author search was made for nits or live insects on the hair of the head and body and on the bedclothes and for scratch marks on the skin which might suggest infestation; at the same time other members of the family were inspected and the environment was surveyed with the same purpose in view. With two or three exceptions, the results have been entirely negative; the proportion is no larger than might be encountered in any disease.

While this evidence does not in any single case exclude the possibility that the patient may have been bitten by one or more lice prior to the onset of the disease, or may have had a light infestation which was not discovered, it does suffice to definitely establish that *the disease was not associated with lousiness.* This much is, indeed, sufficiently well established by the geographic and social distribution of the disease, a considerable proportion of the cases having occurred in persons of such habits and living in such an environment that the harboring of lice is not to be suspected.

Discussion

The evidence thus far adduced indicates that there is endemic in the United States a disease which is clinically indistinguishable from the mild typhus occurring during interepidemic periods in the Old World and in Mexico. The relationship of this disease to typhus is further borne out by serological similarities. The Weil-Felix reaction is positive. The value of this observation in establishing the relationship of the disease in this country with that of the Old World has been modified by the recent discovery that the Weil-Felix reaction is positive in Rocky Mountain spotted fever, a disease which, though it belongs to the typhus group, is immunologically distinct.

Observations in experimental animals are interpreted as meaning that the endemic typhus of the United States has common origin with the tabardillo of Mexico. The typhus which has been occurring in our eastern seaports does not depend upon direct importation from across the sea. It belongs to the North American continent.

In addition to the peculiarities of the virus, the disease in this country manifests certain epidemiological characteristics which are in contrast with those generally attributed to the typhus of the Old World. They relate principally to the mode of transmission. These considerations have led to a tentative rejection of the human louse as the principal vector and of man as the principal reservoir of the disease in this part of the United States and the search for some other mode of transmission.

In typhus fever it has been shown by Nicolle and others that beside the chimpanzee and the monkey certain small rodents are susceptible to the virus, i.e., guinea pigs, rabbits, rats (white and gray), mice (white), and the gerbille. In a recent publication Nicolle (1926) reports a second series of passages of typhus virus through 12 generations of white rats.

The question arises whether in the endemic typhus of the southeastern United States a reservoir of the disease may not exist other than in man, a rodent reservoir with accidental transmission to man through the bite of some parasitic bloodsucking insect or arachnid. Such a hypothesis is compatible with the epidemiological characteristics which have been presented, namely, 1) the uneven focal distribution of the disease; 2) its sporadic occurrence; 3) its apparent lack of direct communicability from an infected person; 4) its association with the place of business rather than with the home, particularly with those premises upon which foodstuffs are handled or stored; 5) the recurrence of cases on the same premises after considerable intervals of time; and 6) its seasonal incidence.

Obviously, the rodents upon which suspicion immediately falls are rats and mice, and the parasitic intermediaries which are first suspected are fleas, mites, or possibly ticks.

Summary

In summary, there is endemic in the United States a disease which resembles typhus and gives a positive Weil-Felix reaction. The virus of this disease has been identified with that of tabardillo in Mexico, and both have been shown to be closely related to the virus of Old World typhus by immunological tests. The North American strain appears to be originally derived from Old World sources.

The epidemiology of the typhus of the United States is not compatible with man-to-man transmission by the louse. It suggests the existence of some other mechanism for the propagation of the virus. From a consideration of what is known of this group of diseases, the rickettsioses, and specifically with regard to the susceptibility of rodents to typhus virus, it seems probable that a reservoir may exist apart from man. A reservoir in rats or mice, with accidental transmission to man through the bite of some bloodsucking parasite, would be consistent with the known facts.

Note

This paper was read at the Twenty-seventh Annual Conference of State and Territorial Health Officers with the United States Public Health Service, Washington, D.C., June 4, 1929.

1932
Clara Nigg and K. Landsteiner

Studies on the Cultivation of the Typhus Fever Rickettsia in the Presence of Live Tissue

The earlier reports of researchers contained only suggestive evidence on the multiplication of rickettsiae in tissue fragments maintained *in vitro*. The definitive demonstration of the propagation and continued serial passage of rickettsiae in tissue culture, reported briefly in a previous communication (1) is described in detail by these investigators in this 1932 paper. Their initial findings were quickly confirmed by K. Sato (2) and by Pinkerton and Hass (3).

Unfortunately, many years elapsed before the potential of the tissue culture system for rickettsial research was fully exploited. In the 1950's the development of novel techniques for cell cultivation and the dramatic advances that ensued in the field of virology created a renascence of interest in the use of this sysem for rickettsial studies. In the past decade the use of tissue culture for the propagation and production of rickettsiae has made available abundant quantities of the microorganisms that are relatively free of contaminating materials and in a state suitable for purification. This has facilitated the analyses of their physical and chemical properties and the extraction of antigens for use in serological tests. In addition, it has made possible the study of mechanisms involved in rickettsial invasion and replication at the cellular level, and most important, the use of the system has helped establish the existence of metabolic activities of rickettsiae and enlarged our understanding of the relations of the enzyme systems of host cells to rickettsial infections.

This description was prompted by the recent significant work of Mooser on the Mexican type of typhus fever. The results on the cultivation of the rickettsia of typhus fever which have already been briefly presented in a preliminary communication (1) are reported in detail in this paper.

Various attempts had previously been made by other workers [Kuczynski (2), Krontowski and Hach (3), Wolbach and Schlesinger (4), Rix (5), Zinsser and Batchelder (6)—cf. Zinsser and Castaneda (7)], to cultivate typhus fever rickettsiae. Some of these experiments indicated multiplication of the organisms but none led to the establishment of strains which could be maintained indefinitely *in vitro*. The methods used were practically the same; namely, the cultivation in homologous plasma of tissues (generally brain and spleen) from typhus-infected guinea pigs. In such cultures Kuczynski, Wolbach and Schlesinger, and Zinsser and Batchelder were able to demonstrate rickettsiae morphologically, and Wolbach and Schlesinger succeeded in setting up a second generation, which was done by transferring the same piece of tissue into fresh medium.

Since our preliminary article, Sato (8) reported the cultivation of the virus of typhus fever through thirteen generations, using infected, along with normal Descemet's membrane of rabbits, in a medium consisting of aqueous humor and plasma. The liquid was changed every 2 days and the tissue itself transferred to fresh medium when growth ceased, as it did after from 4 to 10 days. The virulence of such cultures was tested by injecting a suspension of cultivated tissue fragments intracardially. Such injections were followed by fever, monocytosis, and pathological changes consisting of dark red discoloration and edema of the spleen, as well as typhus nodules in the brain, liver, and heart muscle. The author was never able to demonstrate rickettsiae morphologically in his cultures, but described cell inclusion bodies ["*monokokkenförmige Körperchen*"] which he identified with the etiological agent in typhus, considering them to be a peculiar form of rickettsia which does not stain with Giemsa or at most very slightly.

Still more recently Pinkerton and Hass (9) described the cultivation of typhus rickettsiae from the testicle of an infected guinea pig. They used as explant material, small fragments of the membranous exudate imbedded in 1 drop of plasma coagulated by 1 drop of embryonic guinea pig tissue extract. The cultures were transplanted every 2 or 4 days by transferring a portion of the tissue into fresh medium. Rickettsiae were demonstrated morphologically in these cultures in histological sections. They state that in the majority of cases, the rickettsiae, whilst numerous in the first generation cultures, disappeared quite rapidly in successive transfers, but in one group of cultures rickettsiae were found in very great numbers in the fourth and fifth generations after 16 and 21 days *in vitro*.

In the following, a description is given of the technic and the media which have been used in carrying cultures of typhus fever rickettsiae for months *in vitro* without diminution either in virulence or in the number of organisms.

Technic

Typhus Virus. The strain of typhus organisms used in these studies (unless otherwise indicated) was isolated from a case in the southeastern

Cultivation of the Typhus Fever Rickettsia

United States by the U.S. Public Health Service in Washington, D.C.*
It is in all respects quite similar to the Mexican strain of Mooser. A few
experiments were also made with a strain from Nicolle's laboratory in
Tunis.† We have carried the latter strain for some months, transferring
sometimes with brain emulsions and sometimes with tunica washings.
It may be noted parenthetically, in confirmation of Pinkerton's (10)
observations on Wolbach's European strain, that in our hands the
Nicolle strain produced, although irregularly, scrotal inflammation of
slight to moderate intensity, indistinguishable from that produced by
the Mexican type. Rickettsiae, although few in number, could also be
demonstrated in the testicular exudate when such was present.

Media and Cultures. Two types of tissue media have been used with
equal success. One was adapted from that employed by Rivers, Haagen,
and Muckenfuss (11) who used tissue cultures of rabbit cornea in
coagulated plasma for the cultivation of the viruses of vaccinia and
herpes. For our cultures, pieces (from 2–5 mm. square) of normal
tunica from half-grown guinea pigs were soaked in the inoculum
suspension, prepared as described below, for 20–30 minutes in order to
insure intimate contact between virus and tissue; then, one to three
pieces were imbedded, according to the directions given by Rivers,
Haagen, and Muckenfuss (11), in large tubes (10 cm. long and 2.3 cm.
wide) in a small amount of heparinized guinea pig plasma coagulated
by means of Ringer solution extracts of normal guinea pig spleen.

The second medium was based on that used by Maitland and Maitland (12), Rivers, Haagen, and Muckenfuss (13), and others for the
cultivation of vaccinia virus. This medium consists of Tyrode solution,
serum, and minced tissue. For our work, cultures were prepared as
follows: minced normal tunica from half-grown guinea pigs was soaked
in a few drops of inoculum for some minutes, after which Tyrode
solution and guinea pig serum were added in the ratio of two parts of
the former to one of the latter and the mixture distributed in amounts
of about 3 c.c. into 25 c.c. Erlenmeyer flasks.

The tubes and flasks were closed with rubber stoppers and sealed
with paraffin to prevent evaporation.

The cultures were incubated at 37.5°C. and transferred at 8–10 day
intervals.

* We wish to express our gratitude for this material to Dr. G. W. McCoy, Director
of the U.S. Public Health Service.

† This material was furnished us through the courtesy of Dr. Harry Plotz and
Miss Helen Van Sant, to whom we are greatly indebted.

Inoculum for the Cultures.   To initiate cultures, the tunica containing rickettsiae from an infected guinea pig was scraped in a few cc of Ringer or Tyrode solution, or ground in a heavy Pyrex 50 cc centrifuge tube with a glass rod (inserted through a sterile gauze stopper) terminating in a ball deeply cross-hatched to make an effective grinding surface. The slightly turbid fluid thus obtained was used for inoculation. To transfer the cultures from one generation to the next, part of the tissue was removed from the medium and scraped or ground as above with a few drops of the fluid, and the cloudy suspension used to inoculate fresh tissue for several cultures. Tissue fragments were never transferred, only the suspension obtained by scraping.

Stained Preparations.   Preparations for staining were made from the cultures by scraping a bit of tissue on a slide with a cataract knife, then spreading the resulting small amount of turbid liquid into a film which was allowed to dry, fixed in methyl alcohol for 2–3 minutes, again dried and stained with alkaline Giemsa in jars. Good staining was obtained in 15–20 minutes, after which time the slides were washed in running tap water, then rinsed with ethyl alcohol and xylene.

Although the Castaneda stain (14) was found to be excellent for demonstrating rickettsiae in the testicular exudate of infected guinea pigs, where the organisms are found largely within the cellular cytoplasm, it did not give as clear pictures with the scrapings of culture material where there were few or no tissue elements serving as background of contrasting color.

Tests for Virulence.   To test the virulence of the cultures, tissue was removed from the medium and ground with a small amount of liquid. This, along with the tissue debris, was injected intraperitoneally into guinea pigs. Marked scrotal swelling, characteristic temperature curve, and the subsequent demonstration of rickettsiae in the testicular exudate were used as indications of the virulence of the cultures.

Cultivation

It is apparently quite easy to establish cultures of typhus rickettsiae *in vitro* by means of either of the methods described; namely, the coagulated plasma medium or the serum Tyrode medium. All of six strains initiated by the former method and seven of thirteen by the latter were successful. With more careful selection of infectious material from lesions, the failures could doubtless be considerably reduced.

The tissue fragments imbedded in coagulated plasma began to show outgrowths within 2 or 3 days, reaching the maximum in 5–6 days, the

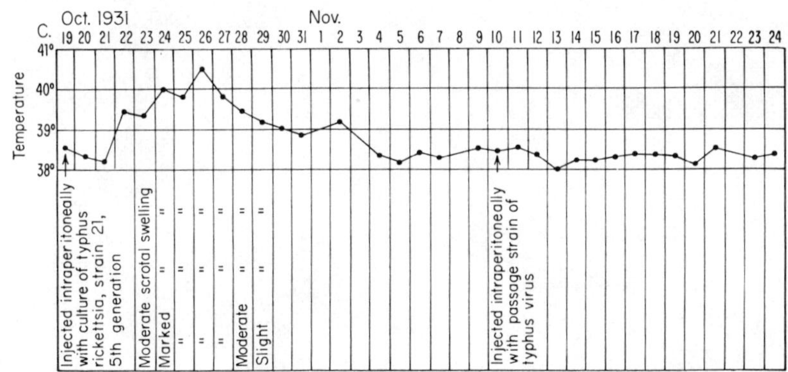

Chart *1*. *Temperature curve of a characteristic infection with cultivated typhus rickettsiae, showing subsequent immunity to passage strain.*

final growth being plainly visible to the naked eye as a halo 1–1.5 m.m. wide, surrounding the tissue.

Maitland and Maitland (12) originally believed that their serum Tyrode medium does not contain living cells. Rivers, Haagen, and Muckenfuss (13) have shown that the tissue, although it did not proliferate, was none the less viable for at least 5 days, and capable of proliferation when transplanted into a suitable medium. While it is uncertain whether the tissue in the typhus cultures was still viable at the end of 10 days, the incubation period which was commonly used, the rickettsiae certainly were. No systematic experiments have been made to determine precisely how long the organisms can survive without transfer.

Inasmuch as the coagulated plasma method is somewhat more arduous, it was discontinued in favor of the serum Tyrode medium after the latter was found to support growth as satisfactorily as the former. Cultures have been carried in the latter medium through twenty generations covering a period of 6 months, without diminution in numbers or virulence, and there seems to be little doubt that they can be carried indefinitely as any bacteriological culture.

Chart 1 shows the course of a characteristic infection with the cultivated rickettsiae and indicates the subsequent immunity to the passage strain.

Few to fairly numerous rickettsiae could always be demonstrated in stained preparations from the first generations in both types of cultures, their number increasing in later generations, although there was considerable variation in the number of organisms. Figure 1 shows the characteristic microscopic picture of the rickettsiae in culture.

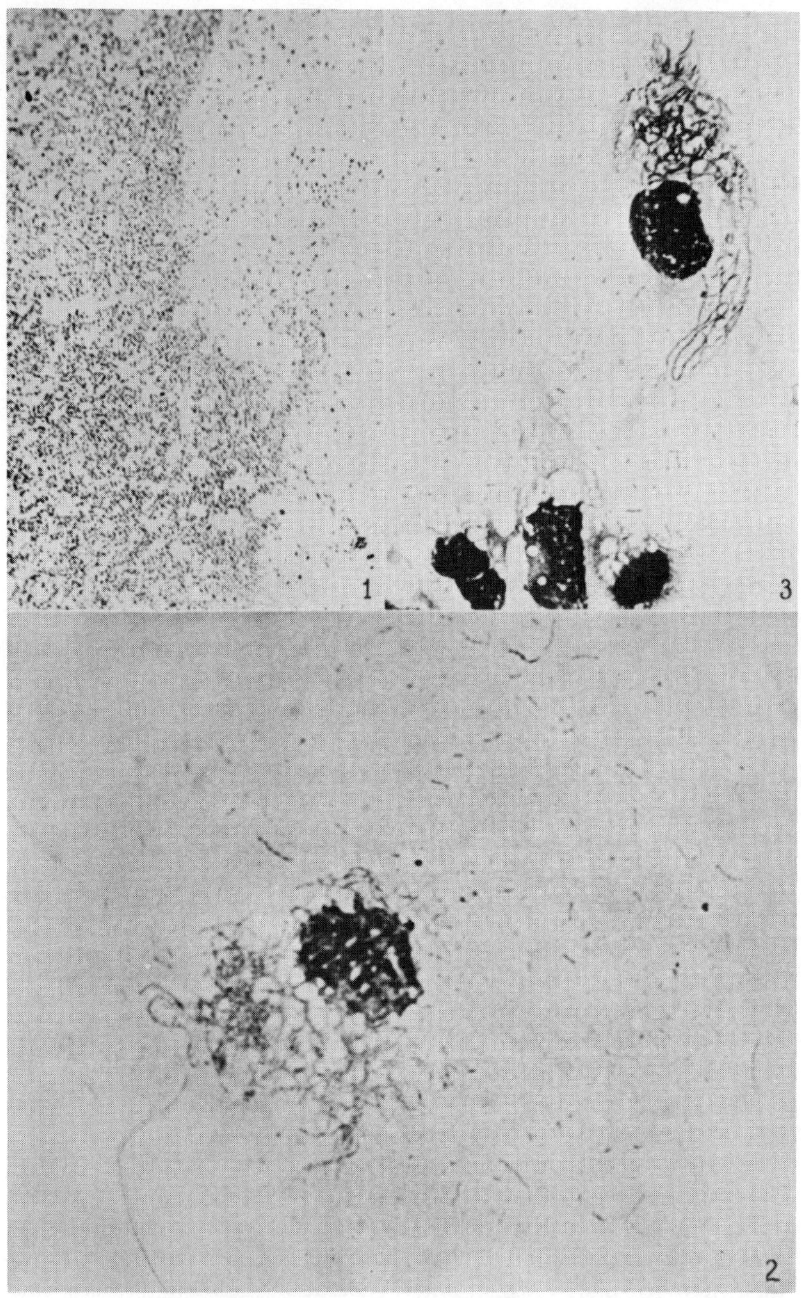

Fig. 1. Typhus rickettsiae in culture, sixth generation. Giemsa. × 1000.
Fig. 2. From a culture of European typhus, fourth generation, showing chains intra- and extracellularly. Giemsa. × 1500.
Fig. 3. From a culture of European typhus, sixth generation, showing long chains intracellularly. Giemsa. × 1000.

Cultivation of the Typhus Fever Rickettsia

The rickettsiae of European typhus were also successfully cultivated from tunica scrapings of an infected guinea pig in the serum Tyrode medium. In the first generations the rickettsiae in these cultures showed a different morphology (see Figs. 2 and 3), viz., a tendency to form chains of varying length, somewhat resembling minute streptococci, resulting in a picture which raises doubt as to the identity of these organisms. However, apart from the fact that there was no growth in the liquid part of the medium, slides from several of the later generations were in all respects similar to those of the Mexican type, and the strain proved to be fully and characteristically virulent on injection into guinea pigs. No growth was obtained on ordinary media with material from this or the Mexican strain.

The fact that the organisms could be demonstrated morphologically in the serum Tyrode medium only in the scrapings from the tissue fragments, and never in the supernatant liquid, would seem to indicate a parasitism of the rickettsiae for the tissue. Guinea pig tests for the infectiousness of the supernatant liquid were equivocal. In this respect the cultures differ from those of some filterable viruses grown in similar media, in that the latter can be transferred by using the liquid [Maitland and Maitland (12), Li and Rivers (15), Rivers (16)].

Experiments with Anaerobiosis and with
Heated and Frozen Tissues

The significance of live tissue is indicated in the results of the following experiments in which heating, freezing, and anaerobiosis were studied as to their influence on the cultures.

The tests for virulence were made with the second generation cultures in the various media, since there was the possibility of a survival of rickettsiae in the inoculum of the first generation.

1. Minced tunica, suspended in a small amount of Tyrode solution, was heated in a water bath maintained at 50°C. for 15 minutes [cf. Pincus and Fischer (17)]. This heated tissue was subsequently inoculated and distributed in flasks in the usual manner. Appropriate controls were prepared simultaneously. The tests and controls were transferred after 10 days' incubation, the former again to heated tissue medium, and the latter to unheated tissue medium. Giemsa-stained preparations were made at the time of transfer and again at the end of the second incubation period of 10 days, at which time animals were injected. The results of these experiments are given in Charts 2*a* and *b*. The numbers in parentheses indicate the generations of the strain.

107

Cultures
with Heated Tissue
Strain 21
(3) R. fairly numerous
to numerous
(4) R. absent
(5) R. absent
(5) R. absent
Guinea Pig 64
No infection. Not immune
to passage strain
(4) R. absent
(5) R. absent
(5) R. absent
Guinea Pig 63
No apparent infection but
immune to
passage strain
R. = rickettsiae.
Control Cultures with
Normal Tissues
Strain 21
(3) R. fairly numerous
to numerous
(4) R. fairly
numerous
(4) R. fairly
numerous
(5) R. numerous
(5) R. few to
fairly
numerous
Guinea Pig 65
Characteristic
infection with
subsequent
immunity
(4) R. numerous
to very
numerous

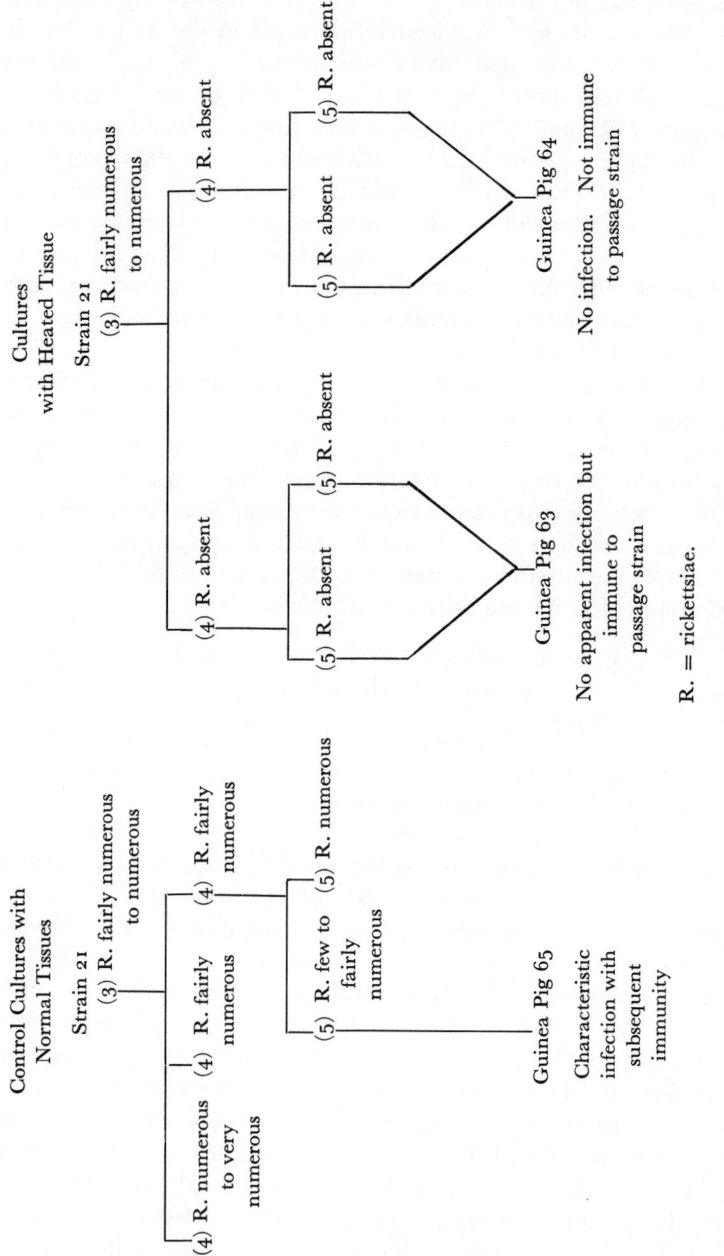

Chart 2a.

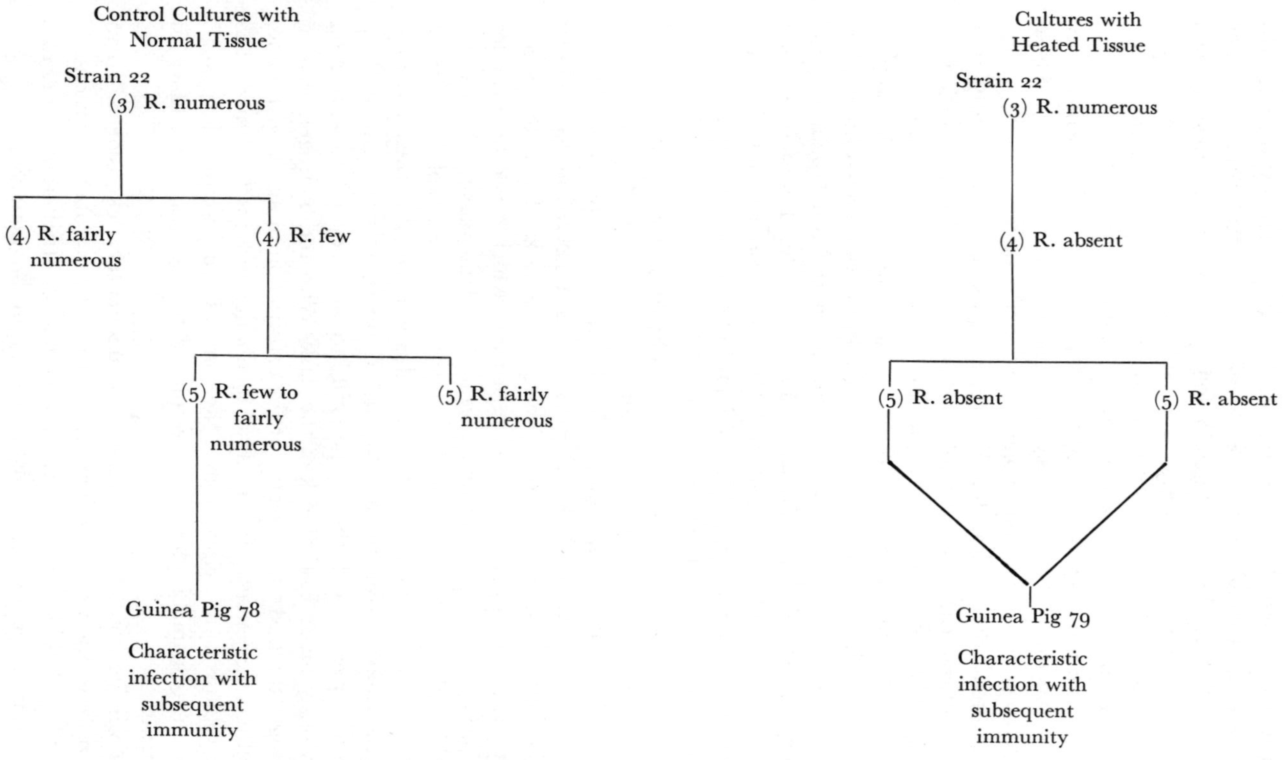

Chart 2b.   Charts 2a and 2b.   Effect of heating the tissue in the culture medium.

It will be noted that rickettsiae could not be demonstrated microscopically in any of the cultures prepared with heated tissue, either after the first or the second generation. However, of the three guinea pigs inoculated with material from second generations, one had a typical infection and was subsequently shown to be immune to the passage strain. A second guinea pig showed no reaction but was later found to be immune, indicating an unapparent infection, whilst only one of the three showed no signs of infection nor immunity. These results suggest two possible explanations: firstly, that heating at 50° for 15 minutes is slightly less than lethal for the tissue used; secondly, that the rickettsiae can remain viable without apparent multiplication for 20 days after being transferred into the heated tissue medium.

2. Minced tunica, suspended in a small amount of Tyrode solution, was frozen with CO_2 snow and alcohol and thawed, fifteen times, after which it was inoculated and distributed in the usual manner. Appropriate controls were prepared simultaneously. Transfers, stained preparations, and guinea pig injections were carried out as in the previous experiments with heated tissue. The microscopic findings and the results of animal tests are shown in Chart 3.

It is seen that tissue killed by repeated freezing and thawing failed to support the growth of the rickettsiae.

3. Normal tunica inoculated in the usual manner was divided between two series of flasks. One series was stoppered and paraffined in the usual manner to serve as controls. The flasks of the other series were identical except for a longer neck into which a two-hole rubber stopper was fitted, carrying one short and one long glass tube, the latter reaching almost to the surface of the medium. Air was replaced in these flasks by passing hydrogen gas through the long tube, the short tube serving as exit. After the air was driven out (5–10 minutes), the long tube was raised (with the stopper still in place) beyond a constriction previously made in the neck of the flask. With the hydrogen passing through, the flasks were sealed at the constriction in an oxygen flame. Transfers were made after 10 days' incubation into media subjected to anaerobiosis as described above, the controls being prepared as usual. The microscopic findings and results of animal tests are shown in Chart 4.

It will be noted that in these experiments the rickettsiae failed to multiply in the tissue medium under strictly anaerobic conditions. If this effect should prove to be constant, it may be attributable either to a deleterious effect on the tissue or directly on the organisms.

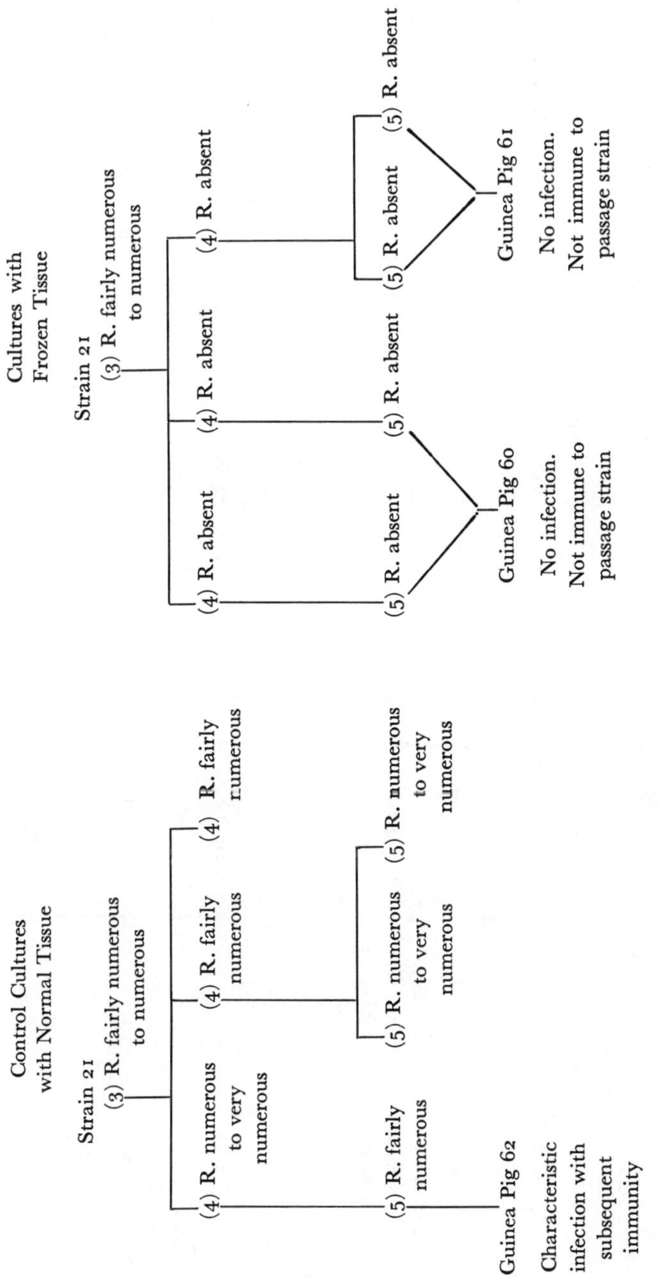

Chart 3. Effect of freezing the tissue in the culture medium. Other experiments with frozen tissue gave identical results.

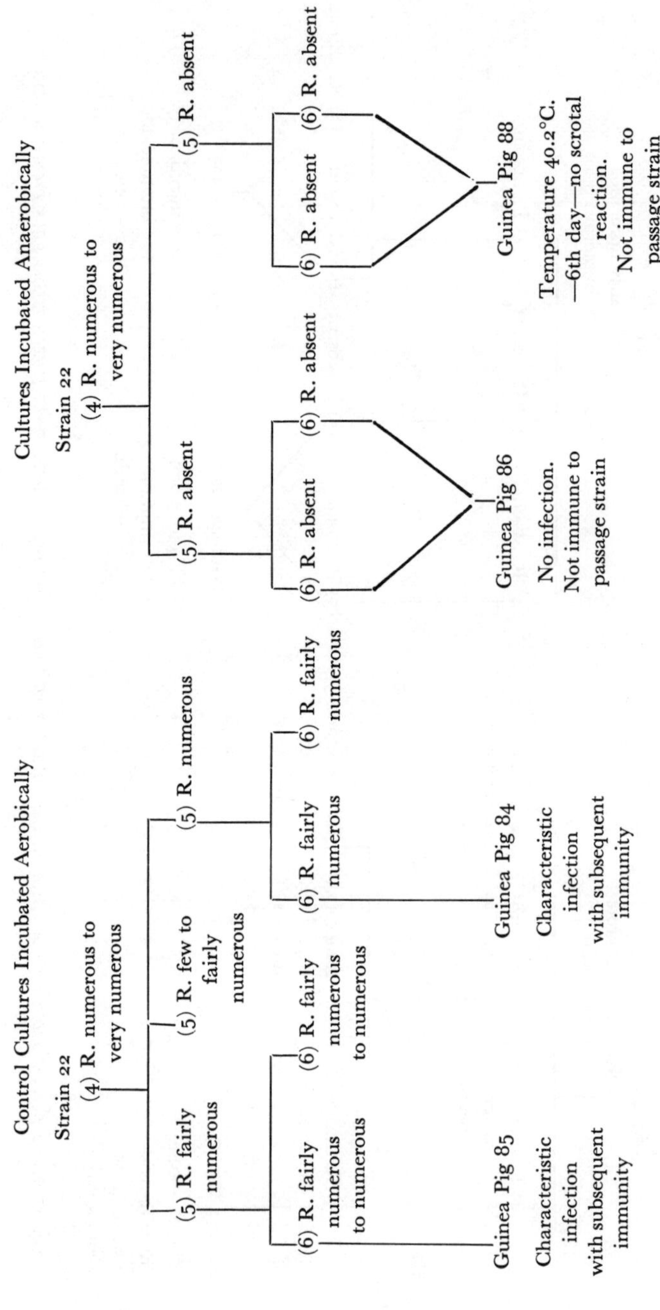

Chart 4. Effect of anaerobiosis on cultures.

Cultivation of the Typhus Fever Rickettsia

Some preliminary experiments were made in order to study further the conditions necessary for cultivation.

It was found that of several tissues tested, only tunica and peritoneum gave satisfactory results in the medium described. The peritoneum, because of its greater surface, offers technical advantages in preparing rickettsia cultures on a larger scale.

A few attempts to cultivate the typhus organisms in a cell-free medium similar to that applied by Eagles and McClean (18) for vaccinia virus, were carried out with centrifuged Tyrode extracts of guinea pig kidney. So far these attempts have been unsuccessful inasmuch as no rickettsiae could be found and no infections could be induced in guinea pigs with these cultures.

Although the preceding results seem to indicate that live tissue is the significant constituent of the media described for the cultivation of the typhus rickettsiae, experiments to maintain cultures in the absence of serum have thus far been unsuccessful. In such experiments a medium was employed consisting only of tissue suspended in Tyrode solution, such as Li and Rivers (15) and Rivers (16) found to be entirely adequate for carrying cultures of vaccine virus. Actually rickettsiae were found in first generations in such a medium but usually reduced in number—and were for the most part absent in the second generations. In one such experiment rickettsiae were demonstrable in two generations, but not in the third. Although serum could not be entirely eliminated from the medium, it was found that the quantity could be reduced to at least half of that used as routine (i.e., one part of serum to five parts of Tyrode solution, instead of one to two parts) without damaging the cultures. It seemed to make little difference whether the serum was diluted with Tyrode, Ringer, or ordinary physiological saline. Whether the function of the serum consists merely in prolonging the viability of the tissue, has not been determined.

Comment

Although the etiological role of *Rickettsia prowazeki* in typhus fever hardly needs further confirmation, it is substantiated by the fact that guinea pigs recovered from infections, entirely typical of experimental typhus, produced by the injection of cultures as herein described, are immune to passage virus. Moreover, rabbits infected with such cultures developed positive Weil-Felix sera.

A significant outcome of the experiments is to be found in the similarity of the growth conditions of *Rickettsia prowazeki* and filterable viruses. In general, the presence of living tissue is considered to be necessary for the cultivation of viruses. This is stressed by Rivers (19) [cf. Dale (20)], and was recently substantiated in a paper by Hallauer (21) on the cultivation of the virus of fowl plague [cf. Landsteiner and Berliner (22)]. This relation of viruses to live tissues has been used as one of the arguments in favor of the view that viruses are not living organisms. It is of interest, therefore, that similar conditions for growth obtain in the cultivation of rickettsiae which, on account of their morphology, certainly must be deemed living microbes.

Summary

1. *Rickettsia prowazeki* can be cultivated for many generations *in vitro*, without diminution in numbers or virulence, in media similar to those described by Maitland, Rivers, and others for the cultivation of certain viruses. In all probability, such cultures can be maintained indefinitely.

2. It has been impossible, thus far, to cultivate the typhus rickettsia without employing living tissue.

1934

Hans Zinsser

Varieties of Typhus Virus and the Epidemiology of the American Form of European Typhus Fever (Brill's Disease)

After the identification of murine typhus, it was believed that Brill's disease was a variation of the former because both diseases closely resembled one another clinically and were endemic in the eastern seacoast cities of the United States. The status of Brill's disease, occurring in the absence of human body lice, yet established as a form of typhus by reciprocal cross-immunity tests with epidemic typhus fever (1), was clarified by Zinsser in his perceptive epidemiological analysis of case histories in the 1934 paper presented here.

In his analysis of 538 cases of Brill's disease occurring in Boston and New York, he found that over 93 per cent of the cases were individuals who came from endemic typhus regions of Europe. Furthermore, the incidence of disease was highest (86 per cent) in members of a single ethnic groups (Jews), and it seemed improbable that a disease, like murine typhus, would be so selective. Zinsser advanced the hypothesis that Brill's disease is actually *a recrudescence of epidemic typhus fever*, in a relatively mild form, in persons who had originally acquired the disease in Europe, where foci of typhus fever existed. This would explain the occurrence of the disease in the absence of lice and belie the role of rats as reservoirs of the disease. He further postulated that epidemic typhus rickettsiae may persist in tissues of human beings for extended periods of time and that lice may become infected by feeding on patients with Brill's disease. This hypothesis would explain the appearance of new epidemics of typhus fever: in Brill's disease man would be the reservoir of infection for both endemic and epidemic outbreaks of typhus fever.

Zinsser's hypothesis was supported by the findings of Murray, Baehr, Shwartzman, Mandelbaum, Rosenthal, Doane, Weiss, Cohen, and Snyder (2) when they recovered seven strains of *R. prowazeki* from 14 cases and infected lice by allowing them to feed on the infected cases. The rickettsiae isolated from these lice were fully virulent and indistinguishable from classic typhus strains (3). Subsequently, the isolation of *R. prowazeki* from lymph glands excised from two asymptomatic patients who had emigrated from an endemic typhus area in Russia 20 years previously (4) added to the validation of Zinsser's theory. This latter observation, however, has not yet been independently confirmed, which may in part be owing to the difficulty in obtaining material from such a select group of patients. In recent years the disease has been recognized in several countries where epidemic typhus fever is not now active, e.g., France, Poland, England, Yugoslavia.

The name Brill-Zinsser was suggested for the disease in recognition of Zinsser's pioneer studies (5).

I

Until 1917 it was the prevailing opinion that there was but one type of typhus virus responsible for this disease in many different parts of the world. At that time, Neill (1) described, in guinea pigs intra-peritoneally inoculated with blood from cases that occurred in Texas, the development of pronounced scrotal swellings not hitherto observed in the experimental disease. These observations made no impression until Mooser (2), in 1928, recognized such swellings as characteristic of the infection of guinea pigs with Mexican virus and found, in the tunica vaginalis of such animals, small Giemsa-staining bodies which he regarded as rickettsiae. This was the beginning of a differentiation between the classical European typhus and a Mexican, or New World variety.

It was subsequently found by a number of observers that the virus obtained from the sporadic typhus cases of the southern United States corresponded, in regard to scrotal swellings and tunica lesions, to the Mexican variety. In an epidemiological study of these cases, Maxcy (3), in 1926, suggested the possibility that the responsible virus was kept alive in an animal reservoir, possibly rodent, and was transmitted to man by some insect other than the louse. This suspicion was corroborated in 1931, when Dyer and his associates (4) of the United States Public Health Service isolated a virus of this type from the fleas of rats trapped in typhus foci in Baltimore; and members of the Harvard staff, together with Mooser (5), obtained a similar virus from the brains of rats caught in the Belem Prison in Mexico City during an epidemic.

Since that time, a large amount of work has been done in many parts of the world on the differentiation of the two types of virus. It is no longer accurate to speak of an "endemic" as contrasted with an "epidemic" virus, since both types can occur both endemically and epidemically. It is, further, no longer correct to designate the two varieties respectively as "European" and "New World," because a "Mexican" type of virus has been found in rats in the Mediterranean basin, isolated strains from Mexico have behaved like the European type, and the Brill's disease virus isolated by us in Boston has shown all the characteristics of the agent which causes the classical European disease.

Before discussing the epidemiological problems which form the primary subject of this paper, it will be helpful to review briefly the similarities and the differences which we believe to be significant in the comparison of the two types of infection. There is an unquestionably close relationship between them which is, of course, of fundamental importance in theoretical and practical immunological investigations. There are, however, experimentally determinable differences which forbid absolute identification.

The significant similarities are the following:

1. Guinea pigs and monkeys convalescent from one variety are immune to the other.

2. Serological tests (6), as carried out by our technique, show cross-agglutination of the two varieties of rickettsia in the sera of convalescent and immunized men and animals. In this connection, one of the most convincing experiments is the one reported by us in which a rabbit, treated with three injections of the killed louse vaccine of Weigl, acquired a Weil-Felix reaction, agglutinated the homologous vaccines up to 1–1000 and the Mexican vaccines up to 1–500; and another rabbit, similarly treated with the killed Mexican rickettsiae of our own vaccines, also acquired a Weil-Felix reaction and developed agglutination for the killed Mexican organisms of 1–1000, and for the European louse organism of 1–100 (slightly 1–200).

3. The vaccination of guinea pigs with killed Mexican rickettsiae vaccines protected regularly against the Mexican virus and 30 per cent to 40 per cent of the animals against the European virus (7).

4. The serum of a horse immunized with the Mexican rickettsiae acquired Weil-Felix reactions up to 1–320 (partial, 1–640) and agglutinated the Weigl louse vaccines up to 1–640 (8).

5. Finally, the occurrence of Weil-Felix reactions in both types of the disease, and the fact that brain lesions indistinguishable from each other occur in guinea pigs infected with either type of virus, add further evidence to their close similarity.

In spite of this established close relationship, the two viruses are not identical. The differentiations may be summarized as follows:

1. The tunica lesions with intracellular rickettsiae and the more rapid development of temperature aroused in guinea pigs by viruses isolated on this continent.

2. The greater virulence of the Mexican-American variety for rats is apparent both in the development of temperature in these animals and by the presence of rickettsiae in the peritoneal cavities and tunicas.*

* This difference of behavior in rats was first noted by Mooser (2) and corroborated by Maxcy.

3. Nicolle and Laigret (9) have found that the "American" virus will survive in rats for a much longer period than will the European, and that it can be carried through much longer series of mouse passages than can the European. This has been confirmed in our own laboratory.

4. In four years of persistent effort in our laboratory, we have never been able to obtain, in rats whose resistance has been diminished by the benzol, X-ray or other methods, the great accumulations of rickettsiae of the European strain which have become a regularly successful routine in the production of our Mexican typhus vaccines.

Considered together, these points of difference suggest that the type of virus isolated from the Mexican-American cases possesses a relatively higher degree of virulence for (is more closely adapted to) rodents. And this view is in perfect accord with what we now know of the epidemiology of the disease in this country—namely, a rat reservoir with rat-flea-man transmission which continues in a man-louse-man cycle only under the circumstances prevailing in heavily louse-infested groups. We are, therefore, inclined to agree with Mooser and with Nicolle in referring to the Mexican-American virus as a "murine" type.

In the study of similarities and differences between the types, it is, of course, of great importance to know to what extent and how permanently it is possible to effect experimental conversion of one variety into the other.

The European virus, like the murine, is preserved in laboratories for years by continuous guinea pig and rat passages and, without special experimental manipulation other than transfer, it remains true to its original characteristics. Moreover, no experimental procedure has so far been devised by which a European strain could be made permanently to assume the behavior of a murine strain.

In an experience of over five years with two European strains, we have never—in spite of persistent efforts—succeeded in more than temporarily modifying the characteristics of these strains in the "murine direction." With all European passage strains, guinea pigs quite frequently develop short-lived scrotal swellings with rickettsiae in small numbers in the tunica cells. Twenty-two of seventy-two recent passage animals of the "Breinl" strain have exhibited such lesions. But these early and moderate lesions, poor in rickettsiae, spontaneously disappear in subsequent generations and serve merely to emphasize the fact that the two types are closely related but not identical. By various methods, such as rat passage, direct intraperitoneal inoculation of tunica scrapings and the artificial suppression of resistance of our passage animals, we have occasionally prolonged and increased the tunica reactions of this European strain for a number of generations. But reversion to the original characteristics has always taken place spontaneously and promptly.

A Tunisian strain, brought to this country by Professor Nicolle, has seemed to lend itself more readily to this type of experiment. Yet even with this strain, no permanent conversion has been possible.

When tissue cultures of this Tunisian virus, grown by the method of Nigg and Landsteiner (10), are injected intraperitoneally into guinea pigs, the first generations may produce the orchitic "murine" reaction, possibly owing to the large numbers of rickettsiae injected. But, in passage, the strain rapidly reverts to its original condition. The same phenomenon is apparent in some recently published observations of Mooser (11). When he passed the Tunisian strain through rats that had received intraperitoneal blood injections, he succeeded in increasing its virulence for rats; and such a rat virus, intraperitoneally injected into guinea pigs, similarly treated with blood, continued to show the orchitic reaction for nine successive passages; but injected into guinea pigs not inoculated with blood, the strain immediately reverted to its original non-orchitic characteristics.

Efforts in the reverse direction—that is, the conversion of the murine type into the classical European variety, have likewise yielded only temporary modifications. Just as the European virus infection of guinea pigs occasionally produces the orchitic type of lesion, so occasional "murine" passage animals fail to cause these lesions. But in subsequent passages, the strains invariably revert.

When the Mexican virus is subcutaneously inoculated in a series of guinea pigs, a condition develops which is—in type of temperature reaction and absence of scrotal lesions—identical with that which characterizes the European. But whenever such a virus is again intraperitoneally injected, it reverts to the typical murine type.

Experiment in the laboratory, however, has thrown less light on this phase of the problem than have observations on strains isolated from Mexican epidemics. In 1930, our associate, Dr. Castaneda (12), brought to this laboratory a typhus virus which he had isolated during an epidemic in Jilotzingo. This strain, carried on by him in guinea pigs for twenty-five generations, behaved like the European variety—that is, gave no tunica and scrotal swellings in most of the animals through which it was passed, and in a few of them only were rickettsiae found in the tunica cells. Eventually, however, after louse passage, it reverted to the murine type, and so continued. Mooser, from another epidemic, isolated four strains, all of which at first behaved like the typical European virus. One of them, sent to us, reverted promptly to the murine type, with scrotal swellings and plentiful rickettsiae in the tunica cells, after seventeen and twenty-three days, respectively, in rats. Three of these strains, retained by Mooser, were similarly converted by him without difficulty by passage through rats which had received intraperitoneal injections of blood. One of his strains has not yet reverted, but retains the characteristics of not causing fever in rats, and showing only occasional rickettsiae-infected cells.† Since other strains isolated from the same and other Mexican epidemics behave, from the beginning, in the typical "murine" manner, it is logical to suppose that these European-similar strains have been altered by a succession of louse-man-louse passages, away from their original murine condition.

From such observations, it would seem not unjustified to conclude that a modification of the murine virus in the direction of the European, by passage through man, takes place more readily and profoundly than a reverse change, when the European strain is passed through rodents. And it is not unlikely from this that these two closely related infectious agents represent variants—one, the "murine," adapted to rodents; the other, the European, adapted to the human host, or "humanized." It is, of course, possible and even probable that both types of virus originated in a single "murine" type. Such a common rat origin obviously suggested by experimental evidence, is discussed at length by Mooser (11) in his recent paper. It might even be logical, considering what we know of rickettsiae, that the original stock strain was an infectious agent of insects. However, such views are difficult to prove conclusively. The point of importance is the fact that, whatever view one may hold concerning a common origin, failure—up to the present time—in producing permanent reversion of the European "humanized" form to the "murine," suggests that the slight, but definite differences between the two are well established, biologically deep-seated and, therefore, probably of remote origin. The bearing of this on epidemiology is obvious.

During the last twelve months, we have become increasingly interested in this problem, because we have isolated from Brill's disease cases in Boston three typhus strains which have so far corresponded in

† Since this paper was written this strain, too, has reverted. (Personal communication.)

every respect to what we have spoken of as the "humanized" European type. One of them, strain "B," has—at the present writing—been maintained for ten months in guinea pigs without showing any signs of conversion to the murine type. Two others have been similarly maintained for two and four months, respectively, with the same results. A detailed study of the first strain has been reported. The others will be reported in a separate communication. In no case have we observed more than the occasional scrotal swelling seen in the typical "humanized" European strains, and in no case have there been more than a very few rickettsiae discoverable in the tunica cells. Temperature curves have been similarly characteristic, and intraperitoneal inoculation into X-rayed rats has never yielded the "murine" type of reaction.

Brill's disease is an urban condition seen in the northeast coastal cities of the United States, and has occurred chiefly in immigrant populations. This, together with the characteristics of the strains, naturally suggests the possibility that this form of typhus fever is the imported classical variety; and it is therefore an obvious thought that, if it were possible to obtain some information concerning the epidemiology of Brill's disease, such information would throw considerable light on the epidemiology of the disease as it has occurred for centuries in the typhus regions of southeastern Europe.

II

The epidemiological studies which we have been able to make in Boston were facilitated by the cooperation of the Staff of the Beth Israel Hospital. The large material from New York was made available for analysis by the generous cooperation of Professor Haven Emerson of Columbia, who placed at our disposal his statistician, Miss Dochterman; and by the unselfish collaboration of Doctors George Baehr and Frederick H. King of the Mt. Sinai Hospital of New York.‡

Nativity

It has been obvious to everyone who has studied Brill's disease that this malady occurs most frequently in the Russian-Jewish populations of our large cities. Table 1 consolidates the nativity records of all the cases of which we have information.

‡ We are also indebted to Dr. Benjamin Alexander for collecting data in the homes of some of the Boston patients.

Table 1. All cases

City	Totals	Born in United States	Not stated	Foreign-born	Percentage foreign-born
New York	494	18	13	463	96.2
Boston	44	4	0	40	90.9
Totals	538	22	13	503	94.8

Table 2. Comparison of Jewish and non-Jewish hospitals[a]

Hospital	Totals	Born in United States	Not stated	Foreign-born	Percentage foreign-born
Jewish	430	12	13	405	97.1
Non-Jewish	64	6	0	58	90.6

[a] Jewish: Mt. Sinai, Jewish Hospital.
Non-Jewish: New York, Bellevue, Presbyterian, Post Graduate, Long Island College.

The percentages of foreign-born are thus extraordinarily high. In New York, while the percentage of Brill's disease cases consisted of 96.2 per cent of foreign-born, the percentage of foreign-born to the total population throughout these years fluctuated between 37 and 41 per cent.

The records from New York included cases from two Jewish Hospitals (the Mt. Sinai and the Jewish) and from five non-Jewish hospitals (the New York Hospital, the Presbyterian, the Bellevue, the Post Graduate and the Long Island College Hospital). Since the former are almost selectively occupied with the foreign-born population it was of obvious importance to determine how these hospitals compared with the non-Jewish ones in regard to nativity of Brill's disease cases.

In computing these percentages we eliminated the 13 of which nativity was not stated.

It will be seen (Table 2) that there was no significant difference between the two types of hospital.

Mass immigration to the United States practically ceased in 1914. The percentage of foreign-born in New York dropped from 41 per cent in 1910 to 34 per cent in 1930. In Boston the foreign-born white population was 28 per cent in 1930. It was of interest to compare the percentage of incidence of Brill's disease in foreign-born for the earlier and the later periods of which we have records (Tables 3 and 4).

Table 3. Comparison of early decades with later periods
New York cases

Period	Totals	Born in United States	Not stated	Foreign-born	Percentage foreign-born
1910–20	300	6	8	286	97.9
1921–33	194	12	5	177	93.6

Table 4. Boston cases

Period	Totals	Born in United States	Not stated	Foreign-born	Percentage foreign-born
1902–12[a]	28	3	0	25	89.2
1929–34[b]	16	1	0	15	93.7

[a] Dr. R. I. Lee from Massachussetts General Hospital (13).

[b] Beth Israel Hospital [Ten of these cases have formed the subject of a paper by Doctors Ernstene and Riseman (14).]

There was thus no significant difference in the distribution of Brill's disease between the native and foreign-born groups in the course of twenty-three years, although there must have been a considerable relative increase, during this time, of the native-born living under conditions identical with those experienced by the individuals who contracted the disease.§

A disproportionate selection of foreign-born by a disease is obviously incompatible with transmission by agencies to which the population as a whole is exposed. In this instance such selection cannot be reconciled with the assumption of rat- and rat-flea transmission. But alone these figures are not conclusive since foreign-born populations are generally poor, badly housed and perhaps disproportionately more

§ No figures are available to show this relationship for the Jewish population of New York. For Russians and Poles, however, Dr. G. J. Drolet has kindly furnished us the following records:

1910: Total Russians and Poles in New York 312,490
    Number of these foreign-born.. .'............... 188,074 or 60.2 per cent
    Natives of foreign parentage.................... 124,416 or 39.8 per cent

1930: Total Russians and Poles in New York........... 1,403,445
    Number of these foreign-born.................. 680,770 or 48.5 per cent
    Natives of foreign parentage.................... 722,683 or 51.5 per cent

Table 5. Jewish and non-Jewish cases

Period	Total cases	Jewish cases	Percentage Jewish cases	Percentage Jews in total pop. of N.Y.
1910–20	300	291	97	26–29
1921–33	194	178	91	29–27.1

Table 6. Comparison of foreign-born and native Jewish cases[a]

Period	Total Jewish cases	Foreign-born Jewish cases	Percentage foreign-born
1910–20	291	287	95.2
1921–33	178	170	94.9

[a] Unfortunately there are no available records which show what percentages of the total Jewish population of New York were native and of foreign birth, respectively.

exposed to environmental conditions favorable to all transmitting agencies. It was necessary, therefore, to carry our analysis into greater detail.

One of the outstanding features of the records is the large percentage of Jews. Epidemiological observations all over the world exclude the supposition that there is a racial susceptibility that renders Jews more likely to contract this disease. Typhus, when it becomes epidemic, spreads equally among Jews and Gentiles, wherever it occurs. The large percentage of Jews in these statistics means merely that the immigration from typhus endemic foci to the United States has largely consisted of the Jewish population of these regions, and the large percentage of Russians means almost entirely Russian Jews.

It is of considerable interest therefore, to examine how many of our cases occurred in members of the Jewish race.

Of the total of 494 New York cases, 469 or 94.9 per cent were Jews.

Of the earlier 28 Boston cases we have no racial records, but if, as seems justified, we classify the 18 Russians and 2 Poles of this group as Jews, we have, of the total of 44 cases, 36 or 82 per cent Jews.

For reasons stated when we were dealing with analyses of the foreign-born, it seemed desirable again to compare earlier and later decades. Tables 5 and 6 present the figures for New York—first as to the percentage of cases occurring in members of the Jewish population as a whole—then the percentage of such cases occurring in foreign-born Jews as contrasted with native Jews.

Table 7. Twenty years old and younger

Period	Foreign-born	Native
1910–20	17	3
1921–33	3	4
Total	20	7

Combining the records of the two tables we find that, from 1910 to 1933, 97 per cent of all cases in New York were in Jews and 92.3 per cent of all cases were in Jews of *foreign birth.* And in the period 1921–33, when a considerable proportion of the total Jewish population in New York were of native birth, 91 per cent of all cases were in Jews and 86.4 per cent of all cases were still in Jews of *foreign birth.*

For Boston these relations are still more striking since in 1929–33, when foreign-born Jews (Russians) were to native-born Jews (Russians) roughly as 3.1 is to 3.6, the typhus cases (all but one in Russian Jews) were foreign-born 15 to native-born 1.

Since, of course, the foreign- and native-born lived together in the same quarters, houses, families and conditions, this is a state of affairs incompatible with familial transmission, common factors of housing, hygiene or exposure to common insect or animal reservoirs.

In commenting on these figures a possible source of error suggests itself. This disease is far more severe in the adult than it is in the young. It is conceivable, therefore, that many mild cases in the younger native-born group might have escaped hospitalization and consequently finding no statistical representation, might have created a purely fictitious preponderance of the older foreign-born group.

Such a possibility is almost completely counterbalanced by the consideration that we have, as controls on the foreign-born Jewish population, the large groups of similar age represented by the foreign-born of other races and by the native-born living under comparable environmental circumstances.

Moreover the records show that a good many cases under twenty years of age were hospitalized and that of these the majority were of foreign birth (Table 7).

Information bearing on the point can further be obtained by examining the age distribution of cases for the two periods, remembering that between 1921 and 1933 a large number of the native-born must have reached the ages (21 to 40) in which, in both periods, over 50 per cent of the cases occurred (Table 8).

Table 8. Age distribution[a]

Age	1910–20 (per cent)	1921–33 (per cent)
10–20	7.5	4.16
21–30	27.9	17.65
31–40	37.1	34.37
41–50	19.1	23.43
51–60	7.5	13.54
61+	0.6	6.70

[a] Percentages are of total for each period.

A shift to an older level is apparent in the later period corresponding to the aging of the foreign-born population.

If, now, we analyze all our cases by country of origin, tabulating first those countries which may be regarded as endemic foci of the classical European typhus fever (Austria is included in these since all those marked Austrian were Jews by race and can justifiably, for the most part, be classified as coming from Austrian Poland) we obtain the information shown in Table 9.

The importance of this tabulation lies in the fact that, of the 502 cases known to be of foreign birth, 471 or 93.6 per cent were born in the endemic typhus regions of Europe; and 404 or 80.4 per cent were born in Russia alone.

The total number of typhus cases reported is of course a very small fraction of the Jewish population of the cities. And since the virus isolated from Brill's disease cases by us resembles the European type, it becomes important to make sure that this preponderance of the foreign-born Jewish patients is not due to a constant influx of infected cases from abroad. This point is easily checked by examining the length of time elapsed between arrival in America and occurrence of the disease. This has been done for us for New York cases in which this information was available, by Miss Dochterman. Her tables show records of 126 cases:

> 2 were on incoming vessels.
> 29 had been in the United States 1 to 10 years.
> 47 had been in the United States 10 to 20 years.
> 35 had been in the United States 20 to 30 years.
> 13 had been in the United States over 30 years.

Epidemiology of Brill's Disease

Table 9. Place of birth

| Country | New York cases | | Boston cases | Totals |
	Jewish hospitals	Non-Jewish hospitals		
Russia	338	33	33	404
Austria	32	5	1	38
Poland	12	1	2	15
Rumania	9	1	0	10
Hungary	3	1	0	4
Germany	2	0	1	3
Lithuania	1	0	0	1
Ireland	1	0	3	4
England	3	2	0	5
Scotland	1	0	0	1
Denmark	0	1	0	1
Sweden	0	1	0	1
Finland	0	1	0	1
France	1	0	0	1
Italy	1	5	0	6
Spain	0	2	0	2
Greece	0	2	0	2
Armenia	0	1	0	1
Turkey	1	1	0	2
Not stated	13	0	0	13
United States	12	6	4	22
Totals	430	63[a]	44	537

[a] One Puerto Rican omitted.
New York Records—One group from 1910–33.
Boston Records—Two groups (1) 28 from 1902–12, (2) 16 from 1929–34.

The Boston figures, as far as available, indicate a similar state of affairs.

In view of the "European" or "human" characteristics of the virus, it is of importance to note that two of the cases were on incoming vessels. And three cases at the Boston City Hospital described by Dr. Berlin and by Dr. Shattuck (not used in our tabulation) had been in the country only ten days when hospitalized. This evidence to the effect that for a considerable period the disease was being imported agrees with the experimentally determined nature of the virus.

Table 10. New York cases occurring in the same house

1.	Sam K.	1920
	Sarah G.	1928
2.	Lem T.	1921
	Isidor W.	1916
3.	Ida W.	1915
	Louis Y.	1922
4.	Aaron W.	1913
	Jennie D.	1912
5.	Isaac H.	1918
	David W.	1914
6.	Max B.	1912
	Charles B.	1910
7.	Barnett K.	June, 1910
	Lena R.	August, 1910
8.	Abraham Z.	1911
	Lena T.	1910

Familial Distribution

The next matter of importance is distribution in families, time and place. For the New York cases, such information can only be obtained at a time much later than occurrence, by family name, address and date. In working this out, it is striking that of the 494 cases of which we have records from 1910 to 1933, there are only eight instances of more than one case in the same house, the houses being largely tenement houses. In none of these did the patients bear the same name, and in only one instance did the cases occur in the same year, and then three months apart. We tabulate these in Table 10 omitting names and addresses for obvious reasons.

The above record quite excludes a traceable transmission relationship in the New York cases.

As far as the Boston cases are concerned, the 28 of Dr. Roger Lee, spread over ten years, were scattered over five districts in Boston and six suburbs. There were no two cases of the same name or in the same house. The sixteen later cases, including the ten reported by Ernstene and Riseman and six additional ones seen at the Beth Israel since 1932,

Table 11. Occupation—Boston cases

Males	Females
5 tailors	15 housewives
3 salesmen	2 shirtwaist makers
2 lawyers	1 seamstress
2 harness makers	1 stenographer
2 peddlers	1 tailoress
1 junk dealer	1 wife who aided in store
1 shirt maker	
1 brakeman	
1 cabinet man	
1 schoolboy	
1 baker	
1 bakery wagon driver	
1 laundry wagon driver	
1 waiter	
Total 23	21

again had no two in the same family and were widely scattered over the city and suburbs.

Occupations

There being no possible transmission relationship in regard to family, time or domicile, it might still be possible that there existed an occupational relationship by which the cases could be traced to contact through food handling or to individual shops in which a great many of the patients had worked. For New York, this is an extremely difficult thing to determine, since so many of the men were primarily engaged in the garment trades, or were owners of stores. However, some light is shed on this problem by the fact that, with an absence of familial relationship, there was an almost equal division between men and women. Of the total of 538 cases of which we have records, 290 were males, and 248 females. According to Miss Dochterman, who collected the initial data for us for New York, a majority of the women were housewives.

For Boston we have definite records of occupation in every case, and these figures are tabulated in Table 11 since this matter is of such great importance.

It is apparent from this that the occupational distribution showed no common factors of epidemiological significance.

Seasonal Occurrence

A study of seasonal occurrence for all our cases indicates a sharp rise for the months of June, July, and August, the peak in July. We omit chart for economy of space. This corresponds with the seasonal curve of the endemic disease in the southern United States (Maxcy) but is quite at variance with European typhus curves, which rise to peaks usually during the winter months.

No final conclusions as to the reason for this state of affairs can be drawn. The endemic in the southern United States is, undoubtedly, in the majority of cases, of rat–rat-flea origin. In Mexico proper however, where a rat reservoir is also known to exist and where the virus strains correspond to those obtained in the southern United States, the peak of typhus is usually in the winter months, thus resembling the European. It appears probable therefore, that winter peaks merely indicate epidemic man-louse-man accumulations during the season of maximum louse infestation and have no significance in regard to original source of the initial cases.

Discussion

The classical European typhus and the Mexican (or endemic American) disease are caused by infectious agents which resemble each other so closely that they may be regarded as slightly divergent variants of the same original stock. The fundamental similarities between them are evident in cross-immunity, widely overlapping serological reactions, identical adaptation to a man-louse-man epidemic cycle and relations to the Weil-Felix reaction. Nevertheless the two are not identical. Animal experiment with virus isolated in Mexico and in the United States indicates that these strains possess a higher infectiousness (closer adaptation) for certain rodents than do similar strains isolated from cases on the European Continent and in North Africa. These findings are consistent with the fact now established for both Mexico and the southern United States that the typhus virus of these regions is inter-epidemically preserved in rats. Information obtained from the "J" strain of Castaneda and from recently isolated epidemic strains in Mexico by Mooser suggest that the typical "murine" or rat virus may temporarily assume the characteristics of the European type by relatively few passages through man. But the experimental reversibility of such strains to the original murine type indicates that the primary sources of such epidemics were "murine." Years of experimental effort in our laboratory to transform a typical European strain into a murine have so far been unsuccessful. But even if this were eventually accomplished it would still be true that the observed differences of behavior in guinea pigs and rats are not superficial divergences rapidly acquired or reversed, but have become moderately stabilized. For these reasons we regard the differential nomenclature, i.e., "murine" and "humanized" virus as useful and, in the light of present knowledge, probably consistent with facts.

The Brill's disease viruses behave in laboratory animals like the European type. That European typhus has actually been imported with immigrants hospitalized within the incubation time after debarkation is a matter of record. We therefore regard Brill's disease as representing the European disease, established in America in endemic form and distinct from the southeastern disease described by Maxcy as well as from the tabardillo of Mexico.

While the interepidemic reservoir of the last named disease is known to exist in rats, the interepidemic reservoir of the continental European virus is still unknown. The former opinion that typhus in Europe was preserved in human carriers has been questioned on the logical grounds that such an explanation necessitates the assumption of an uninterrupted chain of man-louse-man transmissions for long years between epidemics, a supposition which appears unlikely in view of the facts that the virus is present in the blood of cases for a short time only, that infected lice usually die inside of two weeks and that there is no hereditary infectivity of lice.

Brill's disease appeared to offer an extraordinary opportunity for the study of the interepidemic reservoir of the European typhus virus, since it is obviously easier to make exact epidemiological studies when cases are constant but few, than when a multitude of intersecting trails obliterate each other.

The salient points of our epidemiological studies are the following:

1. Of 538 cases occurring in New York and Boston in the course of about thirty years, 94.8 per cent occurred in individuals of foreign birth.

2. Over 90 per cent of all the cases occurred in a single racial group and, within this group 95 per cent of the cases were in the foreign-born members of this group. Calculated for the New York cases as a whole this means that in 1910–20, 92.3 per cent; and 1921–33, 86.4 per cent of *all* cases occurred in *foreign-born* members of the Jewish race although these individuals were living intimately together with a constantly increasing number of native-born of the same race. Large control

groups of foreign-born of other races and nations and of native-born of the same cities were practically exempt.

3. Ninety-three and six-tenths per cent of all the cases were born in those regions of southeastern Europe in which typhus is endemic and often epidemic. Eighty and four-tenths per cent came from Russia alone.

4. Of 126 cases about which data were available 75.6 per cent had been in this country for over ten years; the remainder from one to ten years. In two only could the origin of infection be attributed to foreign sources.

5. No connection whatever could be traced between cases. There was no domiciliary or occupational relationship. There were no two cases in the same family. A few only were food handlers.

It seems obvious that these simple facts are incompatible with any hypothesis of transmission which involves a virus reservoir in domestic animals or in insects. Although it is possible and even probable that a reservoir of murine typhus may coexist and give rise to an occasional case, such a source of infection could not explain the incidence of Brill's disease. It would be impossible to reconcile a common source of infection such as rats and rat-fleas with the almost exclusive selection of the foreign-born of a single racial group.

Surveying our evidence as a whole and correlating our studies on the nature of the virus with epidemiological data we must consider the hypothesis that the Brill's disease virus is maintained in the bodies of the infected human beings. In appraising this possibility we are forced to a conclusion which we have attempted, by much scrutiny of our data, to escape because of its divergence from accepted views.

If there were an uninterrupted chain of mild cases with man-louse-man transmission it would be difficult to reconcile this with the almost complete exemption of the native-born of the afflicted racial group and with the complete absence of familial, domiciliary or occupational relationship. Incidentally it may be mentioned that careful scrutiny of many of the Boston cases failed to reveal lousiness in families, with only one case in adult groups of from three to five members. And rat studies were negative when made.

The only assumption which is compatible with all the data is that the cases of Brill's disease which have occurred in New York and Boston are recrudescences of typhus fever acquired at an earlier time of life in endemic typhus foci of Europe.

This view implies the premise that the virus of typhus, once acquired, remains latent for many years in an indeterminable number of individuals and may become active in a fraction of these under circumstances of fading immunity. In this respect the condition would resemble that held for a number of other infections and, however divergent from opinion hitherto held on typhus epidemiology, seems forced upon us by observed facts.

This would imply a relatively small percentage of recrudescences if one considers that there were only twenty-two recorded hospitalized cases of Brill's disease in 1910 in New York, with a total Jewish population of over 1,200,000, a considerable proportion of whom were native-born. It is also in harmony with the progressive abatement of the disease, 300 cases in 1910–20; 194 cases, 1921–33, in the face of a total increase of the Jewish population to over 1,800,000 but a relative decrease of the foreign-born. One is justified in expecting a spontaneous extinction of the disease with the gradual cessation of immigration, under American conditions of hygiene.

Finally the biological attributes of the virus are compatible with the assumption of a human reservoir.

Conclusions

1. Brill's disease is an imported form of the classical European typhus fever.

2. The cases observed in New York and Boston represent recrudescences of old infections originally acquired in European foci.

3. In communities not heavily louse-infected such cases remain sporadic but in louse-infested and crowded areas such recrudescent cases may furnish foci for the origin of small or large outbreaks according to circumstances. The recrudescent cases may thus serve to maintain endemic prevalence by bridging breaks in the chain of man-louse-man propagation.

It is suggested that this is the manner in which the European virus has been maintained in continental foci for centuries.

4. Rat reservoirs are thus not necessary for the endemic continuance of the disease, though they probably coexist.

E. H. Derrick

"Q" Fever, a New Fever Entity: Clinical Features, Diagnosis, and Laboratory Investigation

The Australian physician E. H. Derrick was the first to recognize Q fever as a distinct disease entity. In a now historic paper (1937) he reported on an outbreak of a fever of unknown origin that had occurred two years earlier among abattoir workers in Queensland, Australia. His report clinically describes nine typical cases and records his studies on the isolation and the nature of the causative agent. Derrick named the disease "Q" fever, the "Q" denoting "Query," not "Queensland." In the same year, 1937, the etiological agent of the disease was identified and classified as a rickettsia by Burnet and Freeman (1); it was subsequently named *Rickettsia burneti* after Burnet (2).

Halfway around the world but almost at the same time a similar organism was isolated by Davis and Cox (3) at the Rocky Mountain Laboratory at Hamilton, Montana, from ticks (*Dermacentor anderson*) collected near Nine Mile Creek, Montana. Because the organism was filterable it was called *R. diaporica* (4), and the disease that was produced in animals was provisionally named Nine Mile fever. On the basis of clinical similarity between Q fever and Nine Mile fever, and complete cross-immunity, Dyer suggested that both diseases were identical (5); this was confirmed by Cox (6) and by Burnet and Freeman (7). Because of certain unique properties possessed by the agent of Q fever, the name *Coxiella burnetii* was proposed to designate the agent as the prototype of a new genus (8).

The ubiquity and diverse epidemiological patterns of Q fever are direct consequences of the distinctive features of its etiological agent. *C. burnetii* is the only rickettsial agent that is definitely known to infect man naturally by the airborne route. In contrast, the bite of an infected arthropod vector is the common mode of transmission of other rickettsial infections to man. The great resistance of the Q fever agent to the external environment, e.g., heat, sunlight, drying, is a factor assuring its survival in aerosols and its epidemiological spread. It has broad tissue tropisms, growing well in the reproductive tract of the cow and sheep, the intestines of ticks, and the respiratory tract of man. In widely separated geographical areas the rickettsiae have been recovered from air samples and from a variety of domestic animals, fowls, ticks, mites, and body lice. That a natural reservoir for the disease exists is suggested by studies wherein *C. burnetii* has been recovered from wild animals and fowls. Man is only accidentally involved in the complex natural cycle of the etiological agent; the infection of man is not a vital stage in the cycle. Q fever appears to be a disease of nature adapted to arthropod transmission and capable of explosive but noncontagious attack on local groups of susceptible people, possibly invading victims through the respiratory tract.

Q fever was initially thought to be indigenous to Australia; its worldwide distribution was unsuspected until a few years after its discovery. In the winter of 1944 and the spring of 1945 the disease occurred among Allied troops serving in the Mediterranean theater of operations. Robbins and his associates, in a series of papers, thoroughly and accurately described the outbreaks (9). Q fever was subsequently found to exist sporadically and endemically on a global scale; *C. burnetii* has been found in 67 countries on six continents (10).

Since Derrick's original report appeared, a voluminous body of literature has accumulated on Q fever which attests to the worldwide research carried on by investigators in several biological disciplines on the manifold facets of this unique rickettsial infection. Because Q fever may assume a multiplicity of epidemiological patterns, its control has been difficult to achieve and it remains a continual threat to world health.

Introduction

In August, 1935, the occurrence of a number of cases of fever among workers in a large meatworks in Brisbane was brought to the notice of the Director-General of Health and Medical Services for Queensland, Sir Raphael Cilento, who directed me to investigate the matter. It appeared that the cases which incited the inquiry had begun to occur early in 1933. Since then there had been about 20 cases—not indeed a large number among 800 employees. Most of the cases resembled in a general way the nine cases to be described in this paper. The type of fever was a continued one of seven to twenty-four days' duration. There were certain features about the cases which caused the medical attendants to believe that they constituted a distinct clinical entity. The most outstanding feature was the uniform failure of blood cultures and agglutination tests to throw light on the diagnosis.

Further cases have occurred from time to time, and the courtesy of many practitioners has enabled me to investigate them directly. When the inquiry began, a number of diseases came to mind as possible causes: typhus, which in several forms is endemic in Queensland; undulant fever, a recognized occupational disease of meat workers; aberrant typhoid and paratyphoid fevers; and leptospirosis. All the tests for these, however, gave negative results. The commoner animal diseases were next considered and excluded. Then the suspicion arose and gradually grew into a conviction that we were here dealing with a type of fever which had not previously been described. It became necessary to give it a name, and "Q" fever was chosen to denote it until fuller knowledge should allow a better name.

One line of investigation, guinea pig inoculation, has been particularly fruitful. Guinea pigs acquire the disease readily by injection of blood or urine from a patient. Their subsequent immunity permits a specific diagnosis to be made, and has rendered it possible to prove that "Q" fever is a pathological as well as a clinical entity.

As no organism could be seen in or cultivated from human or guinea pig material, it appeared likely that the infecting agent was a virus. Infected guinea pig liver was thereupon sent to Dr. F. M. Burnet, of Melbourne, who, transferring the infection to mice, was successful in discovering rickettsial bodies in their spleens.

As the work proceeded, its scope had to be extended. Cases of fever of doubtful causation were found to occur from time to time in and around Brisbane apart from meat workers. When these were investigated some of them proved to be due to "Q" fever. The cases now to be described include, therefore, in addition to five from the abattoir, two from other parts of Brisbane, one from Gympie and one from Pomona.

While much about the disease is still obscure, the time is ripe for a general review of present knowledge.

Clinical Features

Nine cases of illness have been proved to be "Q" fever by guinea pig inoculation and immunity tests. The number is small, but it is hoped that from them an idea of the clinical picture of the disease may be obtained. A general description will be given here, and the details of the cases in the next section.

The patients were all men; their ages were 50, 29, 45, 18, 17, 37, 36, 33, and 55 years.

Incubation Period. In case VI the incubation period could be deduced as fifteen days or less.

Onset. The onset of the illness in all cases was acute. Within a few days of the first premonitory symptoms the victims were in bed quite ill. The first complaints were usually malaise, anorexia, headache, pains in the back and limbs, and feverishness.

Course of the Illness. As the illness developed, the symptoms became more severe and the general condition of the patient worse. The headache was troublesome and persistent, and often interfered with sleep. The face was flushed or pale, the eyes were closed and the tongue was coated. In the more severe infections the patient became drowsy, even stuporous, and passed on into a typhoid state. The symptoms gradually abated as the temperature fell. With those patients running the shorter course the improvement, once it started, was rapid.

Fever. The temperature rose rapidly and remained high. The daily maxima were usually between 39 and 40°C. (102 to 104°F.). Some of the charts show large daily remissions. These may be due in part to the use of antipyretic drugs for the relief of headache, but this may not explain them all. The course of the fever varied considerably. There were two fairly distinct types. In case II (Fig. 2), IV (Fig. 4), V, and VI the fever lasted from six to nine days. Its subsidence was rapid, case II showing a definite crisis. These cases had much the same type of fever as that characteristic of urban or murine typhus.

In other cases the course was more prolonged, with a gradual defervescence. In case I (Fig. 1) the primary fever lasted fourteen days, and after two days' interval there was a relapse lasting another eight days. In case III (Fig. 3) there were at least seventeen days of fever, and in case IX (Fig. 6), twenty-four days. The course in case VII (Fig. 5) was extremely prolonged. The fastigium of the fever lasted till the twenty-third day, and the fall thereafter was very gradual, so gradual that one could not decide the precise day of ending. There was still a slight evening rise of temperature in the ninth week.

Pulse Rate. One of the features of these cases was the slow rate of the pulse at the beginning of the illness in comparison with the height of the fever. This is shown well in Fig. 6, in which the pulse rate curve hardly leaves the base line, and in Figs. 2 and 3. Case VII was the only one in this series in which the pulse rate exceeded 100 to any great extent. The slow pulse rate is of some help in the diagnosis, but its value is limited by the occurrence of a slow pulse rate also in typhoid and typhus fevers and in Weil's disease.

Headache. The outstanding symptom was headache. It was present in every case but one, and was the chief complaint of most of the patients. The terms severe, intense and raging were used in the notes to describe it. If often persisted for some days after admission of the patient to hospital, and called for special treatment.

Shivers and Sweats. Four patients noticed shivers at the onset. Two patients had a rigor, one on the third and the other on the seventh day of illness. Some had profuse sweating at night. This may have been due in part to the headache drugs.

Rash. A rash is not a feature of "Q" fever. Six of the nine patients had no sign of a rash. In cases I and VIII a few indefinite red spots were found when the abdomen was examined at the time of the patient's admission to hospital. They would hardly have been thought worthy of record except for the endeavor to make a clinical diagnosis. Only one of the nine, patient VII, had a definite rash. It appeared on the fourteenth day of illness as a punctate red rash, first on the back, then on the chest and abdomen. It had partly faded by the next morning and had gone the morning after.

The absence of a characteristic rash during the first week in "Q" fever is of importance in distinguishing the disease from urban typhus. The occasional case of typhus that occurs in Brisbane almost always has a well-marked rash which appears about the fifth day and is a striking feature of the illness. It is to be borne in mind, however, that there are atypical cases of fever belonging to the typhus group, particularly in certain places, which run their course without a rash.

Jaundice. Only one patient in this series became jaundiced. This was number VII, the most severely affected of them all. The jaundice appeared on the thirteenth day of the illness, deepened during the next week, and disappeared in another ten days. Its presence raised a problem in diagnosis which is discussed later.

Conjunctival Congestion. One patient (number I) had severe congestion of the conjunctivae, which lasted till at least the eleventh day. The associated photophobia continued throughout the illness. At least one other patient had bloodshot eyes at the onset. Photophobia was a prominent symptom.

Congestion of the conjunctivae is regarded, and rightly so, as a valuable help in the differential diagnosis of the leptospiroses. "The injection of the conjunctivae is almost pathognomonic" [Manson-Bahr (1)]. The presence of this sign in two of our cases of "Q" fever, as well as its occurrence in various types of typhus fever, is a reminder that it is not an absolute sign of a leptospirosis.

The Spleen. In none of the nine cases was the spleen recorded as definitely palpable. This was surprising, for infected guinea pigs and mice invariably have enlarged spleens; and in the series of cases of undiagnosed fever in abattoir workers previous to the occurrence of these nine, many of whom must have had "Q" fever, about a quarter had palpable spleens. I feel that the spleen must be enlarged to some extent in human cases of "Q" fever, and that in a more extensive series it would sometimes be found large enough to be palpated.

The Blood. Blood examinations were made in four cases (Table 1). In one case there was a definite anemia. In each of the examinations the

Table 1. "Q" Fever Cases, Blood Examinations[a]

Case number	Day of illness	Number per cubic millimeter	Appearance	Hemoglobin. Percentage	Number per cubic millimeter	Neutrophile cells		Lymphocytes		Eosinophile cells. Percentage
						Percentage	Total	Percentage	Total	
I	5	4,480,000	Anisocytosis	88	9,300	74	6,882	26	2,418	
	26	4,490,000	Anisocytosis	88	6,300	62	3,906	38	2,394	
II	10	5,300,000	Normal	104	5,700	35	1,995	65	3,705	
IV	14	5,040,000	Normal	100	8,900	38	3,382	61	5,429	1
VII	11				9,000	56	5,040	44	3,960	
	28				8,500	68	5,780	32	2,720	
	32	3,600,000	Hypochromia, polychromasia, slight basophilia	67		46		54		

[a] These examinations were made by the staff of the pathological laboratories of the Brisbane General Hospital and the Mater Misericordiae Public Hospital, and are quoted by courtesy of Dr. J. V. Duhig and Dr. G. Taylor.

total of the white cells was within normal limits. In three cases there was a relative and absolute lymphocytosis. In two of these the counts that disclosed the lymphocytosis were made after the temperature had fallen to normal.

Other Signs and Symptoms. Vomiting was present in three cases; in two it was persistent. Two patients had some abdominal distension. Constipation was the rule. No patient had diarrhea. Two had a slight cough. Three had epistaxis; in one of them it was severe and repeated. At the beginning of the illness albuminuria was found almost invariably, clearing up before long. The finding of granular casts in the urine is recorded twice. Enlargement of lymph glands was not noticed in any case.

Convalescence. During convalescence the strength and sense of wellbeing returned at varying rates. Those patients whose fever had run the shorter course improved rapidly after it was over. Some of them returned to work as soon as 16, 18 and 20 days after the illness began. In others the restoration to health was slower. Patient VII was still away from work after five months, the convalescence being delayed by anemia, corneal ulcer, and neck stiffness. Individual patients complained of "nerves," pain in the thigh, numbness in the hand, insomnia, and

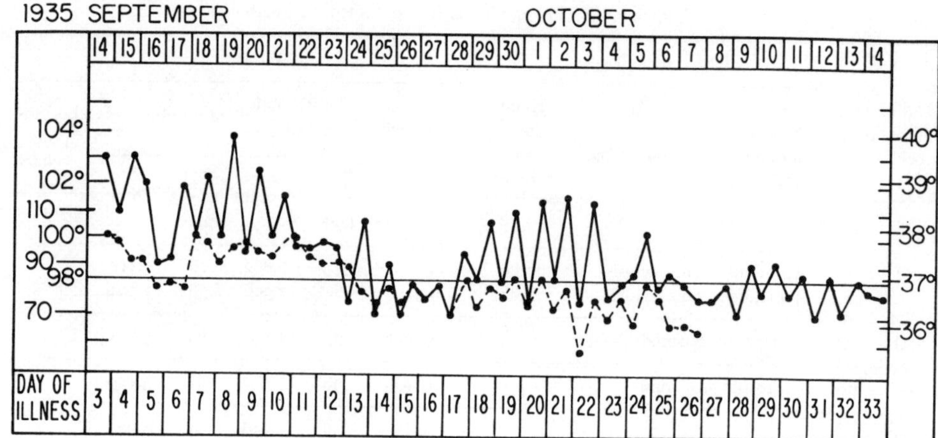

Fig. 1. Chart of G.N. (case I). Continuous line = temperature; broken line = pulse rate.

thinning of the hair, as well as of the general weakness and weakness of the legs which are to be expected after a serious illness.

Case Histories

In these cases, following Osler's practice in discussing typhoid fever, I have taken the day on which the patient went to bed, as far as that information could be accurately obtained, as the first day of the illness. It is necessary to make this definition, as frequent reference will be made to the day of illness on which events occurred. If the illness was to be counted from the day of the first symptom, the duration would be several days longer.

Case I

The notes of case I are published by courtesy of Dr. L. A. Little and Dr. P. J. Kelly.

G. N., aged fifty years, a worker among hides at the abattoir, was admitted to the Mater Misericordiae Public Hospital on September 14, 1935. He said that he had been ill about a week with headache, shivers, pains across the back and in various places. He remained at work, however, until September 12, which date I have taken as the beginning of the illness. At the time of his admission to hospital there was a severe congestion of the conjunctivae with photophobia. The tongue was coated. The abdomen was slightly distended and showed a number of small red spots of doubtful significance. They disappeared in the course of a few days. The spleen was not palpable at the time of admission. A few crepitations were heard at the base of the right lung.

The fever was of a remittent type and terminated by lysis, the primary fever lasting fourteen days (Fig. 1). After two days' interval there was a relapse lasting eight days, and even after this there was a tendency for the temperature to rise slightly in the evenings. The pulse was comparatively slow during the fever, the rate never exceeding 100. The patient was quite ill for a time, drowsy, and lying in a typhoid state. His condition improved somewhat as the temperature fell the first time, and more definitely when the relapse was over. No signs were found in lungs or kidneys or elsewhere to explain the secondary fever. The conjunctivitis was troublesome till at least the eleventh day, and there was still some photophobia on the twenty-ninth day. The patient sat up on October 26 and was discharged from hospital on November 3.

Blood taken on the third day of illness was injected into a guinea pig which probably acquired "Q" fever. Urine was injected into guinea pigs on the twelfth and twenty-ninth days. Both samples contained the infecting agent, and the strain obtained from the latter sample was continued through sixteen passages in guinea pigs.

Case II

The notes of case II are published by courtesy of Dr. E. G. Thomson and Dr. C. Shellshear.

F. L., aged twenty-nine years, meat inspector examining mutton and beef, became ill on September 7, 1935, with headache, lumbar backache, shivers, and cough with a little phlegm. There was some loss of weight. His bowels were constipated (as usual). He was admitted to the Brisbane General Hospital on September 13. The headache was still present and was his chief complaint. The skin was pale and moist, the tongue thickly furred, but raw at the tip. There were a few rhonchi in the lungs and a doubtful area of dullness at the right base.

The fever remained high till the ninth day of illness, when it terminated with a crisis (Fig. 2). The pulse rate at no time exceeded 100. The respiratory rate was practically normal. The patient's general condition improved rapidly with the fall of the temperature. He was discharged from hospital on September 21, and, though not quite well, resumed work on September 25.

The infecting agent was not obtained from urine tested on the

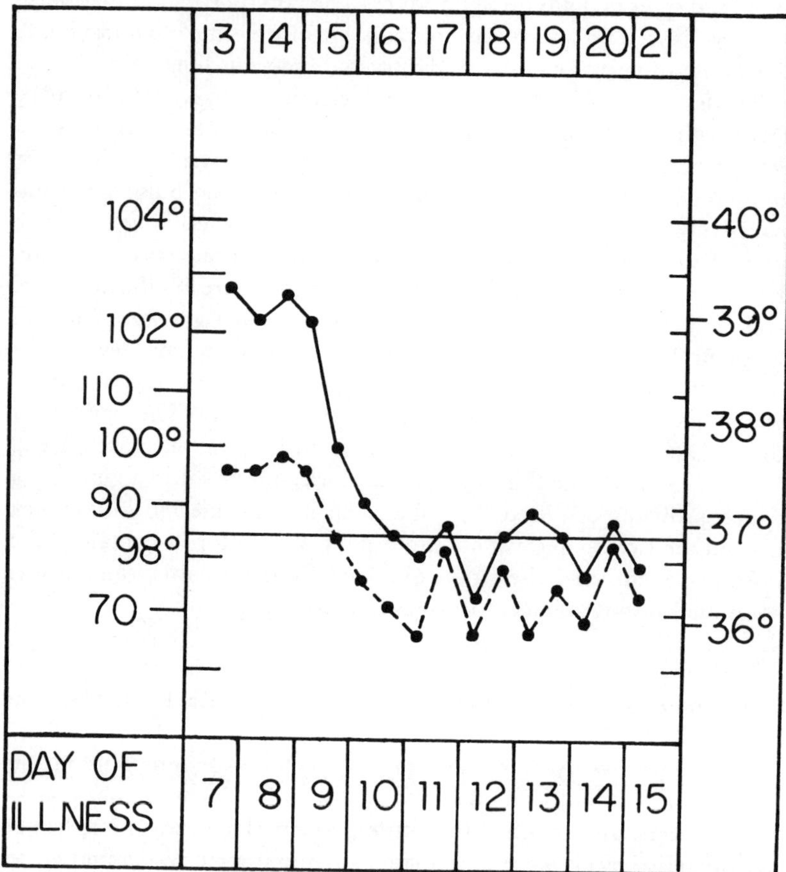

Fig. 2. Chart of F.L. (case II). Continuous line = temperature; broken line = pulse rate.

eleventh day of illness, but was obtained from urine on the twenty-eighth day, that is, the nineteenth day after the fever was over, and over a week after the return to work.

Case III

The notes of case III are published by courtesy of Dr. V. Beresford Taylor.

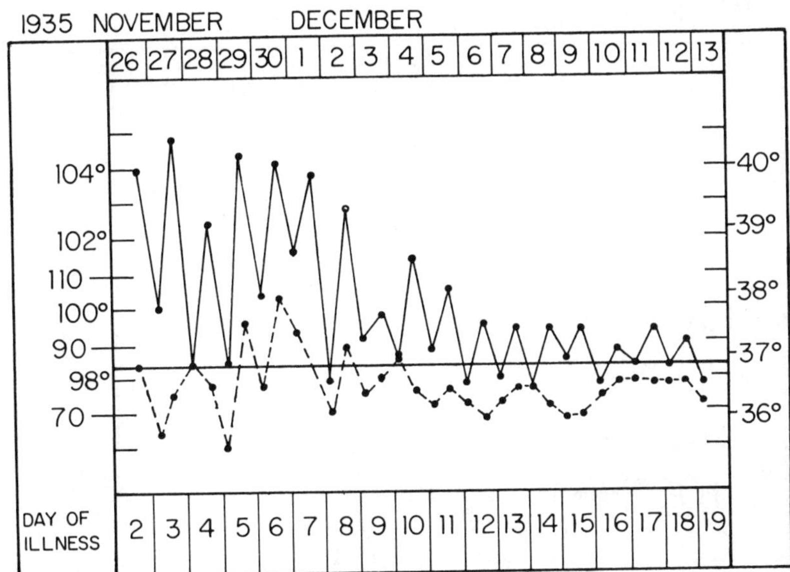

Fig. 3. Chart of A.M. (case III). Continuous line = temperature; broken line = pulse rate.

A. M., aged forty-five years, dairy farmer near Brisbane, first felt ill on November 24, 1935. Next morning he delivered some milk, but went to bed in the evening with a raging headache and a temperature of 38.9°C. He was admitted the next day to a private hospital. The headache was intense, sometimes frontal, sometimes occipital. It continued till the seventh day. The spleen was not palpable. There was no rash.

The temperature was high for eight days, then fell by lysis (Fig. 3). The large remissions may have been due to the use of drugs to relieve the headache. The pulse rate was comparatively slow, only once exceeding 96. The patient left hospital on the nineteenth day, still inclined to have a slight evening rise of temperature, but improving daily in his general condition. Insomnia was a trouble throughout, even persisting into convalescence.

On the fourth day of the illness blood was inoculated into a guinea pig, a mouse and a rabbit. The guinea pig acquired the infection and it was continued through eleven passages in guinea pigs. The mouse became quite ill on the eighth day and had a subnormal temperature, and then recovered. The rabbit showed no definite effect. A guinea pig

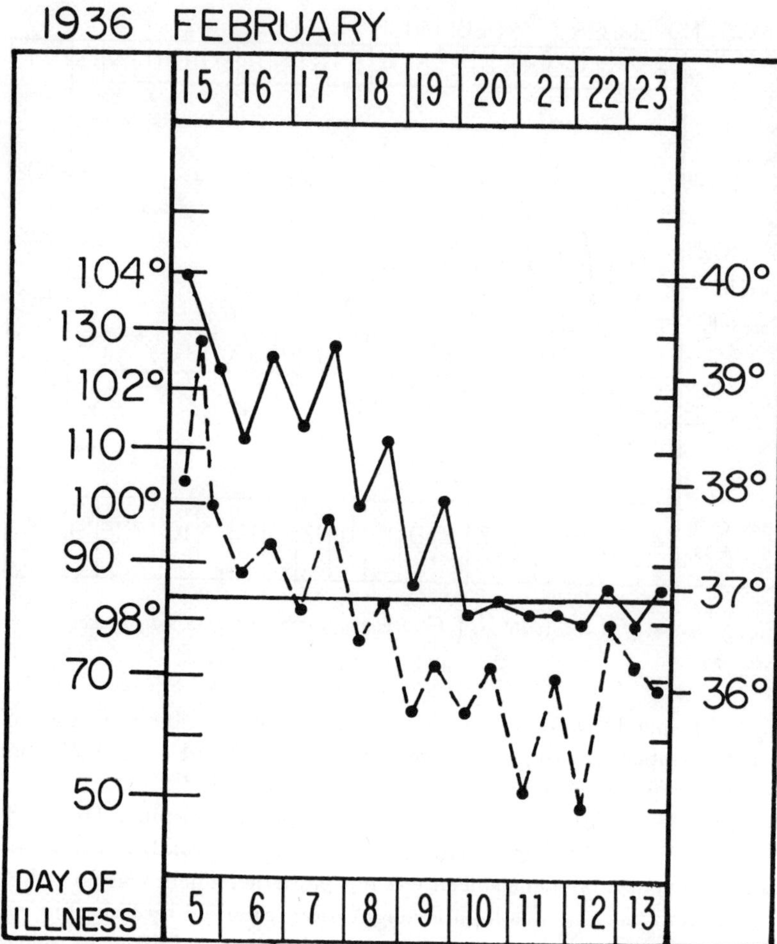

Fig. 4. Chart of E.K. (case IV). Continuous line = temperature; broken line = pulse rate.

injected with urine on the same day was unaffected. This sample of urine showed a cloud of albumin and a trace of acetone, and on microscopic examination numerous granular casts.

Case IV

The notes of case IV are published by courtesy of Dr. A. W. St. Ledger and Dr. P. J. Kelly.

E. K., aged eighteen years, a worker on the beef slaughter floor at the abattoir, became definitely ill on February 11, 1936, with pains in the legs, arms and lumbar region, headache and nausea. There had been lassitude for the previous two days. There was some vomiting and a slight cough. He was admitted to the Mater Misericordiae Public Hospital on February 15, as his condition was not improving. He was then fairly ill.

The vomiting and the lumbar pain continued for a few days more. After that improvement was rapid. The temperature came down quickly (Fig. 4). Except on the day of the patient's admission to hospital the pulse was comparatively slow. The urine showed no abnormality. He was discharged from hospital on March 4 and went back to work on March 30.

Blood taken on the ninth (and last) day of fever was injected into a guinea pig. This animal acquired a latent infection which became obvious on passage. Another sample of blood taken on the fourteenth day of illness (that is, the fifth day of convalescence) and two samples of urine passed during convalescence all failed to infect guinea pigs.

Case V

The notes of case V are published by courtesy of Dr. A. J. Lynch.

J. J., aged seventeen years, beef gutter, became ill on May 9, 1936. There had previously been feverishness, nausea and lassitude for three days, but not of sufficient degree to prevent his working. The head ached severely for several days after the onset. There were weakness, giddiness and loss of appetite. The eyes became bloodshot and could hardly be opened. The face was flushed, the tongue very dirty. The temperature rose and continued high, reaching 40°C. on several occasions. It became normal on May 17. The pulse rate kept at about 90 during the fever. There was no rash. The spleen was not palpable. The patient resumed work on May 25.

The virus was obtained by guinea pig inoculation of blood taken on the fifth day of illness, and the infection has been continued through thirty passages in guinea pigs. Guinea pigs injected with urine on three occasions remained unaffected. Another sample of blood was taken four months after the illness for agglutination tests.

Case VI

The notes of case VI are published by courtesy of Dr. R. Malcolm. J. C., aged thirty-seven years, mutton slaughterman, noticed an "influenza" feeling and pain in the back first on May 10, 1936. He continued to work, however, till May 12. There was a fairly high temperature, at about 38.7°C., for four days, with sweats each night. The pulse was comparatively slow. There were no spots and no epistaxis. On the morning of May 16 the temperature had fallen to 37.2°C., the headache was less severe, and the tongue, although dry, was beginning to clear. There was a big sweat the same night. The temperature was quite normal on May 18. He returned to work on June 1.

A guinea pig was injected with blood on the third day of illness and developed "Q" fever; another was injected with urine on the eighth day without result.

This patient had had two rather similar febrile attacks in the previous four months. In view of the immunity conferred on a guinea pig by one attack of "Q" fever, it is likely that the previous attacks were due to other causes. The patient had returned to work on Monday, April 27, after a fortnight at the seaside. This permits an estimation of the incubation period as fifteen days or less.

Case VII

The notes of case VII are published by courtesy of Dr. E. R. Row and Dr. A. Murphy.

M. D., aged thirty-six years, braceman employed on new sewerage construction, became ill on August 30, 1936, with malaise and pains and aches all over, especially round the hips. Next day he was feverish and had shivers. The following day he began to vomit and vomited two or three times a day for the next week. The bowels were costive. There was no headache and no dysuria. There was a slight cough.

He was admitted to the Brisbane General Hospital on September 8. His temperature was then 39.6°C., his pulse rate 104. He was lethargic, his face was flushed, his tongue was furred and moist. The abdomen was slightly distended. On September 10 there was a very severe epistaxis. The nose was packed and ten mils of Congo red solution were given intravenously. Next day jaundice appeared and became deep during the following week. All this time the patient was very ill, very drowsy, semidelirious, hicupping, and incontinent of urine and feces. The liver was definitely enlarged, but the spleen was not palpable at any time. On September 12, the fourteenth day of the illness, a punctate red rash came out on the back, then on the chest and abdomen. It had partly faded by the next morning and had gone on September 14. On

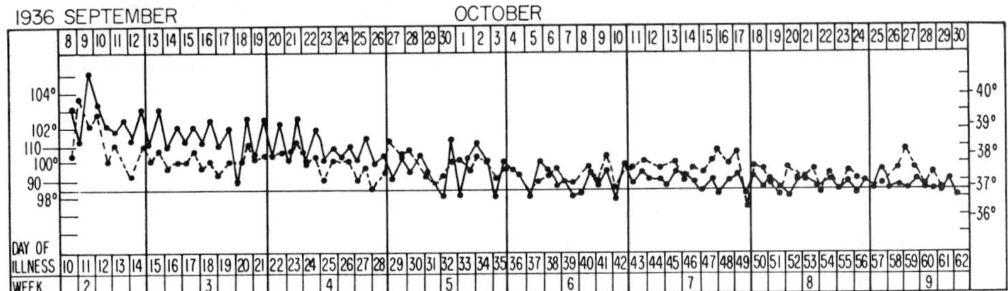

Fig. 5. Chart of M.D. (case VII). Continuous line = temperature; broken line = pulse rate.

September 16 he was given ten mils of calcium gluconate solution intramuscularly, and next day 0.9 gram of sodium thiosulphate intravenously.

On September 18, the twentieth day of illness, there was a definite improvement in the general condition and the jaundice was less. It had practically disappeared in another ten days. After the twenty-third day the temperature came down very gradually, becoming apparently normal on the thirty-ninth day. (See Fig. 5.) A slight degree of fever persisted, however, especially in the evenings, up till the time of his discharge from hospital. The lungs appeared clear throughout. The urine contained much albumin at the beginning of the illness; this soon cleared up. There was no sign of a urinary infection. He became anemic, the red cell count on the thirty-second day being 3,600,000 per cubic millimeter and the hemoglobin value 67 per cent. He slowly improved, sat out of bed on the fifty-fifth day, and was discharged from hospital on the sixty-second day. His convalescence was very prolonged. He was just about fit to resume work when, on December 31, an old corneal ulcer recurred, which further delayed him.

Blood was injected into guinea pigs on two occasions, that injected on the thirteenth day producing "Q" fever, that injected on the thirty-seventh day not producing "Q" fever. Urine was injected four times. The virus was obtained from the urine on the twenty-third and fifty-third days, but not on the thirteenth and seventy-ninth days.

This case was different in many respects from the others—in the severity of the illness, its prolonged duration and the development of jaundice. The diagnosis was very interesting. During the second week, when epistaxis occurred and jaundice developed, the condition seemed clinically to be a typical one of Weil's disease. The tests for leptospirae,

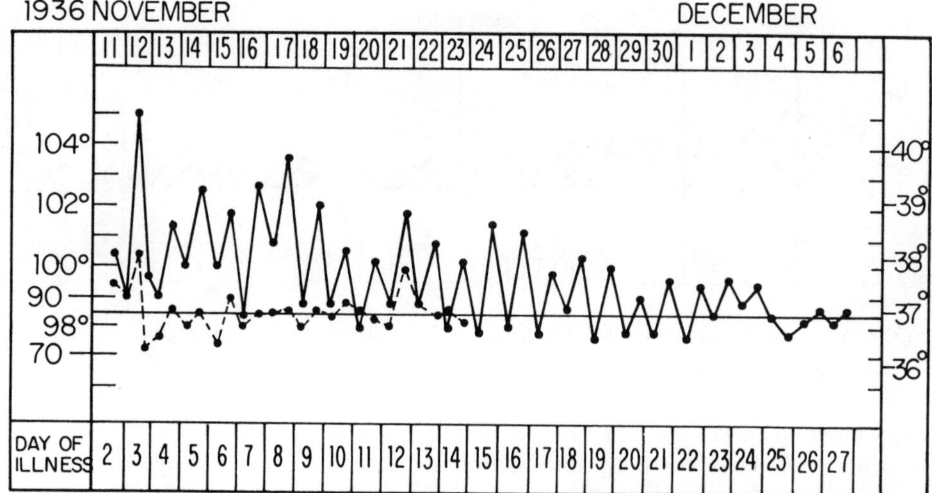

Fig. 6. Chart of J.H. (case IX). Continuous line = temperature; broken line = pulse rate.

however, all gave negative results, and to our surprise the inoculated guinea pigs developed "Q" fever.

Case VIII

The notes of case VIII are published by courtesy of Dr. K. S. McGregor.

L. T., aged thirty-three years, was admitted to Gympie Hospital on November 11, 1936, with a history of headache, pains all over, constipation, one attack of epistaxis and fever of four days' duration. There were a few spots on the abdomen suspicious of typhoid. The spleen was not palpable. The temperature ran an irregular course.

Blood was taken on November 12, and the clot was injected into a guinea pig. The animal developed "Q" fever. The blood serum taken on November 20 did not agglutinate the usual test organisms.

Case IX

The notes of case IX are published by courtesy of Dr. G. E. B. Clayton.

J. H., aged fifty-five years, dairy farmer near Pomona, took to bed on November 10, 1936, with shivery attacks and very severe headache. There had been prodromal symptoms for the previous two days. On November 11 he was admitted to hospital. Next day there was a severe

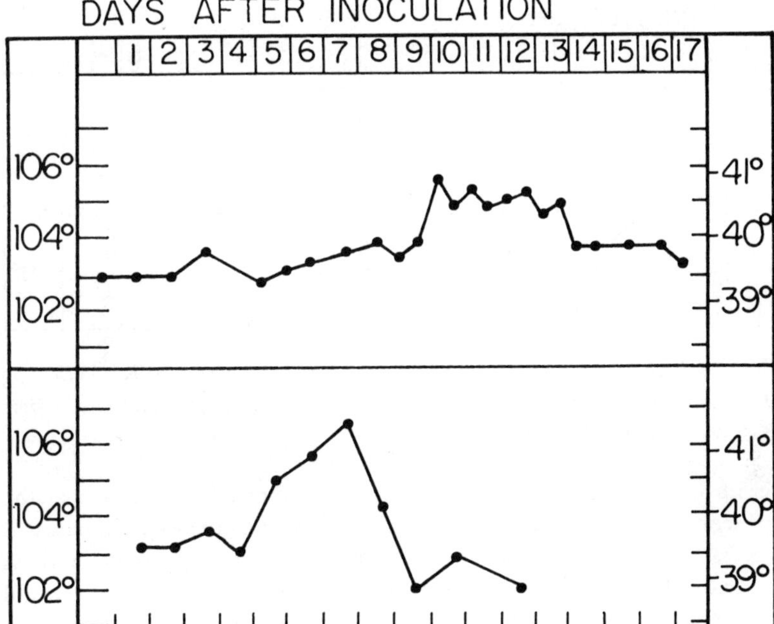

Fig. 7. Two temperature charts illustrating "Q" fever in guinea pigs.

rigor. He had the typical typhoid facies for fourteen days. The headache was severe for four or five days, but not thereafter. There were scattered pains in the abdomen. There was a mild epistaxis once. There was no vomiting. The tongue was very furred in the early stages. The eyes were not injected, the spleen was not palpable, there was no rash of any kind, the stools showed nothing noteworthy.

The fever lasted for twenty-four days, terminating by a very gradual lysis. (See Fig. 6.) The pulse rate remained practically normal while the fever was high. There was a faint cloud of albumin in the urine at the beginning. A sample of blood taken on the fourth day of illness gave "Q" fever to a guinea pig. Another sample taken on the eleventh day was used for routine agglutination tests.

"Q" Fever in Guinea Pigs

Guinea pigs are susceptible to infection with "Q" fever. They may be infected with blood or urine from human patients, or with blood or

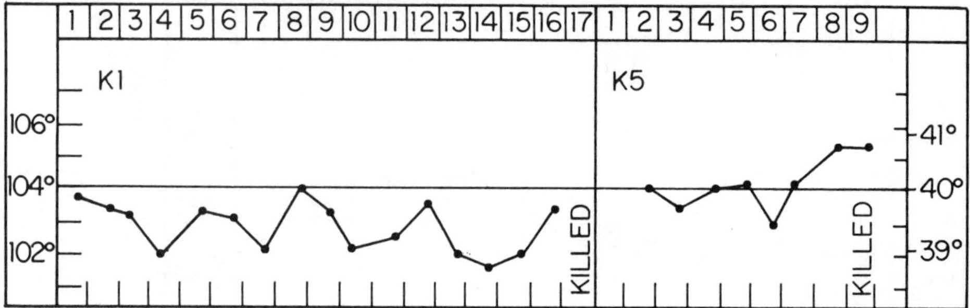

Fig. 8. Inapparent infection with "Q" fever of guinea pig K1 following injection of blood from E.K. (case IV). Guinea pig K5, injected with liver from K1, reacted typically.

organ emulsion from infected laboratory animals. As so much of the present knowledge of the fever depends on guinea pig experiment, it is necessary at this stage to describe the effects of "Q" fever in these animals. The description is based on the study of over 190 successful inoculations. The guinea pigs used were mostly between 200 and 400 grams in weight.

Incubation Period

The incubation period varied from two to eighteen days. It tended to be longer when a smaller infecting dose was used. With ten guinea pigs successfully inoculated with human material, that is, with a comparatively small dose of unadapted virus, the incubation period varied from eight to fourteen days with an average of 10.5 days. With much larger doses of adapted virus, as when guinea pig liver was used for transmission, the incubation period might be as short as two days and was usually less then eight. (See Table 9.) The longest incubation periods were seen when minimal infecting doses were given, as in titration experiments. With these minimal doses the resulting infection might even be inapparent and an incubation period not ascertainable.

Signs and Symptoms

The fever lasted usually about four to six days, sometimes for as short a period as one day, or for as many as eight. Its type was usually characteristic. (See Fig. 7.) The fever typically began and ended abruptly. The temperature might reach 42°C., the average maximum

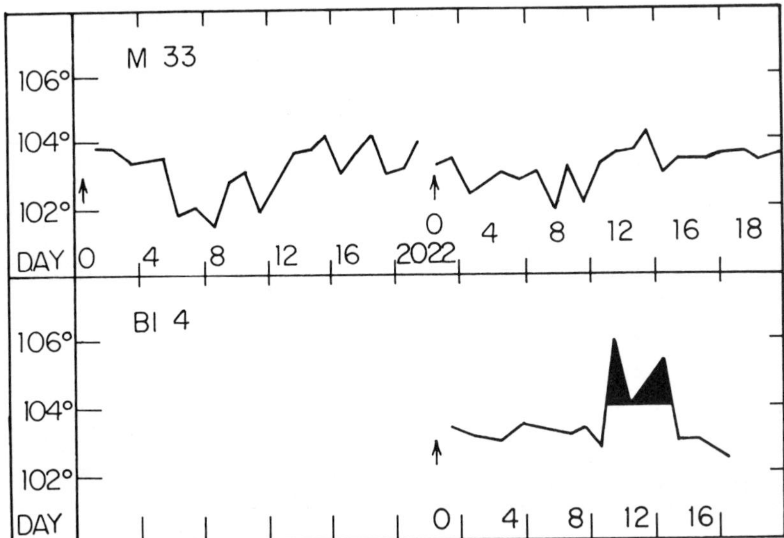

Fig. 9. Inapparent infection with "Q" fever of guinea pig M33 following inoculation with a minimal dose of virus. When given a potent test dose of liver emulsion twenty-two days later, it proved immune. Control guinea pig Bl 4, given the same test dose, reacted well.

of 50 cases being 40.9°C. Recurrence of the fever has not been observed.*

During the time of fever the guinea pig became limp and lost appetite, and the hair stood out. There was rarely any obvious loss of weight, but there was as a rule for several weeks a failure of the normal increase in weight. The signs were not striking and the animal did not as a rule appear very ill. There was no pallor. The mortality was nil.

Very occasionally the infection in a guinea pig was inapparent. The animal remained apparently well and afebrile. That infection had actually occurred was shown in one of two ways: (i) its blood or tissues about two weeks after inoculation transmitted the infection (Fig. 8), or (ii) it was found afterwards to be immune (Fig. 9).

* The temperature of normal guinea pigs varies considerably. There may be a difference of one degree Centigrade or more between temperatures taken in the morning and afternoon, or before and after a meal. The temperature of our guinea pigs was taken as a rule once a day, as far as possible in the afternoon. It is considered that under the conditions of these experiments an afternoon temperature is not abnormally raised unless it exceeds 40°C. Occasionally, on a specially hot and humid day, the temperature of a normal guinea pig may somewhat exceed this.

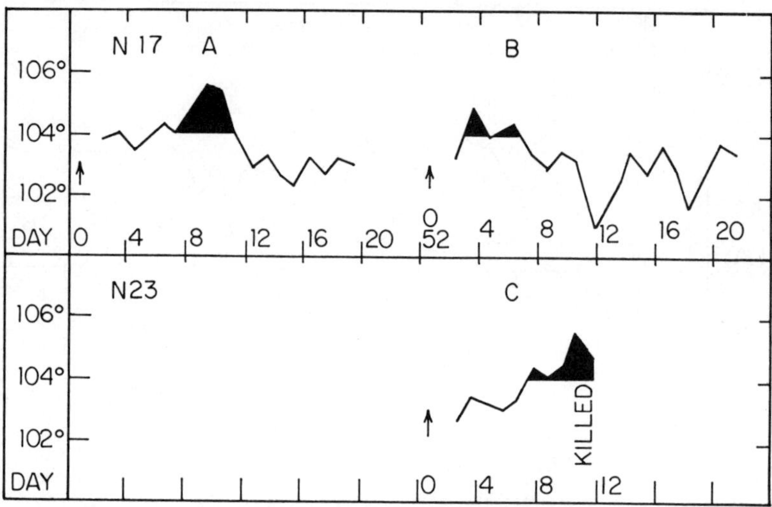

Fig. 10. Immunity test. The temperature charts illustrate: A, an attack of "Q" fever in guinea pig N17. B, immunity of N17 to a test inoculation 52 days later; the mild immediate reaction has no significance. C, definite reaction in control guinea pig N23 to the same test dose.

Morbid Anatomy

With animals killed during the fever, post-mortem abnormalities were few. The spleen was always definitely enlarged. In the severe cases there were petechiae in the wall of the cecum. Otherwise the organs showed no obvious abnormalities to the naked eye. Jaundice was never seen. There was no congestion or enlargement of the lymph glands. There was no sign of a scrotal reaction, nor was there, in guinea pigs inoculated subcutaneously, any particular local reaction at the site of inoculation.

Immunity

In the guinea pig one attack of "Q" fever confers immunity. This was first demonstrated in experiments with the *N* strain of "Q" fever virus, isolated from patient I.

Three guinea pigs were taken which at various times had been injected with this strain and had had a febrile attack. They were reinjected with it 24, 52, and 68 days respectively after the first injection. On these occasions each guinea pig remained afebrile for twenty-one days, except for a reaction in two of them shortly after the injection. Control guinea pigs injected at the same time ran the typical course of "Q" fever (Fig. 10).

Likewise four guinea pigs, after being first injected with the *M* strain of the virus (isolated from patient III), were found immune to a second injection of the same strain 23, 23, 27 and 30 days later.

It was next shown that there was a cross-immunity between the *N* and *M* strains. Three guinea pigs, *N4*, *N7*, and *N11* were first injected with *N* strain and tested by injection with the *M* strain 88, 45, and 31 days later respectively. Two remained completely afebrile. One pig, *N11*, had a mild rise of temperature (to 40.3°C.) on one day only, the tenth. This was most likely without significance. Even if it was to be ascribed to a second attack of "Q" fever, it was a much milder attack than the control guinea pig had—five days of fever, rising to 41°C., after an incubation period of six days. Guinea pig *N11* had a considerable, if not a complete, immunity.

Similarly, six guinea pigs first infected with *M* strain were tested with the *N* strain 17, 24, 24, 24, 31, and 31 days later, and were all found immune.

The results of the cross-immunity tests demonstrated that the *N* and *M* strains were identical. As each subsequent strain was isolated in guinea pigs, it was tested in the same way against one or more of the earlier strains. All the nine patients of this series were in this way proved to have been infected with the same virus.

The immunity of the guinea pig conferred by one attack of "Q" fever is therefore of the greatest importance. It has provided a method of specific diagnosis for individual cases, and it has established "Q" fever as a pathological entity, thus confirming the opinion of physicians that it was a clinical entity. The use of the test in the diagnosis of human infections will be referred to again later.

The immunity lasts at least six months. Two guinea pigs, tested after this interval, were found to be completely immune. Another guinea pig was found immune after twelve months.

Treatment of Infected Guinea Pigs

Only one experiment in treatment has been made. Seven guinea pigs were taken, varying in weight between 200 and 350 grams. They were all inoculated with "Q" fever. As soon as the temperature rose, four of them were each given an intramuscular injection of 0.003 gram of

Table 2. Experimental "Q" Fever in Rats[a]

Serial number of rat	Species[a]	Weight in grams	Temperature reaction	Spleen	Day after infection on which killed	Rat material injected into guinea pig	Result of injection into guinea pig
29	R.r.	145	None	Small	14	Liver	+
56	R.n.	125	None	Very small	22	Liver and kidney	−
73	R.n.	270	None			Blood 0.7 mil on thirteenth day	−
				Rather large (1.75 grams)	28	Liver and lung	−
83	R.n.	235	None	Small	14	Liver and kidney	+
89		102	None	Rather large	18	Liver and kidney	+
96	R.n.	208	39°C. on fourth day 39.2°C. on fifth day	Rather large	12	Liver and kidney	+
108	R.r.	170	39.8°C. on fourth day	Normal (0.84 grams)	18	Liver and spleen	+
97	R.n.	132	None	Large (1.22 grams)	15	Liver and spleen	−

[a] R.n. = *Rattus norvegicus*; R.r. = *Rattus rattus*.

sulpharsphenamine. The other three served as controls. There was no apparent improvement as the result of the treatment.

"Q" Fever in Other Laboratory Animals

Rats. Eleven rats caught wild in Brisbane have been inoculated with "Q" fever material. With three the effects were complicated by the presence of rat-bite fever. The results with the other eight are given in Table 2.

Of the eight rats inoculated, at least five became infected, as shown by the further transmission of the infection to guinea pigs. The transmission failed with the two rats that were not killed until three and four weeks after infection. The temperature reaction of the rats was insignificant, only two showing any rise, and then an evanescent one. The only abnormality to be found in the rats at post-mortem examination was enlargement of the spleen in some of them.

Two unsuccessful attempts were made to raise the virulence of the virus for rats by a series of passages from rat to rat. In the first series the second passage rat failed to transmit the infection to the third. The second series was spoiled by the intrusion of rat-bite fever.

These experiments show that wild rats, both *Rattus norvegicus* and

Rattus rattus, may be infected with "Q" fever, and that in them infection is usually of the inapparent form.

Mice. Only a few experiments were made with mice. In view of Dr. Burnet's work these need not be detailed.

Rabbits. Five rabbits have at different times been inoculated with "Q" fever virus.

One was injected with human blood, two with defibrinated guinea pig blood, and two with guinea pig liver. In every case the material used for injection was proved by guinea pig inoculation to be virulent. There was no definite temperature reaction in any rabbit. Only one attempt was made to transmit the infection back from a rabbit to a guinea pig. This was made with blood taken from rabbit VI on the sixteenth day after inoculation. The inoculated guinea pig was not infected.

Rabbit I was inoculated into the anterior chamber of the eye following the technique of Nagayo and his coworkers (2). There was an immediate local reaction lasting about four days, but no later reaction as occurs with Japanese river fever virus. Descemet's membrane was not examined for rickettsiae, as the rabbit was preserved to see if it developed a Weil-Felix reaction.

The serum of each of the rabbits was tested with *Proteus* X-19 and *Proteus* X-K on various days after inoculation, as shown in Table 3. In no case was any agglutination found. The tests were made with emulsions of living *Proteus* organisms, some with "H" and some with "O" cultures.

The Specific Diagnosis of "Q" Fever

The diagnosis in each of the nine cases was made by inoculation of guinea pigs with blood or urine from the patient, by the development of the characteristic fever reaction in them and by confirmation by immunity tests.

In the earlier cases the blood was citrated to simplify its subsequent injection into guinea pigs. Later I preferred not to use the sodium citrate and to allow the blood to clot. The serum was drawn off and preserved, the clot was ground up and injected. There are good grounds for believing that when blood coagulates, the contained virus passes into the clot. By injecting the clot only, one avoids injecting as well any antibodies that may be present in the serum; and the serum is available for agglutination work. In most cases some of the clot was cultured in broth.

Table 3. Weil-Felix Tests with Inoculated Rabbits

Serial number of rabbit	How inoculated	Weil-Felix Test			
		Day after inoculation	Proteus X-19	Proteus X-K	Proteus X-2
1	Intraocularly with 0.15 mil of defibrinated guinea pig blood, *N* strain	19	−(H)	−(H)	−(H)
2	Intraperitoneally with 2 mils of defibrinated guinea pig blood, *N* strain	19 46	−(H) −(H, O)	−(H) −(H, O)	−(H)
4	Subcutaneously with 3 mils of citrated blood from patient III, *M* strain	12 60	−(H, O) −(H, O)	−(H) −(H, O)	
5	Intraperitoneally with 10 mils of guinea pig liver emulsion, *M* strain	40	−(H, O)	−(H, O)	
6	Intraperitoneally with 10 mils of guinea pig liver emulsion, *K* strain	14	−(O)	−(O)	

When urine was used, it was injected as fresh as possible, in nearly every case within an hour of being passed. In the earlier cases 10 to 40 mils of urine were centrifuged and the deposit was injected, suspended in a small amount of urine. In the later cases 3 to 5 mils of urine were injected directly.

If the temperature of the injected guinea pig rose, either it was killed and a liver emulsion was prepared, or blood was obtained from it by heart puncture. The liver emulsion or blood was then injected partly into a new guinea pig and partly into one that had already had "Q" fever, and was therefore immune. If the new guinea pig developed a typical fever and the immune one remained afebrile for three weeks, the diagnosis of "Q" fever was made. If the original guinea pig was not killed during its fever, its immunity was tested after its recovery as a further check.

For example, 1.5 mils of blood clot from patient IX were injected into guinea pig *B1* 64 on November 17, 1936. The animal became

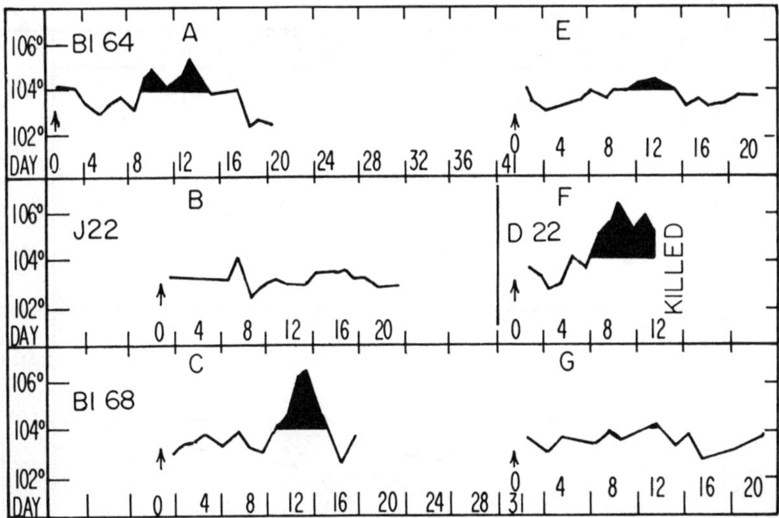

Fig. 11. Temperature charts of guinea pigs illustrating the diagnosis of case IX. A: Febrile reaction in guinea pig Bl 64 after injection of 1.5 mils of blood clot from the patient. B: No reaction in immune guinea pig J22, injected with 0.3 mil of blood from Bl 64. C: typical "Q" fever reaction in new guinea pig Bl 68, injected with 0.2 mil of blood from Bl 64. Compare with curve B. E: No definite reaction in guinea pig Bl 64 to a test dose of the D strain of virus 41 days after the first injection. Compare with curve F. F: Characteristic "Q" fever response in guinea pig D22. It was injected with less than half the test dose given to Bl 64. G: Complete immunity of guinea pig Bl 68 to a test dose of the J strain of virus. A control guinea pig (not illustrated here) reacted typically.

febrile on November 26 and had six days of fever. (See Fig. 11.) Blood was withdrawn from it on November 27, 0.2 mil being injected into a new pig, *B1* 68, and 0.3 mil into an immune pig, *J* 22. *B1* 68 had a typical fever reaction, *J* 22 had no rise in temperature. Finally, *B1* 64 and *B1* 68 were both tested and found immune, the former to *D* strain, the latter to *J*.

A shortened method of diagnosis is exemplified in the case of patient V. A sample of blood was taken from him into sodium citrate solution on the fifth day of the illness. One mil of the mixture (representing 0.8 mil of blood) was injected into a new guinea pig *J* 1, and the same dose into guinea pig *N* 39, immune by virtue of previous infection with the *N* virus. *J* 1 went through the characteristic course of "Q" fever; *N* 39's

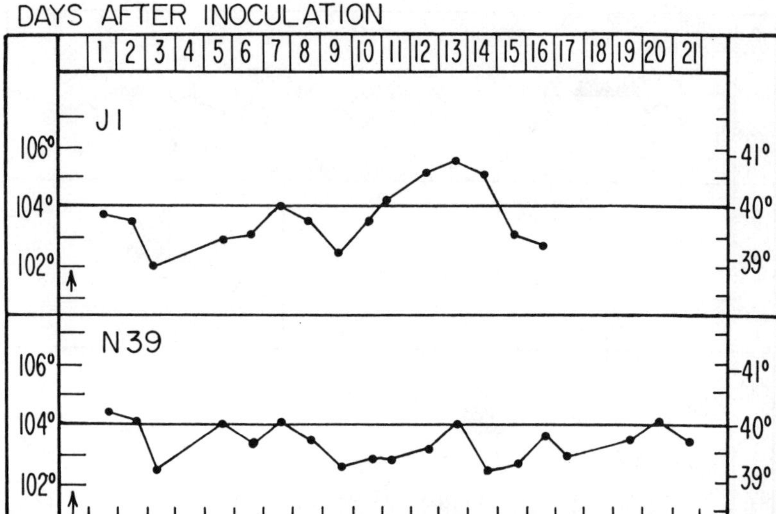

Fig. 12. Temperature charts of guinea pigs J1 and N39, illustrating the diagnosis of case V. Each guinea pig was injected with 0.8 mil of blood from the patient. J1, a new guinea pig, reacted with four days' fever; N39, already immune to "Q" fever, remained afebrile.

temperature remained normal, except for a slight reaction on the first day after injection. (See Fig. 12.) In this case the diagnosis was made in fourteen days as against twenty-four with case IX.

The shortened method is recommended if there is a moderate likelihood that the patient is suffering from "Q" fever, and if the blood is obtained early in the illness so that it contains abundant virus.

The Virus in Human Blood

Table 4 shows that the virus was found in the blood of the eight "Q" fever patients tested during the febrile period. Most of the tests were made with blood quite early in the illness while the temperature was high.

In case IV the blood was taken on the last (ninth) day of fever. There could not have been much virus circulating then, or it was largely neutralized by antibodies, for the infection in the guinea pig was inapparent and became obvious only on passage. Another specimen of blood taken from the same patient during convalescence failed to infect a guinea pig. The blood of patient VII was found infective on the

Table 4. Results of Inoculation of Blood of "Q" Fever Patients into Guinea Pigs

Case number	Date blood taken	Day of illness	Date blood injected	Amount of blood injected	Result in guinea pig	Remarks
I	9/14/35	3	9/14/35	2.5 mils	Probably positive	
II						Not tested
III	11/28/35	4	11/28/35	1.8 mils	Positive	Virus maintained through 11 passages
IV	2/19/36	9	2/19/36	0.25 mil	Positive	Inapparent infection of first pig, obvious infection on passage
	2/24/36	14	2/24/36	1.0 mil	Negative	This sample of blood was taken during convalescence.
V	5/13/36	5	5/13/36	0.8 mil	Positive	Virus maintained through 30 passages
VI	5/14/36	3	5/14/36	About 0.3 mil	Positive	
VII	9/11/36	13	9/11/36	Clot, 2.0 mils	Positive	Virus maintained
	10/5/36	37	10/5/36	Clot, 2.0 mils	Negative	through 5 passages
VIII	11/12/36	6	11/14/36	Clot, 1.0 mil	Positive	
IX	11/13/36	4	11/17/36	Clot, 1.5 mils	Positive	

thirteenth day of illness, but not on the thirty-seventh day when the temperature was approaching normal.

It cannot be assumed from the almost uniformly successful results in these eight cases that inoculation of blood from patients with "Q" fever will always reproduce the fever in guinea pigs. While this series was being collected, 23 other patients with fever of various kinds were investigated in this way. The negative results do not appear in this report, and one cannot say how many "Q" fever cases, if any, were

Table 5. Results of Inoculation of Urine of "Q" Fever Patients into Guinea Pigs

Case number	Date urine obtained and injected	Day of illness	Day of convalescence	Amount injected	Result in guinea pig	Remarks
I	9/23/35	12		?	Positive	Inapparent infection of first pig, obvious infection on passage
	10/10/35	29	5	Deposit	Positive	Virus maintained through 16 passages
II	9/17/35	11	2	Deposit	Negative	
	10/4/35	28	19	Deposit	Positive	
III	11/28/35	4		5.0 mils	Negative	
IV	2/24/36	14	5	Deposit	Negative	
	4/1/36	51	42	Deposit	Negative	
V	5/13/36	5		3.0 mils	Negative	
	5/19/36	11	3	3.0 mils	Negative	
	5/29/36	21	13	3.0 mils	Negative	
VI	5/19/36	8	2	3.0 mils	Negative	
VII	9/11/36	13		4.0 mils	Negative	
	9/21/36	23		4.0 mils	Positive	Virus maintained through 9 passages
	10/21/36	53		3.0 mils	Positive	
	11/16/36	79	?	3.5 mils	Negative	
VIII						Not tested
IX						Not tested

represented among them. On the other hand, the blood of infected guinea pigs, when 0.1 mil or more was injected, only failed once in 33 tests to transmit the infection, and on occasion much smaller doses succeeded. If an analogy can be drawn from the infectivity of guinea pig's blood, it is likely that most human infections may be diagnosed by the inoculation of blood into guinea pigs.

The last two patients lived some distance from Brisbane. With case VIII there was an interval of two days between the taking of the blood and its injection into the guinea pig. With case IX, owing to the week-end intervening, there was an interval of four days. The samples were in the refrigerator for only a part of these times. Yet in each case the virus was still active.

This shows that it is practicable to send blood from a distant center for "Q" fever diagnosis.

The Virus in Human Urine

Table 5 shows the results of inoculating guinea pigs with the urine of seven of the patients. It will be observed that the results with urine were much less consistent than with blood, the virus being obtained in only three of the seven. It is a noteworthy feature that the successful results with urine were obtained late in the illness or during convalescence. Patient II still had the virus in the urine after being afebrile for nineteen days and actually back at work.

Further Observations on the Guinea Pig Immunity Test

It has already been mentioned that a minimal dose of virus may give a latent infection. This occurred in case IV. (See Fig. 8.) There was no apparent reaction in guinea pig K 1, injected with the patient's blood. When K 1 was killed and passaged, the next pig, K 5, became obviously infected. If, therefore, the guinea pig inoculated with human material remained apparently normal for fourteen days, it was then killed and an emulsion of the liver (perhaps with spleen and kidney also) was injected into a fresh guinea pig. This procedure may be expected to detect an occasional case of "Q" fever that would otherwise be missed.

Occasionally in a test the immune guinea pig has shown a slight reaction. This occurred in case VII, and is illustrated in Fig. 13.

Injection of the patient's blood gave a febrile reaction in guinea pig D 2. A liver-kidney emulsion of D 2 was injected into a new pig, D 5, which ran a typical fever curve beginning four days after injection, and into an immune pig, J 30. J 30 had two days of fever beginning fourteen days after injection.

It is possible that this had nothing to do with "Q" fever, for blood obtained by heart puncture on the second febrile day failed to infect another guinea pig. In any case the reaction in the immune pig is not to be compared with the reaction in the new pig, D 5, and there can be no doubt about the reading of the result—J 30's previous infection with

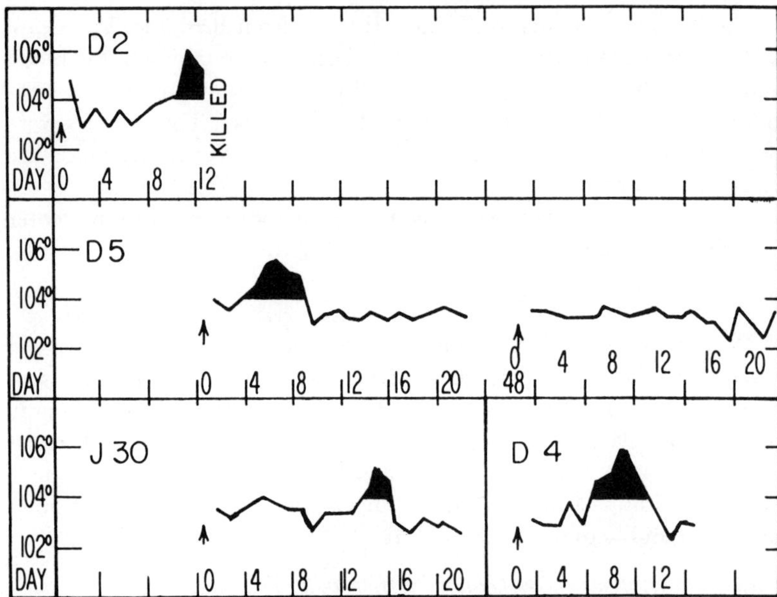

Fig. 13. Temperature charts of guinea pigs illustrating the diagnosis of case VII. Guinea pig D2, injected with two mils of blood clot from the patient, reacted with fever. Guinea pig D5, injected with a liver-kidney emulsion from D2, reacted strongly and rapidly; it proved immune to a test injection of the J strain of virus 48 days later. Immune guinea pig J30, injected in the same way from D2, showed only a mild delayed reaction of doubtful significance. Control guinea pig D4 showed a vigorous "Q" fever reaction, although it was injected with only a tenth of the test dose given to D5.

the *J* strain of virus had given it a considerable, if not a complete, immunity to the amount of *D* strain injected. The identity of the *J* and *D* viruses was fully confirmed by subsequent tests, in all of which the immunity to the test dose was complete.

If a new guinea pig used in a test happened to be insusceptible to "Q" fever, the test would fail. A guinea pig insusceptible in the terms of the dosage used in this work must be a rarity, if indeed it exists. In the long series of inoculations, no new guinea pig has failed to react when inoculated with guinea pig liver obtained during the period of fever. One guinea pig, already referred to, inoculated with guinea pig blood unexpectedly failed to become infected. There may have been some reason other than insusceptibility to explain this result. However,

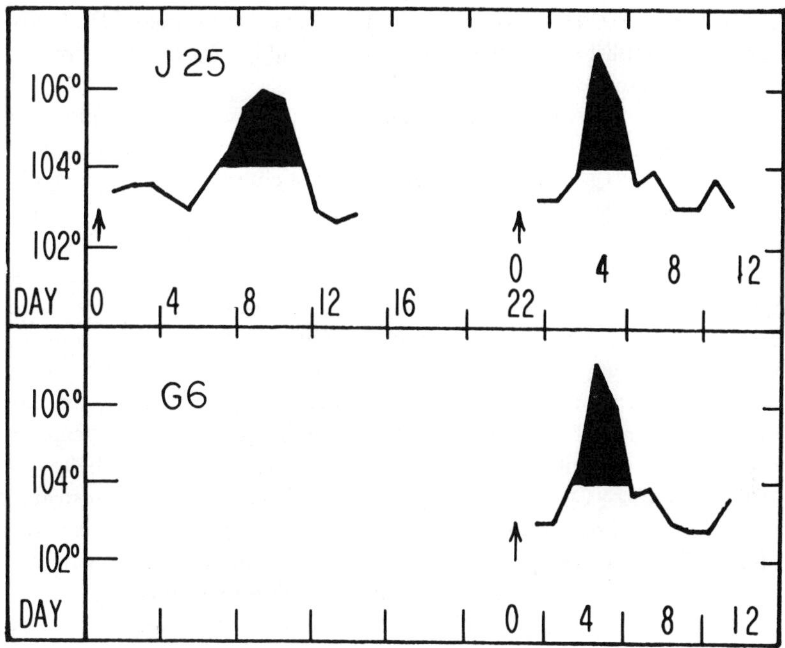

Fig. 14. Temperature charts of guinea pigs, showing the absence of cross-immunity between "Q" fever and leptospirosis of the Pomona type. Guinea pig J25 was first given "Q" fever, to which it reacted typically. Twenty-two days later it was given leptospirosis, to which it reacted just as well as the control guinea pig G6, which had never had "Q" fever.

in view of this failure, and the occasional cases in which immunity to the test dose appeared to be partial only (immunity being always relative), and the possibility of a raised temperature in a test animal being due to a concurrent infection, it has been thought advisable not to depend in any experiment upon the results with one pair of guinea pigs only.

During this investigation the blood of twenty-three febrile patients, other than the nine of this series and one with leptospirosis, was inoculated into guinea pigs. Most of the guinea pigs did not react at all; a few showed fever of indefinite type, which either could not be reproduced in passage or which did not make the guinea pig immune to "Q" fever. The illnesses of some of these twenty-three patients were afterwards diagnosed definitely as typhoid fever, septicemia, pneumonia and tuberculosis. In no case in which a diagnosis of one of these diseases was established did the corresponding guinea pig react in the way characteristic of "Q" fever.

There are, however, many infections to which guinea pigs are susceptible. A febrile reaction by itself would not be sufficient to sustain a diagnosis of "Q" fever, although a fever of characteristic type would be strongly suggestive. It is necessary to test further in a "Q"-immune guinea pig any infection obtained.

The immunity given to a guinea pig by an attack of "Q" fever is specific as far as it has been investigated. The specificity has been tested by inoculating a pair of guinea pigs, one new and one "Q"-immune, with the infecting agent of each of the following diseases: leptospirosis of three types (Pomona, Ballico and classical Weil's disease), rat-bite fever, undulant (abortus) fever and caseous lymphadenitis of sheep. In each experiment both guinea pigs reacted with fever, and the behavior of the new and "Q"-immune pigs was identical. One test is illustrated in Fig. 14. No cross-immunity was found between "Q" fever and any of these diseases. An opportunity has not yet come to find out whether there is any cross-immunity with murine typhus or psittacosis.

A positive diagnosis of "Q" fever based on guinea pig immunity may therefore be accepted as reliable. A negative result would not exclude "Q" fever. It should be added that in most of the nine cases diagnosed as "Q" fever in this way, no alternate diagnosis was possible. Culture of the blood and tests for agglutination with the organisms of the common fevers all gave negative results (Table 6).

The guinea pig immunity test has been of great value in detecting these nine cases, in studying the disease and in establishing "Q" fever as an entity. However, the long time that it takes—two to four weeks—greatly limits its clinical value.

The Clinical Differential Diagnosis

A satisfactory discussion of this subject must await fuller knowledge and be based on the clinical study of a larger series of cases. At this stage, however, a reference will be made to points that may assist in the making of a clinical diagnosis early in the illness.

The possibility of "Q" fever is to be borne in mind in the presence of a high fever of acute onset, accompanied by a severe headache, a comparatively slow pulse rate, and no other obvious localizing symptoms.

The other fevers to be considered are influenza, the typhoid-paratyphoid group, typhus and the leptospiroses.

Table 6. Results of Blood Culture and Serum Agglutination Tests

Case number	Day of illness	Blood culture	Serum agglutination tests									
			Eberthella typhosa	Salmonella paratyphi	Salmonella schott-mülleri	Salmonella hirsch-feldii	Proteus X-19	Proteus X-K	Proteus X-2	Proteus X-L	Brucella abortus	Pseudomonas aeruginosa
I	7	− [a]	−	−	−		− (H)	− (H)			−	−
	14	−	−	−	−	−	− (H)	− (H)			−	−
	29		−	−	−		− (H)	− (H)			−	−
II	11		−	−	−		− (H)	− (H)			−	−
III	4	−										
	22		−	−	−	−	− (H, O)	− (H, O)			−	−
IV	14						− (H, O)	− (H, O)	− (H)			
V	5	−										
	132		−	−	−	−	− (O)	− (O)			−	
VI												
VII	11	− [b]	− [b]	− [b]	− [b]							
	23		−	−	−	−	− (O)	− (O)				
	33		− [b]	− [b]	− [b]							
	37						− (O)[c]	− (O)[c]	− (O)[c]	− (O)[c]		
VIII	14		−	−	−		− (O)	− (O)			−	
IX	11		−	−	−		− (O)	− (O)			−	

[a] Means that the result of the test was negative.
[b] These tests were done in the laboratory of the Brisbane General Hospital (Dr. G. C. Taylor, Acting Pathologist).
[c] These tests were done by Dr. R. Y. Mathew, Commonwealth Health Laboratory, Cairns.
The Weil-Felix tests were at first done with motile (H) cultures, later with nonmotile living (O) cultures.

"Q" fever is to be distinguished from influenza by the mildness or absence in the former of localized respiratory symptoms (coryza, sore throat, cough), by the comparatively slow pulse rate, and by the sporadic distribution. Nevertheless in some of the cases of "Q" fever mild respiratory symptoms were present, and these patients were naturally regarded as suffering from influenza until the continuance of the fever excluded it. If cases of "Q" fever should occur with a very short course, they would be hard to distinguish from influenza.

From typhoid and paratyphoid fevers, "Q" fever may perhaps be distinguished by its more acute onset and the absence of diarrhea. But the clinical state of the patient with "Q" fever may appear very similar to that of a typhoid patient. Later in the illness the failure of the specific tests and, if it occurs, an abrupt defervescence will exclude the typhoid group.

The absence of a distinctive rash in the first week of a fever will speak strongly against typhus, and the absence of a Weil-Felix reaction in the second week will practically exclude it. The distribution of cases and the nature of onset are rather similar in "Q" fever and urban typhus.

In one case (case VII), in which jaundice was present, there was a close resemblance clinically to Weil's disease, the final diagnosis of "Q" fever depending on the pathological tests. Of the nonicteric leptospiroses the form most likely to be encountered in south Queensland is seven-day fever. Congestion of the conjunctivae at the onset, shorter duration of the fever, and a special incidence in summer and autumn would strongly suggest this diagnosis.

The Virus of "Q" Fever

Strains

The first strain of the virus to become established in the laboratory was the *N* strain obtained from the urine of patient I. It was maintained through sixteen passages in guinea pigs. The next strain, *M*, from the blood of patient III, was maintained for eleven passages. The earlier studies were made with these two strains. For economy of guinea pigs, passage of the *N* strain was stopped. Shortly afterward the *M* strain was lost through storing too long the liver emulsion containing it.

The *J* strain, from the blood of patient V, has been maintained by passage in guinea pigs ever since it was obtained in May, 1936. It has now (April, 1937) undergone thirty passages. Most of the later work on the virus has been done with this strain. It does not appear to have altered in virulence or in any other way while under observation.

"Q" Fever

The first *D* strain was obtained from the blood of patient VII. An emulsion of the liver of the third-passage guinea pig (*D*6) was sent in ice to Dr. F. M. Burnet in October, 1936. The strain kept in Brisbane unfortunately died out after five passages. The fifth-passage pig (*D*11) ran the typical course of "Q" fever. On the second day of fever 0.6 mil of blood was taken from it and injected intraperitoneally into guinea pig *D*15. *D*15 unexpectedly failed to react, and the series terminated. This is the example already mentioned of failure of transmission with blood. Another *D* strain from the same patient's urine went through ten passages and its transmission was then discontinued.

The strains from the other patients were kept going only long enough to establish their identity with the stock strains.

For the future it has been decided to maintain one strain only of the "Q" fever virus—the *J* strain.

Attempts to Cultivate and Detect the Infecting Agent

The blood of four of the patients was cultured in various media without success. The blood and spleen of infected guinea pigs were repeatedly inoculated into a variety of media and incubated aerobically, anaerobically and in an atmosphere with 10 per cent carbon dioxide. Quite a number of organisms have grown on these media, but all have proved harmless when reinjected into guinea pigs. The infecting agent of "Q" fever has not been cultivated.

Smears of blood and organs of infected guinea pigs have been stained in various ways, but no significant microorganism has yet been seen in them. Nor has one been recognized by dark-ground examination. This work was done on guinea pig tissues only. Reference may here be made to Dr. Burnet's success in finding rickettsial bodies in the spleens of infected mice.

Resistance of the Virus

The virus contained in a liver emulsion may maintain its infectivity for several months if kept in the refrigerator at a temperature of about 5°C. Table 7 shows the results of a number of observations on this point. It will be seen that the emulsion prepared from the liver of guinea pig *M*9 was still potent after three months of storage, but was inert after four months. The *M*38 emulsion infected a guinea pig after 47 days, but not after 64. Three other emulsions lasted at least 20 to 28 days.

167

Table 7. Preservation of the Virus by Storage at 5°C

Material injected	Dose	Time stored at 5°C. (days)	Guinea pig injected	Result	Incubation period (days)	Duration of fever (days)
Liver emulsion $M9$	0.1 mil	0	$M22$	+	10	2
		32	Bl 2	+	10	3
		59	$M44$	+	10	4
		92	$M45$	+	12	6
		123	$M51$	−		0
Liver emulsion $M38$	0.5 mil	6	$M36$	+	6	4
		6	$M39$	+	6	4
		37	$N40$	+	8	4
		37	$M46$	+	8	4
		37	$M47$	+	12	6
		47	$M49$	+	12	6
		64	$M50$	−		0
		85	$M52$	−		0
Liver emulsion $N36$	0.2 mil	0	$N29$	+	12	4
		20	$M34$	+	11	6
		20	Bl 4	+	11	4
		20	Bl 6	+	12	5
Liver emulsion $J1$	2.8 mils	28	$J9$	+	9	At least 3
Liver emulsion $K8$ and $K9$ mixed	0.5 mil	24	$K11$	+	11	At least 3
		24	$K18$	+	11	5
		81	Bl 24	−		0
		81	Bl 28	−		0
		81	$J4$	−		0

[a] + means that the guinea pig became infected; − means that it did not.

No doubt the loss of potency with storage is a gradual one. Quantitative experiments to investigate this have not been done, but a gradual loss of potency of the $M38$ emulsion is hinted at by the increase in the incubation period of the test animals concurrently with the length of storage.

It was too hastily assumed that, because the $M9$ emulsion lasted three months, other emulsions would do the same. Passage of the M strain in guinea pigs was therefore suspended during a rush of other work, and

Table 8. Titration of Virus in Blood and Liver of Guinea Pigs

Donor guinea pig	Material injected	Dose	Recipient guinea pig						Result
			Number	Incubation period (days)	Duration of fever (days)	Maximum temperature (°C.)	Subsequent immunity		
*M*10, killed on second day of fever	Whole blood	2.5 mils	*M*12	9	3	40.9	Immune		+
		0.1 mil	*M*13	9	5	40.9	Not tested		+
		0.01 mil	*M*14	10	At least 5	41.3	Killed and passaged		+
		0.001 mil	*M*15	11	1	40.2	Not tested		+
	Liver	0.5 gram	*M*16	6	At least 1	40.9	Killed and passaged		+
		0.03 gram	*M*17	9	4	41.2	Immune		+
		0.003 gram	*M*18	8	At least 3	41.7	Killed and passaged		+
		0.0003 gram	*M*19	13	4	40.7	Immune		+
*J*9 killed on third day of fever	Blood plasma	0.01 mil	*J*10	9	6	41.7	Not tested		+
		0.001 mil	*J*11		0		Not immune		−
		0.0001 mil	*J*12		0		Not immune		−
		0.00001 mil	*J*13		0		Not tested		−
	Liver	0.1 gram	*J*4	4	7	40.9	Not tested		+
		0.01 gram	*J*8[a]	8	2	41.2	Not tested		+
		0.001 gram	*J*18	7	5	41.2	Not tested		+
		0.0001 gram	*J*19	7	5	41.3	Not tested		+
		0.00001 gram	*J*20	8	6	41.0	Immune		+

[a] Guinea pig *J*8, 475 grams, was much larger than the other guinea pigs.

the *M*38 emulsion was stored, in the expectation of resuming the series of passages later. But when this was attempted after 64 days the emulsion was inert, and the *M* strain was lost.

In spite of this unfortunate occurrence the fact that the virus may be preserved in the refrigerator for a month or more has been of great help in the work. For instance, when the *M* strain was lost, recourse was had to a stored liver emulsion from guinea pig *J*1. This was apparently unimpaired by a storage of twenty-eight days, and a new series of passages was begun. Frequently material has been stored for a few days to suit the convenience of the work.

One experiment only has been made to test the resistance of the virus to glycerol. An infective liver emulsion was mixed with an equal part of glycerol and stored at 5°C. After twenty-one days it was still infective.

Table 9. Comparative Incubation Periods in Guinea Pigs Infected with Blood and Liver

Injection material	Dose	Number of cases	Incubation period (days)		
			Shortest	Longest	Average
Blood	0.5 mil or more	9	5	9	7.1
	0.1 to 0.4 mil	19	5	13	9.4
	Total: 0.1 mil or more	28	5	13	8.6
Liver emulsion	0.5 mil or more	46	2	8	5.4
	0.1 to 0.4 mil	28	3	11	6.5
	Total: 0.1 mil or more	74	2	11	5.8

[a] One mil of liver emulsion would represent roughly 0.1 gram of liver.

The Distribution of Virus in the Tissues

It has already been seen that the virus may be found in the blood of human patients during the fever, and less commonly in the urine late in the illness or during convalescence.

With infected guinea pigs also the virus is present in the blood during the fever. On 32 out of 33 occasions in which at least 0.1 mil of such blood was inoculated into new guinea pigs, the infection was transmitted.

The liver of a guinea pig is an even more potent source of the virus than the blood. Liver emulsions were prepared by crushing the liver in a mortar or a Griffith's tube with about five to ten times its volume of saline solution and lightly centrifuging to remove the larger particles. In quantitative work the piece of liver was weighed and then ground thoroughly with sand. Emulsion of infected liver in a dose of at least 0.1 mil was injected at various times into 75 new guinea pigs. All became infected, though in one case the infection was latent only.

A complete quantitative estimation of the relative concentration of virus in the different organs has been out of the question because of the large number of guinea pigs that would be required. Titrations of blood and liver have been made twice, and the results are shown in Table 8.

The table indicates that as the infecting dose became smaller, the incubation period as a rule became longer. With the $M10$ material the incubation periods show that the minimum infective doses of both blood and liver were almost reached with the highest dilutions. With the liver of *J*9, however, it would appear that still smaller doses might have been successfully given. The first liver contained at least 3,000, the second at least 100,000, minimum infecting doses per gram.

That the virus is more concentrated in the liver than in the blood is confirmed by the shorter incubation period on the average in guinea pigs infected with liver (Tables 8 and 9).

Blood and liver may already be infective in the latter part of the incubation period.

For instance, guinea pig *N*19 was killed on the ninth day after injection, before there was any rise of temperature. Two mils of its blood infected guinea pig *N*20. Guinea pig *J*26 was accidentally killed eight days after inoculation and before any reaction occurred. An emulsion of its liver infected *J*27.

The infectivity of guinea pig blood and liver may persist for at least seven days after the fever is over. Some observations on this point are given in Table 10.

The persistence of the virus allows the full course of the fever to be observed in a test guinea pig and the same animal then to be used for passage. No doubt the amount of virus is rapidly decreasing during this time. The long incubation periods in the successful cases in Table 10 show that only a small amount was present a week after the fever was over.

Only four attempts have been made to find the virus in guinea pig urine. In two the urine was taken during the fever, in the others during convalescence. All the attempts failed.

Epidemiology

Despite considerable work, much about the epidemiological aspect of "Q" fever remains obscure. Some information of epidemiological interest is given in Table 11.

No predilection for any particular season of the year is apparent, either in the present series of nine cases or in a previous series of twenty probable but unproved cases.

Six of the patients were domiciled in Brisbane, another one near by. There was one patient each from Pomona and Gympie, 86 and 106 miles respectively north of Brisbane. "Q" fever appears likely, therefore, to have a wide distribution in the south of Queensland.

"Q" Fever and the Typhus Group

"Q" fever as here described does not correspond with any fever of which I am aware. The nearest relationships are with psittacosis and the typhus group. To typhus it has been necessary to make frequent reference in the text. It is convenient now to summarize the resemblances and divergences between "Q" fever and the typhus group.

The course of the fever in some of the "Q" fever cases—continuously high, then rapidly falling early in the second week (Figs. 2 and 4)—is rather similar to the course of urban typhus. The longer type of "Q" fever terminating by lysis (Figs. 3 and 6) may be paralleled by occasional cases of the rural typhus of Malaya (3) and elsewhere, although Malayan typhus, like the *K* typhus of north Queensland, usually terminates within seventeen days.

The febrile and immunological responses of guinea pigs to "Q" fever have a general resemblance to their responses to the typhus viruses. The literature of experimental typhus research has been of great assistance to me in this guinea pig work. The immunity experiments here described are similar to those performed, for instance, at the Institute for Medical Research, Kuala Lumpur, on tropical typhus, and described in the "Annual Reports" and other publications. And the method of setting out the results of the immunity tests (Figs. 9, 10, 11, 13, and 14) I have copied from an article by Pijper and Dau on the typhus-like fevers of South Africa (4). It has not yet been possible to test for any cross-immunity between "Q" fever and fevers of the typhus group.

On the other hand, there are important differences in the guinea pig reactions. For example, "Q" fever differs from rural typhus in the much greater susceptibility of the guinea pig to the former, and it differs from urban or murine typhus in the absence of the characteristic scrotal reaction.

Dr. Burnet's discovery of a rickettsial organism as the cause of "Q" fever provides another resemblance to the typhus group.

Because of these resemblances, a Weil-Felix reaction has been carefully looked for with "Q" fever. But no reaction could be obtained, either in the human cases (Table 6) or in rabbits inoculated with three strains of "Q" virus (Table 3). In view of the importance of the point, I took advantage of Dr. R. Y. Mathew's large experience with the best at the Commonwealth Health Laboratory, Cairns. He kindly tested the serum of patient VII (thirty-seventh day) and found no agglutination with the OX-19, OX-K, OX-2, or OX-L strains of *Proteus*.

Another important divergence from the typhus group is the absence of a characteristic rash with "Q" fever. Only one of the nine patients had an obvious rash, and that was a late one, on the fourteenth day.

"Q" Fever

On the other hand, a rash is a striking and characteristic feature of typhus and commonly appears before the end of the first week. Though many patients may run their course without one, a series of typhus cases could hardly fail to include a fair proportion with a rash.

The typhus group of fevers includes many individual varieties. Among them there is considerable diversity in the details of the clinical course, the rash, the degree of guinea pig susceptibility and the Weil-Felix reaction. "Q" fever does not appear to correspond with any of the known varieties. It is certainly quite distinct from the two types endemic in Queensland—the urban or murine typhus of the cities and the rural or *K* typhus of the northern scrubs. In this section comparison of "Q" fever has advisedly been made with the generality of the group. There are some suggestive resemblances, but the divergences are important. The exact relationship, if any, between "Q" fever and the typhus group remains for the future to decide.

Summary

There occurs in Queensland a fever entity of a type not previously differentiated. It has provisionally been named "Q" fever, and nine cases are here described.

"Q" fever does not appear to correspond with any known fever. It has certain resemblances to the typhus group, but is distinguished therefrom in various ways, particularly by the absence of a characteristic rash and by the consistently negative response to the Weil-Felix test.

The onset of the illness is acute. The course and duration of the fever vary. In some cases there is a rapid defervescence after about six to nine days; in others the course is protracted to the third or fourth week or more and the fall of temperature is gradual.

The outstanding symptom is headache. It may be severe and persistent and is in most cases the chief complaint. The pulse rate is comparatively slow.

None of the cases has been fatal.

Guinea pigs are susceptible to "Q" fever, and they were infected by inoculation of blood or urine from each of the nine patients. Infected guinea pigs show as a rule a characteristic fever of about four to six days' duration. Mild infections may be inapparent. The mortality in guinea pigs is nil. If the guinea pig is killed during the fever, the spleen is found to be enlarged.

One attack in a guinea pig confers immunity. The immunity, being specific, has provided a means for the specific diagnosis of "Q" fever.

In this way it has been proved that the infecting agent was the same in each of the nine cases, and therefore that "Q" fever is a definite pathological entity. Its existence as a clinical entity had previously been suspected.

Rats are mildly susceptible to "Q" fever and develop the disease in an inapparent form. Rabbits are insusceptible.

The infecting agent of "Q" fever is present in the blood of human patients during the fever period. It may also be present in the urine in the later stages of the illness and in convalescence. It is also present in the blood and particularly the liver of infected guinea pigs. Minute amounts of these will transmit the infection to other guinea pigs.

The *J* strain of "Q" fever virus has been maintained in the laboratory for nearly a year by passage from guinea pig to guinea pig. It has undergone thirty passages. Other strains were maintained for sixteen and eleven passages.

The virus has not been cultivated on artificial media, nor has it yet been seen by microscopic examination of human or guinea pig tissues.

When material containing the virus is stored in the refrigerator, it retains its virulence for a month or more.

The epidemiology of "Q" fever is obscure. There is no obvious relation to the season. Most of the cases occurred in meat workers or dairy farmers. It is suspected that there may be a reservoir of infection in some animal with a blood-sucking parasite as a vector. Attempts to find such a reservoir have so far failed.

The fevers of the Queensland coast have long provided a complex problem. For many years the composite nature of "coastal fever" has been evident, and recent years have witnessed the culling out from the chaos, one by one, of a number of definite entities. "Q" fever is now the latest to be differentiated; it is not likely to be the last.

Acknowledgments

I am grateful to Sir Raphael Cilento, Director-General of Health and Medical Services, Queensland, for giving me the opportunity to investigate "coastal fever," thereby gratifying a desire of long standing, and for permission to publish this article. To Dr. J. Coffey, Deputy Director-General, I am grateful for assistance in many ways.

The work has been greatly facilitated by the help of many persons. I am specially indebted to those practitioners, already mentioned, who have permitted me to investigate their patients and to quote the histories. Dr. A. W. St. Ledger and Dr. L. A. Little appear to have been the first to appreciate the presence in Brisbane of a new undefined disease. Dr. J. J. Delaney and Dr. A. J. Lynch were also early to recognize it.

Dr. A. D. D. Pye, General Medical Superintendent of the Brisbane and South Coast Hospitals Board, and Dr. S. Julius, Assistant Medical Superintendent, have most courteously given me access to patients and to their records. So also have Dr. Noble, Dr. Robertson and Dr. Pasquarelli, resident medical officers at the Mater Misericordiae Public Hospital. Dr. J. V. Duhig and Dr. G. Taylor, pathologists to the two hospitals, have kindly permitted me to quote some of their pathological results.

To Dr. A. Neave Kingsbury, Director of the Institute for Medical Research, Kuala Lumpur, I am indebted for cultures of *Proteus* OX-19 and OX-K; and to Dr. R. Y. Mathew, Commonwealth Health Laboratory, Cairns, for a culture of *Proteus* OX-L and for performing agglutination tests on the serum of patient VII; also to the late Dr. G. W. F. Paul, Medical Officer of Health for Brisbane, for arranging the supply of wild rats.

I am greatly indebted also to Mr. E. F. Sunners, Chairman of the Queensland Meat Industry Board, and members of his staff for offering me every facility at the abattoir to forward this investigation. Colonel H. Finney, Acting Commonwealth Veterinary Officer for Queensland, has given me much advice and information on veterinary subjects that have arisen.

Mr. H. E. Brown has helped considerably with the technical work throughout these investigations. Mr. D. J. W. Smith, B.Sc., has identified the guinea pig parasites and has assisted with the more recent animal experimentation. The other members of the staff of this laboratory have also assisted in a variety of ways.

Use of Yolk Sac of Developing Chick Embryo as Medium for Growing Rickettsiae of Rocky Mountain Spotted Fever and Typhus Groups

The demonstration by Herald R. Cox that rickettsiae are readily cultivable in the yolk sac of chick embryonated eggs and that these microorganisms can be maintained by serial passage in this host was a tremendous impetus to the advancement of our knowledge of rickettsial infections. Because of its simplicity, and the receptivity of yolk sac tissue in supporting the proliferation of rickettsiae, the technique quickly superseded existing procedures for the propagation of these infectious agents. In addition to the rickettsiae, agents shown by Cox to be cultivable in the yolk sac of embryonated eggs include those of Q fever, Tobia petechial fever of Columbia (spotted fever) and South African tick bite fever (*fièvre boutonneuse*) (1).

The technique not only provided a means for producing rickettsiae in large numbers for experimental studies but it was also useful for the direct isolation of these infectious agents from clinical specimens, the preparation of specific rickettsial antigens for complement fixation and agglutination tests, the assay of infectious preparations, the biological assay of chemotherapeutical agents, and the preparation of potent rickettsial vaccines.

The observations herein reported concern the use of the yolk sac tissue (i.e., the embryonic membrane enclosing the yolk mass) of the developing chick embryo for the cultivation of the infectious agents of Rocky Mountain spotted fever (western Montana strain), endemic typhus (Wilmington strain), European or epidemic typhus (Breinl strain), boutonneuse fever (a Moroccan strain), Brazilian spotted fever,* and an unidentified rickettsial disease recently isolated from *Amblyomma maculatum* (ticks) collected in Texas (referred to later as *maculatum* infection).†

Method and Materials

Fertile eggs that had been incubated at 39°C. for 5 or 6 days were injected in the yolk with infectious material by means of a hypodermic syringe fitted with a 21-gauge needle 1¼ inches long. The inoculum,

---

* Obtained recently through the courtesy of Dr. Octavio Malgahaes, Director of the Ezequiel Dias Institute, Minas Geraes, Brazil.

† Unpublished work of Dr. R. R. Parker, U. S. Public Health Service.

usually 0.5 c.c., was introduced through an opening in the air sac end of the egg just large enough to admit passage of the needle. A greater quantity of material could be introduced through this end of the egg, since the volume of the air sac diminishes to compensate for the material injected. After the hole had been sealed with paraffin, the inoculated egg was incubated at 35°C.

Inoculum. The original inoculum for the eggs of the spotted fever series was defibrinated guinea pig heart blood taken on the third or fourth day of fever, while the inoculum for the other rickettsiae consisted of the testicular washings of guinea pigs sacrificed on the second day of scrotal involvement. For serial passage of the infectious agents in eggs a 10 per cent suspension of yolk sac only, in normal saline, was usually employed. Equally good results were also obtained when a 1:100 or a 1:1000 dilution of the yolk sac was used. The yolk sac was aseptically removed from the infected egg and ground with Alundum in a heavy Pyrex 50-c.c. centrifuge tube fitted with a glass rod (inserted through a gauze stopper) terminating in a ball to make an effective grinding surface.

Tests for infectivity. In determining the titer of infectivity of any one of the embryonic chick tissues, the following procedure was employed: the tissue selected for titration (yolk sac, chorio-allantois, or embryo proper) was completely removed aseptically from three or four eggs of the same series and washed once or twice with sterile saline to remove any of the yolk or other fluids that might be present. The selected tissue material was then drained free from excess moisture, pooled, weighed, and ground in a mortar with the abrasive to a homogeneous suspension. The ground tissue was diluted with saline to make a 10 per cent suspension and the latter was centrifuged (1,500 r.p.m. in an angle centrifuge for 15 minutes) to throw down tissue fragments. The supernatant fluid was carefully pipetted off and diluted decimally with saline, and each dilution was tested by injecting guinea pigs intraperitoneally with 1 c.c. each. The guinea pigs were carefully observed for scrotal swelling. Daily temperatures were taken until death or discharge (after 28 days), and microscopic examinations for the presence of rickettsiae were made of smears prepared from the peritoneal or scrotal exudates of guinea pigs dying or sacrificed *in extremis*.

Results

Maintenance of strains. All of the above-mentioned rickettsial infections have been readily maintained in series passage by the technique previously described.

Table 1. Rocky Mountain Spotted Fever. Records of Guinea Pigs receiving 1 c.c. each of Chick Tissue Suspensions on Apr. 18, 1938

Number of guinea pig:	1	2	3	4	5	6
Inoculum:	10 per cent yolk sac	1 per cent yolk sac	10 per cent chorio-allantois	1 per cent chorio-allantois	10 per cent embryo	1 per cent embryo
Date, 1938	Temperature, °C					
Apr. 19	39.3	39.0	38.0	38.8	38.8	39.5
20	39.0	40.7	38.2	39.3	39.0	38.8
21	40.7[a]	40.3[a]	39.0	39.4	38.8	39.0
22	40.6[a]	40.7[a]	40.1	40.8	40.0	40.3
23	41.0[a]	39.8[b]	40.9	41.0	41.0[a]	41.0
24	40.8[b]	37.8[b]	40.8[a]	40.7[a]	41.2[b]	40.7
25	40.6[b]	[c]	40.6[a]	40.4[b]	40.0[b]	40.8
26	[c]		38.6[a]	38.8[a]	39.2[a]	37.0
27			[c]	[c]	[c]	[c]

[a] Scrotal swelling.
[b] Scrotal hemorrhage.
[c] Dead.

Of two series of spotted fever transfers (same strain), one has been carried through 10 passages and the other through 37. Endemic typhus has been carried through 37 transfers, European (epidemic typhus) through 10, Brazilian spotted fever through 14, and boutonneuse fever and the recently isolated *maculatum* disease through 35 each.

The spotted fever, endemic typhus, boutonneuse fever, and Brazilian spotted fever strains of rickettsiae usually kill the embryo on the third or fourth day. After the death of the embryo the embryonic tissues and membranes rapidly autolyze. Hence, in order to facilitate the complete removal of the infected yolk sacs it has become routine procedure to transfer the strains on the third or fourth day while the embryo is still living or within 24 hours following death.

Infectivity tests. Titration tests carried out with the strains of spotted fever and endemic typhus indicated that the yolk sac was more infectious than other tissues of the developing chick. The infective titers of the yolk sac suspensions have been, as a rule, 100 to 1000 times higher

Table 2. Rocky Mountain Spotted Fever. Titration Test of Fourth Passage Yolk Sac. (Eggs incubated 4 days at 35°C. Each Guinea Pig received 1 c.c. Intraperitoneally on May 12, 1938)

Number of guinea pig:	7	8	9	10	11	12
Dilution of yolk sac used as inoculum:[a]	10^{-1}	10^{-2}	10^{-3}	10^{-4}	10^{-5}	10^{-6}
Date, 1938	Temperature, °C.					
May 13	40.4	40.0	39.3	39.4	39.2	39.0
14	41.0[b]	40.8[b]	39.8	39.6	39.3	39.4
15	40.4[b]	40.8[b]	40.8	39.6	39.4	40.0
16	40.5[c]	40.8[b]	40.3	40.4[b]	39.8	39.6
17	40.8[c]	40.3[c]	40.3[b]	40.8[b]	40.0	40.4
18	40.5[c]	40.0[c]	38.0[b]	40.8[b]	40.7[b]	40.6
19	[d]	39.0[c]	[d]	40.4[b]	41.2[b]	40.4
20		[d]		40.8[b]	41.0[b]	40.4
21				40.2[b]	41.0[b]	40.6
22				[d]	36.0[b]	37.0
23					[d]	[d]

[a] The 10 dilution was not made.
[b] Scrotal swelling.
[c] Scrotal hemorrhage.
[d] Dead.

than those usually obtained with other tissues or with blood or tissue suspensions of infected guinea pigs.

Yolk sac suspensions of all of these infectious agents, with the possible exception of the *maculatum* disease, have produced in guinea pigs a shortened incubation period and, as a rule, a more severe type of infection. The spotted fever strains in particular have been so virulent that of over 90 guinea pigs which showed evidence of infection, not one survived.

In Table 1 are presented the daily records of guinea pigs injected with tissue suspensions representing the first passage of spotted fever in the developing chick.

In Tables 2 and 3 are recorded the results obtained by injecting guinea pigs with diminishing amounts of centrifuged suspension of fourth and seventeenth passage yolk sac.

Table 3. Rocky Mountain Spotted Fever Titration of Seventeenth Passage Yolk Sac.
(Guinea Pigs injected on July 6, 1938. Other Data the same as in Table 2)

Number of guinea pig:	13	14	15	16	17	18	19
Dilution of yolk sac used as inoculum:	10^{-1}	10^{-2}	10^{-3}	10^{-4}	10^{-5}	10^{-6}	10^{-7}
Date, 1938	Temperature, °C.						
July 7	39.3	39.3	39.3	38.5	39.2	38.7	38.2
8	40.7	40.2	39.2	38.5	38.5	38.5	38.0
9	40.5	40.0	38.8	39.0	38.7	38.5	38.2
10	40.6[a]	40.3[a]	39.0	40.2	40.3	39.8	38.4
11	40.4[b]	38.0	40.5	40.2	40.6	41.0	38.4
12	[c]	[c]	40.6	40.6	40.8[a]	40.8	38.4
13			40.8[a]	41.0	40.3[a]	40.8[a]	38.6
14			41.0[a]	41.0[a]	40.0[a]	40.6[a]	39.0
15			40.5[b]	40.8[a]	[c]	40.0[a]	39.0
16			39.8[b]	38.6[a]		[c]	38.4[d]
17			[c]	[c]			

[a] Scrotal swelling.

[b] Scrotal hemorrhage.

[c] Dead

[d] No evidence of infection. Not immune to a subsequent test with spotted fever virus.

Table 3 shows that both the virulence and the infective titer of the spotted fever agent has been readily maintained through at least 17 passages in the yolk sac.

The positive results with yolk sac suspensions of spotted fever in dilutions of 1:1,000,000 represent an infectivity end-point at least 30 times higher than has been reported for mammalian tissues (1), 10 times greater than that which we have been able to obtain with cultures of a modified Maitland or Rivers type,‡ and approach the limits of infectivity reported for tick tissue virus (1).

Table 4 summarizes some of the results obtained in titration tests with spotted fever and endemic typhus, using various tissues of the developing chick embryo.

The data in Table 4 suggests that a higher limit of infectivity is

‡ Unpublished work.

Table 4. Rocky Mountain Spotted Fever and Endemic Typhus. Comparative Titration of Tissues of the Developing Chick

Disease	Number of transfers in the egg	Temperature of incubation of eggs	Tissue titrated	End-point of titration
Spotted fever, series A	2	39°C.	Yolk sac	1:100,000
			Chorio-allantois	1:1000
			Embryo	1:10,000
	4	39°C.	Yolk fluid	1:10,000
			Yolk sac	1:100,000
			Chorio-allantois	1:1000
			Embryo	Less than 1:1000
Spotted fever, series B	4	39°C.	Yolk sac	Less than 1:1000
			Chorio-allantois	Less than 1:1000
			Embryo	Not tested
	4	35°C.	Yolk sac	1:1,000,000
			Chorio-allantois	1:1000
			Embryo	Not tested
Spotted fever series B	17	35°C.	Yolk sac	1:1,000,000
			Chorio-allantois	Not tested
			Embryo	Not tested
	18	35°C.	Yolk sac	1:1,000,000
			Chorio-allantois	1:10,000
			Embryo	Less than 1:100
Endemic typhus	1	35°C.	Yolk sac	1:100,000
			Chorio-allantois	1:1000
			Embryo	1:100
Endemic typhus	18	35°C.	Yolk sac	1:1,000,000
			Chorio-allantois	Not tested
			Embryo	Not tested

obtained when the inoculated eggs are incubated at 35°C. It is also shown that the yolk (fluid) is infectious, and, in the one experiment made, it contained the infectious agent in even greater quantity than the chorio-allantois or embryo proper. Thus far it has not been determined whether the infectious agent multiplies in the yolk or whether its infectivity is due to extruded rickettsiae from cells of the yolk sac.

In another series of experiments the inoculated eggs were incubated at 32°C., but this temperature was found to be too low for development and survival of the embryo.

A few tests were also made in which embryos younger or older than

5 or 6 days were used. Younger embryos were found to be too readily killed either by the infectious agent or by the lower incubation temperature (35°C.) to which they were subsequently subjected, while older embryos (8 or 9 days) gave a lesser yield of rickettsiae.

Microscopic observations.   Material to be examined for rickettsiae was spread in a thin layer on slides and stained with Giemsa or by Macchiavello's method.§

Rickettsiae were rarely or never found in smears from the chorioallantois or from tissues of the embryo proper. On the other hand, rickettsiae of all the diseases studied, with the exception of European typhus, were readily and consistently found in the yolk sac. In the latter case, rickettsiae have not as yet been observed, although yolk sac suspensions have proved to be typically pathogenic for inoculated guinea pigs.

In smear preparations rickettsiae are rarely or never seen intracellularly, but are found scattered extracellularly throughout the yolk sac tissue. In endemic typhus, spotted fever, and boutonneuse fever, large numbers of clumped rickettsiae are sometimes observed in an apparently extracellular position.

Rickettsiae were readily found in the first passage of endemic typhus, spotted fever, boutonneuse fever, and the *maculatum* disease, but they were not observed in Brazilian spotted fever until the third passage.‖

In the *maculatum* disease, it was possible to demonstrate rickettsiae in the yolk sac before they were found in guinea pig tissues (testicular washings and peritoneal exudate). This finding suggests the possibility that the method described may be of value for determining whether or not the diseases of unknown etiology are rickettsial.

Discussion

In 1936 Bradford and Titsler (2) reported successful cultivation of gonococci in the developing chick embryo. Fertile eggs were injected

§ This method, which was devised by Dr. Attilio Macchiavello, has been found to be excellent for the demonstration of rickettsiae. It has advantages over Giemsa in that it takes only 7 or 8 minutes to prepare the slide, and the contrast between organisms and cellular material is sharper. The method is as follows: Fix slide in flame. Flood smear with 0.5 per cent aqueous basic fuchsin with pH 7.2 to 7.5. Stain for 5 minutes. Rinse rapidly with 0.5 per cent citric acid. Wash thoroughly. Counterstain with 1.0 per cent aqueous methylene blue for 1 or 2 minutes. Rinse with water and examine when dry.

‖ The guinea pig that was killed to furnish the inoculum for Brazilian spotted fever had shown only 2 days of fever without any scrotal reaction, and we were unable to demonstrate any rickettsiae in the testicular washings or tunica scrapings.

in the yolk (yolk mass) and serial transfers from egg to egg showed that the organism multiplied in this medium.

More recently Barykine and colleagues (3) described a somewhat similar technique in which "exanthematic" (European) typhus was cultivated in the tissues of the developing chick embryo. However, both of the above methods differed from the method described by us in that the *yolk sac* was not employed for passage or demonstration of the infectious agent.

The technique described here is extremely simple and has proved to afford less chance for contamination than do the methods of Maitland (4), Rivers (5, 6), and Goodpasture (7). In the few instances in which bacterial contamination did occur, the bacteria, as a rule, were found in greater numbers in the yolk sac than in the chorio-allantois or other tissues.

In a single preliminary experiment with the virus of equine encephalomyelitis (eastern strain) titration tests showed the infectious agent to have multiplied at least a thousandfold within 30 hours. The yolk sac, chorio-allantois, and embryo proper contained equivalent quantities of the virus.

These observations suggest that the yolk sac may also prove to be a good medium for the isolation and culture of certain bacteria and viruses.

Summary

A technique is described whereby the yolk sac of the developing chick embryo is used for the cultivation of rickettsiae. By this method the rickettsiae of Rocky Mountain spotted fever, endemic typhus, European (epidemic) typhus, boutonneuse fever, Brazilian spotted fever, and an unidentified rickettsial disease recently isolated from *Amblyomma maculatum* (ticks) have been readily maintained in serial passage.

The yolk sac suspensions of spotted fever and endemic typhus have been as a rule 100 to 1000 times more infective than mammalian tissues or other tissues of the developing chick and approach the limits reported for tick tissues. In addition, in all the diseases studied, with the possible exception of the *maculatum* infection, yolk sac suspensions have produced a more severe infection with a shortened incubation period.

Rickettsiae of all the diseases studied, with the exception of European typhus, were readily and consistently found in the yolk sacs.

It is suggested that the technique, which is very simple and permits a minimum of contamination, may prove of value for the isolation and cultivation of other infectious agents.

1940

R. Lewthwaite and S. R. Savoor

Rickettsia Diseases of Malaya: Identity of Tsutsugamushi and Rural Typhus

A comparatively obscure disease prior to World War II, scrub typhus became an unexpected problem of military importance during operations in the southwest Pacific and China-Burma-India areas among troops engaged in jungle warfare. When man entered the infected "silent" areas where scrub typhus had existed in a rat-mite-rat cycle of infection, he supplanted the rodent as a host of the infected larval mite. As a consequence, human cases increased at an alarming rate, and the most intensive control measures were required to curtail the disease. The price was costly but our understanding of this rickettsial disease was markedly advanced. Ironically, scrub typhus in the Pacific theater and Q fever in the Mediterranean areas were far more distressing to military forces than the notorious epidemic typhus fever. To foster appreciation of the complex problems associated with studies on scrub typhus and of the significance of the following paper, which represents one of many excellent reports on the disease, a brief review is presented of the salient historical developments.

The earliest descriptions of scrub typhus in the medical literature of the Western world were an 1878 report by Theobald A. Palm (1), in which he told of a disease called by the natives of Japan *Shima-mushi*, or "island insect," and a paper (1879) by Baelz and Kawakami on Japanese "flood fever" (2). Natives of the affected regions believed that the disease was caused by the bite of a small insect or mite, *mushi*. The word *tsutsugamushi*, often used synonymously with *scrub typhus*, means disease mite. An excellent account of name origins, of the history of the tsutsugamushi disease, and of the studies of Japanese investigators in the early 1900's on the development cycle of the mite vector, *Trombicula akamushi*, was published in 1945 by Blake, Maxcy, Sadusk, Kohls, and Bell (3).

The similarity of scrub typhus to Rocky Mountain spotted fever was recognized several years before the etiological agent of scrub typhus was identified— as early as 1908—by Asburn and Craig (4) and in a study reported in 1918 by Kitashima and Miyajima (5). No fewer than five investigators vied for the honor of being named discoverer of the causative agent. Credit for the rickettsial etiology of scrub typhus however, is usually given to Nagayo and his colleagues (6), who found minute diplococci and rods in smears from human tissues and in the cells of Descemet's membrane from infected eyes of rabbits. The microorganism was named *Rickettsia orientalis* but Ogata (7) proposed the term of *R. tsutsugamushi*. The latter name is used more often.

The studies of Japanese scientists on tsutsugamushi disease stimulated other investigations on the typhus-like fevers encountered in the Pacific islands and parts of Asia. Dutch investigators in Sumatra and Java differentiated murine (flea-borne) typhus from Sumatran mite fever but were unwilling to concede the identity of the latter with tsutsugamushi disease despite similar reactions in experimental animals and positive cross-protection tests. At the Institute of Medical Research in Kuala Lumpur, English researchers were engaged in studies of typhus-like fevers in the Federated Malay States. In 1929 Fletcher, Lesslar, and Lewthwaite (8), while studying two forms of tropical typhus, discovered a serological difference that proved of great value. They found that serum obtained from cases of rural typhus agglutinated in high dilution suspensions of the Kingsbury (K) strain of *Proteus*. Serum from cases of urban typhus was positive in the Weil-Felix reaction with the standard *Proteus* OX-19 strain whereas the rural form was negative. In subsequent studies Lewthwaite and Savoor (9) proved that the urban type was really murine (flea-borne) typhus, which explained the agglutination with the OX-19 strain, and that the rural type was (mite-borne) scrub typhus.

The paper reprinted here is representative of the many publications that came from their studies. In clinical, pathological, etiological, serological, and epidemiological studies, they explored the etiological relation of tsutsugamushi disease and the rural form of tropical typhus (scrub typhus). They concluded that both diseases resulted from the same causative agent, *R. orientalis*. The information obtained by these English researchers, helping to clarify the status and relations of the different forms of tropical typhus, was to prove invaluable in the control of scrub typhus during the war.

The object of this paper is twofold: to describe tsutsugamushi, which although tropical is closely linked with diseases well known in non-tropical countries; and to try to eradicate the terms *rural typhus* and *scrub typhus*.

Fletcher and Lesslar (1), by serological and epidemiological studies, first proved that typhus-like fevers existed in British Malaya; these differed from classical typhus in that they did not flare up in epidemics and were not louse-borne. The last decade has seen a remarkable increase in knowledge of the typhus-like fevers throughout the world. From almost every British dominion and colony, from at least seven European countries, from the Mediterranean littoral, from North and South America, and from the Far East have come reports of endemic fevers showing characteristics of the typhus group. Gray, Peters, and Davies (2) reported a human infection of this type acquired in the port of Bristol.

These discoveries have led to confusion in classification owing to apparent differences in clinical signs, serology, case-mortality, or epidemiology. By international cooperation between laboratory workers many diagnostic criteria have been established, and the existence of a few cardinal groups of typhus fevers has been demonstrated. Much confusion still remains, however, especially between tsutsugamushi, rural typhus (scrub typhus), Sumatran mite fever, and urban typhus (shop typhus). Urban typhus is a flea-borne endemic disease, of the X-19 serological type, found the world over; we have shown that it belongs to a group of rickettsial diseases differing widely from the tsutsugamushi-rural typhus group (3). A laboratory investigation we have nearly completed suggests that the differences between Sumatran mite-fever and tsutsugamushi are no more than those that may distinguish two strains of any organism.

We are convinced that tsutsugamushi and rural typhus are identical, and that rural typhus can no longer be considered a disease *sui generis*; hence the term should be discarded. We rely largely on our study of 250 patients seen during the past ten years. Of these, 181 were in or near the town of Kuala Lumpur; hence we were able to observe the course of the disease daily to its termination and to investigate it in ward, laboratory, and post-mortem room. The percentages given below refer to these Kuala Lumpur patients. The rest were seen by us in consultation, and were therefore visited less often. Of the total, 15 were Europeans, the rest Asiatics.

Definition

Tsutsugamushi is an acute infection caused by the *Rickettsia orientalis* (*R. nipponica*, *R. tsutsugamushi*). The onset is abrupt, with fever and severe headache; a macular and papular rash appears about the fifth day; and the termination is either by crisis or lysis at the end of the second week. It is conveyed by the bite of a larval trombidiid; a variable dermal lesion develops at the site of inoculation. Clinically it resembles typhus exanthematicus and other typhus-like fevers: in epidemiology it differs from them widely.

Incidence

In Japan the disease has long been endemic, but it is also common in British Malaya and Formosa. The coastal fever of Queensland appears to be identical with tsutsugamushi; Unwin (4) reported a series of 1500 cases, and the clinical, serological, and epidemiological features were so similar to those of tsutsugamushi that his conclusion that the disease was a mite-borne typhus was inevitable. There is little doubt that etiological and cross-protection studies will ultimately prove the identity of this mite-borne typhus with tsutsugamushi and rid the nomenclature of yet another superfluous term. Other endemic foci of tsutsugamushi are Indo-China and the Philippine Islands, and from the Dutch East Indies have been reported some hundreds of cases of pseudo-typhus or Sumatran mite fever.

In Malaya the disease is not seasonal; every month of the year yields cases. It is in a sense occupational, for the victims show one common characteristic: they have been over country covered with lalang (a tall course grass, *Imperata cylindrica*) or with other undergrowth.

Clinical Picture

The few case histories of value in the estimation of the incubation period show it to be eleven to twenty-one days. The onset is usually abrupt, symptoms developing within twenty-four hours of the initial malaise. There is sometimes a prodromal period of general malaise, with mild headache lasting two to three days, rarely five days. Fever, shivering, and headache are almost invariably the first symptoms, accompanied occasionally by vomiting and by pain in the chest or all over the body.

Initial dermal lesion. This can seldom be found. It may be no more than a papule. Only in 14 of our cases did it develop into an ulcer, and the view that the presence of an ulcer is a sine qua non of tsutsugamushi can no longer be upheld. The ulcer is merely a stage in the development of a lesion that is first macular, then papular, and only in a few cases progresses beyond this to become a necrotic ulcer. The papule usually develops and disappears during the incubation period and is therefore seldom visible when the patient seeks advice. Indeed, Schüffner (cited by Wolff [5]) in an early description of tsutsugamushi in Sumatra considered that, since he had seen the primary ulcer in all his European patients its occasional absence in natives might be due to its having already healed.

The ulcer, when present, is typical. It consists of a black crust surrounded by a contiguous hyperemic areola. The crust is slightly depressed below the surface and may be round or oval, measuring about 5 mm. in diameter if round or 4 × 6 mm. if oval; in one case it was only 2 mm. in diameter. The areola is 4–5 mm. broad and has a sharply defined outer margin (Fig. 1). These features are typical of the lesion at the end of the first week of fever, but variations are sometimes seen. During the first three or four days of fever only part of the central

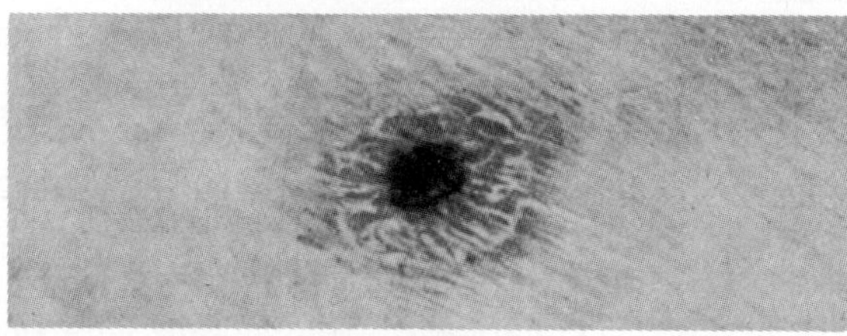

Fig. 1. The initial ulcer in man, on the upper arm, on the tenth day, showing the black scab and surrounding areola.

crust may be black, the rest being gray, and the red areola may shade off into the adjacent skin.

Two European patients had noticed the dermal lesion during the incubation period. One said that two days before the onset of symptoms he saw on his right calf "a tiny red spot," and that "in the center of this spot there developed a bead of white matter that eventually turned black and was surrounded by a narrow red zone." The other, whose lesion was in the scapular region, said that a week before the onset of symptoms he felt on his back "what seemed to be a small boil"; the lesion was then presumably papular.

The dermal lesions of another patient provide strong evidence of the identity of rural typhus and tsutsugamushi.

A European with a fever suspected to be of the typhus group was seen in consultation by one of us. Seven days before the onset of illness he had spent the day shooting among lalang on an estate known to be an endemic focus of both diseases. The typical syndrome of rural typhus and of tsutsugamushi was present. The blood agglutinated the OX-K strain of *Proteus* to a titer of 1 in 680 on the eleventh day. Defervescence by lysis was complete on the fifteenth day; but delirium was progressive, and death from cardiac failure took place on the nineteenth day.

During the first few days of illness there was in the posterior triangle of the neck a tiny red papule, abraded at its apex. The successive involvement of the lymphatic glands of the posterior triangle, anterior triangle, axilla and groin of the same side, and axilla and groin of the opposite side could be clearly followed as the illness progressed, and it left no doubt that the papule marked the portal of entry of the virus. Yet by the eighth day of illness, early in the development of the rash, the small abraded papule had entirely disappeared.

This contradicted the report of the development of the initial lesion in previous cases of tsutsugamushi in Malaya; in these the ulcer persisted with its black necrotic center at least until the end of the third week, even in the mildest case. So insignificant and ephemeral was this lesion that it would almost certainly have escaped detection on the darker skin of an Asiatic patient. At that time the view was held that the presence of a typical black necrotic ulcer differentiated tsutsugamushi from rural typhus; no other type of primary lesion was described. Judged by this criterion the case occupied an intermediate position between the two diseases. Interpreted in the light of our recent experimental work, however, the lesion was consistent with a diagnosis of tsutsugamushi. As will be shown later, papular lesions that do not progress to ulceration have developed at the sites of experimental intradermal inoculations of the virus of tsutsugamushi into monkeys and gibbons, the resulting infections being of maximal severity.

The black crust falls off usually from the third week onwards, although fomentations may effect this earlier. A well-defined pit is left; in one patient it was visible three years later. The site of the ulcer is determined to some extent by the clothing worn. The usual dress of those traversing lalang or jungle includes stockings rolled down below the knee, shorts, and shirt open at the neck; hence the commonest sites are the calf, at the upper margin of the stocking, and the neck. It is clear that the vector, the mite, brushed from lalang to clothing in passing, crawls over the clothing and attaches itself to the first accessible spot. Other sites have been the ankle, the upper arm, and the scapular region.

An apparently similar dermal lesion is found in certain other typhus fevers—e.g., the *fièvre boutonneuse* of the Mediterranean littoral. Professor M. Ciuca, of Bucharest, familiar with this disease, saw one of our cases of tsutsugamushi in consultation and considered that the dermal lesions of the two diseases were indistinguishable.

Lymphatic glands. In 40 per cent of patients in whom a primary ulcer cannot be found the lymphatic glands of both axilla and groin are enlarged. In some the epitrochlear and cervical glands are similarly affected. The enlargement and tenderness are seldom great. In patients with a primary ulcer the lymphatic glands draining the site may be greatly enlarged and extremely tender; but often these glands are no bigger than the glands elsewhere. In the "intermediate" human case described above, the progressive involvement of the groups of glands could be followed until all were affected. It is probable that, when the initial lesion has been inconspicuous and fleeting, the same progressive involvement has taken place but has been proportionately inconspicuous and fleeting, so that when the patient comes under medical care no one group of glands predominates.

Fever. In most of the uncomplicated cases of our series the fever showed the same main features. During the first few days the temperature is about 102°F.; from the seventh to the twelfth day it is at its maximum, reaching 104–105°F.; it then declines by quick lysis to normal or 99°F. by the thirteenth or fourteenth day. A brief rise to 100–101°F. during the next day, falling to normal within twenty-four hours, and often repeated on the following day, marks the end of defervescence. The average duration of fever is thus fourteen to fifteen days. Daily remissions are the rule; they range from one to three degrees Fahrenheit and take place usually in the morning.

There are many variations from this typical curve. The temperature may be very high from the outset. Daily remissions may be either inconsiderable or pronounced; in one instance the temperature fell on the fourth day from 104°F. at 4 A.M. to 98.6°F. at 8 A.M., rising to 101.6°F. twelve hours later. In a few cases complete defervescence took place during twenty-four hours. In others the fever lasted only twelve or thirteen days. A complicating acute bronchitis or bronchopneumonia prolongs the febrile period considerably; in one patient this lasted twenty-three days; in another, twenty-seven days; in another, after a typical defervescence that ended on the fifteenth day, a rise of temperature to 103°F. on the sixteenth day marked the onset of bronchitis, with fever of seven days' duration.

Severity cannot be gauged by the height of the fever. In the graver cases the rise of temperature may be relatively slight, especially in delirious or stuporous patients, a feature noted by Wolbach and his colleagues (6) in Western (louse-borne) typhus. In two such cases in our series which ended fatally the average temperature during the last four or five days was about 99.6°F. In some of the fatal cases there was a terminal hyperpyrexia; in others, a terminal fall to subnormal.

Pulse-rate. Always increased. Usually it is 100–120, but wide variations are found. It may not strictly follow the fluctuation of temperature, though in defervescence it usually declines with it. In one stuporous patient the pulse-rate never exceeded 96 until the day of death; in patients with cardiac failure, on the other hand, the rate may exceed 150. Bradycardia was present in one or two cases during the first few days of convalescence. Where there is acute bronchitis or severe delirium the pulse may become irregular.

Respiration. Slightly accelerated in the milder cases, but in the presence of much pulmonary congestion, acute bronchitis, or delirium the rate exceeds 40.

Headache. Present in 92 per cent of cases; it is most severe during the first week, and passes off as fever declines. Vomiting occurred in 39 per cent of cases at the onset, rarely persisting beyond the first few days. Epistaxis was noted in only 4 patients. Catarrh, present in 28 per cent of cases, is always mild.

Cough. Present in 80 per cent of the series, causing anything from mere discomfort to great distress; expectoration is rare in the absence of complications. The commonest lung affection was a mild congestion. Rales and rhonchi, present in 65 per cent of the patients, were usually few and basal; but in 13 per cent of these an acute bronchitis or bronchopneumonia supervened with consequent dyspnea, cardiac embarrassment, prolongation of illness, and graver prognosis.

Rash. It was rarely possible to make out a rash in the dark-skinned Tamils, who constituted the majority of our patients. In a few one could observe an indefinite subcuticular mottling on close scrutiny of the chest and abdomen. In most of the Sikhs, however, and in all the Europeans the rash was visible. A prodromal rash was noted by Fletcher and Field (7); in one of their cases it was urticarial, affecting the face, and disappeared within twenty-four hours. None of our patients was seen on the first day, and only one on the second day. The rash proper appears between the fourth and sixth day. Its distribution is general, on the chest, abdomen and flanks, limbs, and in some cases the face. Both macules and papules are present, discrete and dusky-red, and fading on pressure; they never become confluent. They are about 1–1.5 cm. in diameter. The papules are just perceptibly raised. In one European one could clearly distinguish an intense red center which shaded off gradually to a less intense periphery. Macules on the face are larger and darker than those on the trunk. Fading begins as a rule on the third day of the eruption and is complete within six or seven days.

In a case described by Fletcher and Field (7) there was a macular rash on the chest and abdomen when the patient was first seen on the seventh day; the macules soon disappeared, but rose spots appeared on the abdomen, lower part of the chest, and front of the arms, suggesting typhoid. In another patient macules were present on the palms and soles. In others some of the macules became purpuric, and in one case they could be detected as a dusky mottling of the abdomen as late as the thirty-third day.

The striking resemblance of the rash to the macular rash of secondary syphilis has been emphasized by Fletcher and Field (7).

Spleen.   Most of the patients had probably had malaria; therefore the splenic enlargement noted in 80 per cent cannot certainly be attributed to tsutsugamushi; moreover, it was present in only 1 of 15 Europeans. But that it may be due to tsutsugamushi is suggested by the many instances of appreciable shrinkage of the spleen during convalescence. Tenderness on palpation of the spleen was present in a few cases.

Deafness.   Some deafness was present early in 66 per cent of patients. In 50 per cent it was slight, in 8 per cent considerable, and in 8 per cent extreme. The waxing and waning of this symptom in the extreme cases is striking. One such patient, whose illness was protracted by an acute bronchitis, was only slightly deaf when seen on the ninth day, and his history was easily elicited. When seen again on the sixteenth and eighteenth days he was stone-deaf; but his hearing had partially returned on the twentieth day, and was again normal on the twenty-seventh.

Eye signs.   The commonest affection of the eyes—present in 40 per cent of our cases—is a peculiar mild suffusion, with photophobia. The eyes are half-closed, somewhat watery and faintly glistening, and give a dulled yet anxious expression to the countenance. Injection is present but usually slight. In the darker-skinned Asiatics the eye condition is a valuable aid to the early diagnosis of mild cases; for in these, apart from raised temperature and pulse-rate, there may be only slight cough and chest pain, slight deafness and headache, and slight enlargement of the glands of the groin. Injection of the conjunctival vessels may be noticeable, but only rarely.

Nervous system.   Mental disturbance was present in 35 per cent of the cases. In the majority it is manifested as delirium, sometimes as stupor of varying degree. The delirium, only slight during the first few days of illness, increases during the second week and subsides with defervescence. It is mainly of an active type, exaggerated at night, and occasionally evident only then; the patient attempts repeatedly to get out of bed, and is liable to wander from hospital unless watched. In some cases there is a low muttering delirium; the patient takes little interest in his surroundings, and though at times he can answer rationally his cerebration is slow. There are tremors of the lips and tongue and twitchings of the face and fingers. Stupor may vary from a mere dulling of the intellect to absolute coma. In the slighter degrees the patient's expression is dull and vacant; his clouded intellect can only imperfectly appreciate questions. The condition is short-lived, appearing late in the fever.

Occasionally, especially where insomnia, headache, and congestion of the lungs have induced great prostration, the patient is irritable toward his condition, the nursing staff, and treatment, and complains bitterly and repeatedly. Slight giddiness is common, often accompanied by headache, and it may be troublesome in those with much pulmonary congestion and consequent bouts of coughing.

Pain. Rarely pronounced. In 40 per cent of patients there was pain across the chest, made worse by coughing and undoubtedly due to congestion of the lungs. A vague aching, described as being all over the body, was present in 2 per cent of cases. Other less common sites of pain are, in order of frequency, joints, lumbar region, glands of groin, back of neck, and throat. In 8 cases there was abdominal discomfort with associated distension. Pain localized to the hepatic and splenic areas was present in 4 and 3 patients respectively, in all of whom pulmonary congestion was severe.

A leaden hue of the face and neck was conspicuous in 2 of the European patients. Edema of the feet was rare. Sore throat and hoarseness were often present in the later stages. Aphonia was rare, except as a terminal event. The tongue was furred in 82 per cent of cases. Looseness of the bowels was present in 34 per cent, but in only 12 per cent could it be termed diarrhea. Retention of urine occurred in only 1 patient; supervening on the ninth day of illness it continued until death on the seventeenth. Incontinence of bladder and rectal sphincters was rare. Appearing late in the disease it is a grave sign; only 1 patient thus affected recovered. Albumin could be demonstrated in the urine of about half the patients. It is never more than a trace and is transient.

Complications

The commonest complication, developing in 13 per cent of our series, was an acute bronchitis or bronchopneumonia, most often supervening during the second week, rarely after defervescence. In 2 cases venous thrombosis and its local sequelae developed, and 1 patient had bilateral parotitis and left facial paralysis. A subdural hemorrhage with resulting hemiplegia was noted once. It took place on the thirteenth day and was the immediate cause of death in a patient comatose from the ninth day onwards.

Course of the Disease

During the first five or six days the disease is usually mild. Apart from fever and headache, the syndrome is characterised by sudden onset, deafness, cough, pain in the chest, suffusion of the eyes, occasional vomiting, and slight enlargement of lymphatic glands; not all of these may be evident. In dark-skinned patients the rash rarely affords help. At this time there is little to indicate whether the infection will prove mild or severe, except in the few cases with early delirium.

As the second week progresses the signs increase, especially deafness, pulmonary congestion, and mental disturbance; and there is some degree of prostration. Should delirium or a lung complication develop, a severe infection is certain and the outcome is always in doubt. In 50–60 per cent of cases, however, neither occurs, and decline of fever brings rapid improvement. Headache, cough, pain and discomfort are lost, the appetite returns, and restlessness gives place to repose; although prostration and occasionally deafness may linger, the patient is fit for discharge from hospital within a further seven or eight days. In a minority of cases toxemia is more intense and the pulse becomes irregular; delirium or lung complications, often both, dominate the picture. Insomnia, discomfort, and cardiac and respiratory embarrassment induce great prostration, and the condition of the patient is critical. Yet recovery, remarkable in its rapidity, often follows; and, as in the less severe cases, convalescence is uneventful, save for protracted physical exhaustion. Death is usually due to intense toxemia and myocardial failure; less often to bronchopneumonia. An acute bronchitis or bronchopneumonia prolongs the course of the disease; otherwise the regularity of the evolution of tsutsugamushi, in sequence of clinical events and duration, is most characteristic.

Case-Mortality

Of the 181 patients under our close observation, 13 died. One of the striking features of tsutsugamushi in Malaya has been the increase in the case-mortality in recent years; in one endemic area, in 1929 it was treble that of 1927. The case-mortality is now about 15 per cent. This rate, though much below that of the more severe epidemics of the louse-borne typhus of Europe, is about equal to the European rate in interepidemic periods and in some of the less severe epidemics. Whether, as in louse-borne typhus, the mortality is higher in the old than in the young is difficult to decide. The incidence is closely bound up with occupation. More than 200 of this series were Tamil laborers, all but 3 or 4 of whom worked on estates; and it is rare for the Tamil laborer to remain in Malaya, and still more so to work on an estate, beyond the age of fifty. Further, the laborer's estimate of his age can rarely be accepted as accurate. About 25 patients were under eighteen; 2 of these died—a girl of eleven and a boy of fifteen. About 20 patients were over forty, and 4 of these died.

Weil-Felix Reaction

The serum of patients convalescent from tsutsugamushi agglutinates the OX-K type of *Proteus* strains but not the OX-19 type. In our series repeated samples were drawn and tested during convalescence, as urged by Fletcher and Lesslar (8), and evidence was thereby obtained of a waxing and waning titer, which constitutes almost certain proof of an active infection. The serological reactions of the first few patients in Malaya with a primary ulcer suggested that their sera agglutinated the OX-K type to low titers only. Felix and Rhodes (9), however, using sera from Japan and Sumatra from patients with a skin lesion, showed that agglutination was constant and often high. We have amply confirmed this finding among our cases in Malaya, readings higher than in 1 in 2000 being common. It may happen, though extremely rarely, that the clinical picture is typical of tsutsugamushi, yet the Weil-Felix reaction is persistently negative. In our series only 2 cases were in this category. It is occasionally asked what is the lowest titer that may be regarded as positive evidence of tsutsugamushi infection. In our experience an arbitrary standard of agglutination in a serum dilution of 1 in 125 may be taken as the lowest limit; but such low titers should be regarded as establishing the diagnosis only when the syndrome of tsutsugamushi is present, since in 2 of 11 cases of leptospirosis (see below) titers of 1 in 480 were recorded. Where successive samples of sera are available, the presence or absence of a waxing and waning agglutination curve simplifies interpretation.

Differential Diagnosis

Three diseases may in their early stages afford difficulty in diagnosis: urban typhus (shop typhus), leptospirosis, and typhoid fever.

Urban typhus. This disease simulates clinically those cases of tsutsugamushi that have no skin lesion when seen by the physician. The disease is conveyed by the rat flea, *Xenopsylla cheopis*; a skin lesion is never visible. Sera from convalescent patients agglutinate only the

OX-19 type of *Proteus* strains. In contrast to tsutsugamushi, it is a disease of the town, especially of the small and congested food shops that abound in every eastern town and village. If blood is drawn early in the fever and inoculated intraperitoneally into male guinea pigs, these will usually develop fever and scrotal swelling; whereas guinea pigs are very insusceptible to inoculation of blood from patients with tsutsugamushi, and the few that react do not, in our experience, develop scrotal swellings.

Leptospirosis. In even moderately severe cases extreme tenderness of the calf muscles and a much greater injection of the eyes than that seen in tsutsugamushi are valuable diagnostic points from the outset. In milder cases, in which muscular pain may be barely appreciable, early differentiation is not easy. The characteristic red or reddish-brown spots, small and closely set, contrast with the larger and more discrete papules and macules of tsutsugamushi. In many cases the rash is absent. The fall of temperature early in the second week, the negative Weil-Felix reaction (in all but rare instances), and the ready experimental reproduction of the disease in guinea pigs make later diagnosis easy.

Typhoid. This disease presents in the early stages two distinguishing features: its insidious onset and its less rapid development. The patient's condition in tsutsugamushi at the beginning of the second week is comparable with that of the third week in typhoid. At the end of the second week the rapid defervescence (in cases uncomplicated by bronchitis) and the rising titers of the Weil-Felix reaction are conclusive of tsutsugamushi.

Rat-bite Fever. This disease merits consideration where no certain history of a bite by a rat is elicited. The ulcer differs, being larger, irregular in outline and painful. On the trunk the elements of the rash are larger. Later, recurrent bouts of fever and other symptoms make diagnosis easy. The *Spirillum minus* is readily found in the blood of guinea pigs infected experimentally. It is worthy of note that we (10, 11) have found that the serum of rabbits inoculated with infected material from two strains agglutinates, often strongly, the OX-K strain of *Proteus.*

II. Morbid Anatomy and Histology

Autopsies were made by one of us in 12 fatal cases (12). All 12 patients had contracted the disease in endemic areas and had had a typical clinical syndrome and a positive Weil-Felix reaction. Naked-eye examination gave no consistent characteristic feature.

Heart: in 5 cases the myocardium was pale; there were subserous petechial hemorrhages beneath the epicardium and endocardium in 4 cases. *Lungs:* there were small punctiform subpleural hemorrhages in 11 cases, bilateral and deep congestion in 7, much edema in 5, and broncho-pneumonia in 3. *Kidney:* in 4 cases cloudy swelling was evident, in 5 there was injection of the surface vessels, and in 1 there were petechial hemorrhages throughout the whole renal substance and pelvis. *Liver:* in 3 cases cloudy swelling was considerable, in 3 subcapsular petechiae were present, in 8 there was considerable fatty degeneration, and in 5 the liver was enlarged. *Lymphatic glands:* in 3 cases there was slight and in 7 considerable enlargement, accompanied by much congestion in 3. The bronchial and the retroperitoneal glands were most affected. *Spleen:* in 11 cases the spleen was enlarged, the weights being two to five times the normal. Most of the patients had probably had one or more attacks of malaria. In 8 cases the spleen was diffluent, in 3 to a degree resembling the acute septic spleen. *Brain:* the only gross change was subdural hemorrhage, which was found in 2 cases. In each it was extensive and unilateral. Minor changes were congestion of the surface vessels in 6 cases and an increase in the cerebrospinal fluid in 5.

Histological examination was limited to the brain, the most important organ in the microscopical diagnosis of human material from the typhus group of fevers. In all, 7 brains were examined; 8 blocks of tissue were taken from each and serial paraffin sections cut and stained by Giemsa's method. Descriptions of the morbid histology of the human brain in typhus exanthematicus and Rocky Mountain spotted fever, reported by many workers, show unanimity in that the typical lesions, however much they may vary in appearance, are related to injury of the capillaries and arterioles of the brain.

In tsutsugamushi the findings in the human brain are meager; but all lesions found in typhus exanthematicus and Rocky Mountain spotted fever have been found in one or other of the 7 brains studied; they differ only in being smaller and fewer. Some pathological change could be found in every brain, but lesions that could be regarded as pathognomonic were absent in 2 and scanty in the other 5. They were found in each of the 8 areas examined but were most numerous in the pons and medulla and least in the cerebellum.

The commonest lesion is a perivascular proliferation of neuroglia cells, one or two cells in depth, along the course of capillaries and arterioles that show swelling of their endothelial cells. Less common is a lesion that is essentially only a greater degree of this perivascular

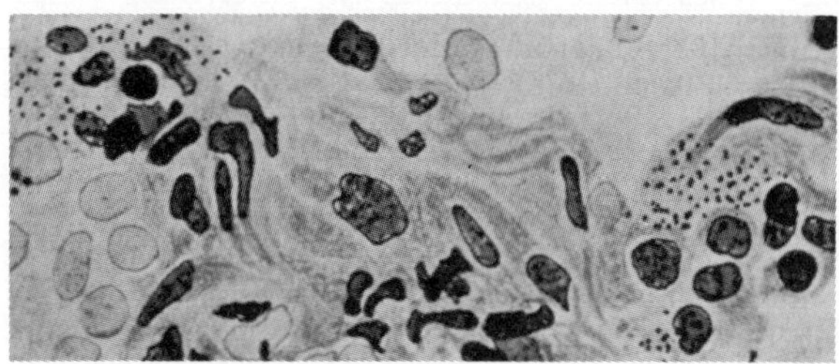

Fig. 2. Human brain. Section of pons. Arteriole shows collapse of lumen, extravasation of blood, and perivascular proliferation. Two clumps of rickettsia bodies are seen, lying close to nuclei. Giemsa. × 1100.

proliferation and includes a few cells indistinguishable from lymphocytes. The proliferation is usually irregularly distributed along the course of the vessel; the lumen may be patent, or vascular injury may have led to extravasation of blood and collapse of the lumen. Again, a thrombus may have formed, with consequent degeneration of the vascular elements, so that the lesion now consists of a clump of neuroglia cells in which lie lymphoid cells, pyknotic fragments of nuclei, and occasionally one or more degenerate erythrocytes or remnants of the lumen of a vessel. Such is the development and structure of the typhus "node."

Besides these hemorrhagic extravasations, small perivascular hemorrhages from capillaries and arterioles were often seen. The endothelial lining of the smallest vessels was often deeply pigmented, presumably owing to phagocytosis of broken-down erythrocytes. Throughout the cerebral cortex there was a general increase of cellular elements, most of which were neuroglia cells, but a few were leukocytes.

Demonstration of rickettsia in the brain. Rickettsia bodies were seen in the vascular lesions in 5 out of the 7 brains. They appear as rounded, ovoid, or lanceolate bodies, usually clearly diplococcal in arrangement. Occasionally, owing to the component elements being set at different depths of focus, there is apparent inequality of size and staining. The size varies appreciably with the intensity of staining, but the average dimensions of the paired organism may be given as 1–1.5 μ long and 0.2–0.3 μ broad. Stained by Giemsa's method they are deep blue with heavy staining or purple with light staining.

The lesions containing undoubted rickettsia bodies are very few, but once they have been found in a lesion which can be followed in serial

sections their study is facilitated. They are found in three situations:
1) most commonly within the cytoplasm of the endothelial cells of the
otherwise uninjured capillaries and smaller arterioles and usually in
pairs in rows parallel with the long axis of the cell; 2) intracellularly or
extracellularly, if shed from the cells as a result of injury (Fig. 2), in the
walls of similar vessels, injury to which has been followed by hemorrhagic extravasation and collapse; and 3) in mononuclear cells of the
perivascular nodes (6), though this is rare. The morphology and staining
of these rickettsia bodies resemble closely those of the rickettsia bodies
which can be found with ease and in abundance in smears from rabbits
and guinea pigs infected experimentally with the tsutsugamushi virus.
They appear to be indistinguishable from the *Rickettsia orientalis* shown
by Nagayo *et al.* (23) to be the causal organism of tsutsugamushi in
Japan.

Epidemiology

Season and climate. British Malaya lies just north of the equator,
between lat. N. 1° and lat. N. 6°. The temperature of the west coast,
whence came all but 7 of the cases in our series, has only a small daily
range, varying from a maximum of about 95°F. to a minimum of about
70°F. There is little appreciable seasonal variation. In Malaya the
disease is apparently not seasonal; every month of the year has its
quota of cases, and there is no consistent preponderance in any one
month. Comparison of incidence with rainfall during twenty-eight
consecutive months did not show any significant correlation. There was
a slight fall in incidence during the driest period of the year—namely,
May to August—but we attach little or no significance to this observation.

Race. Fletcher and Lesslar (1) noted that it was the association with
a particular kind of employment and certain circumscribed areas that
caused the uneven racial incidence. Most of our cases came from oil-
palm estates, and most of the laborers on these estates are Tamils.

Sex and age. Males exceed females by more than two to one. In
children below working age tsutsugamushi is extremely rare, yet the
laborers' hutments abound with children. The incidence falls evenly
among the ten-year age-groups of laborers in an endemic area.

Distribution. Fletcher and Lesslar (1) have described the association
of the virus with waste lalang-covered grazing ground and its persistence in certain circumscribed areas of such land. In one of these areas
overgrown with lalang 6 European soldiers were infected while in

camp; further cases occurred later among carters and cow-herds who pastured their cattle there. From similar grazing land some twenty miles away came the earliest cases of tsutsugamushi in the latter half of 1924. Another case occurred in this area in April, 1927, and 4 more in December 1928; all the patients were either Sikh or Pathan cattle drovers. The most instructive endemic area has been Oil-Palm Estate, which from June 1926 onwards yielded an unbroken succession of cases month by month for some years. During two and a half years we studied intensively certain aspects of the epidemiology of tsutsugamushi on this estate.

Occupation.   Without exception, every victim of tsutsugamushi in our series had had contact with the countryside at some time during the weeks before the illness, especially with land bearing lalang or other undergrowth. More than half our patients were employees of Oil-Palm Estate. The remainder were cow-herds and employees working on rubber estates, roads, or railways; the 4 Europeans who were not planters were a surveyor, a police officer in a rural area, a game-warden, and a man who had been shooting over Oil-Palm Estate a week before the onset of his symptoms. On Oil-Palm Estate the heaviest incidence was among those who worked with the worthless products at the base of the palm trees; the next heaviest was among weeders who worked close to the tree; factory hands and people working in and round the hutments never contracted tsutsugamushi (13). It was evident that the disease could be classed as occupational and that the vector lurked at the foot of the trees among the dead male and female flowers and bunches of overripe fruit that lay there rotting in the damp and shade. Moreover, as the gnawed bunches of fruit testified, rats (the reservoir of the rickettsia) foraged for food at the base of the trees. When the work at the base of the trees in any area was completed, the incidence of tsutsugamushi waned; when work at the base of the trees began, the incidence soared.

The vector.   The principal vectors of the typhus-like fevers throughout the world fall into four main groups: body lice, ticks, rat fleas, and larval mites. Extensive examinations of healthy and sick laborers in areas in which tsutsugamushi was endemic did not discover a single body louse (14); school-children are free from them; victims of tsutsugamushi are nursed in the general wards of hospitals without transference of infection to others; it is certain, therefore, that the body louse plays no part in the transmission of tsutsugamushi.

Ticks are known to be the carriers of typhus-like fevers in North and

South America, South Africa, India, and Europe. We made a series of exhaustive experiments with two species of ticks—namely, the American wood tick, *Dermacentor andersoni*, and the dog tick, *Rhipicephalus sanguineus*. *D. andersoni*, which, so far as is known, is not found in Malaya, is the most important vector of the Rocky Mountain spotted fever. We used it so that, if it should become infected, the tsutsugamushi virus might be sent in the tick to America for comparison with the many typhus strains there available. *R. sanguineus* is the most important vector of the *fièvre boutonneuse* of the Mediterranean littoral and of African tick typhus. Guinea pigs and white rats experimentally infected with tsutsugamushi virus were used as a source of virus. The technique and results have been published elsewhere in full (15). In no case was it possible to recover the virus from a guinea pig or a rat after infection had been attempted by refeeding or inoculation of ticks previously fed on an experimentally infected animal. However, a lessened mortality among the guinea pigs subjected to attempted infection was seen after test inoculation with passage virus; this finding makes it difficult to exclude entirely the possibility that ticks may play a minor part in the epidemiology of tsutsugamushi.

The rat flea, *Xenopsylla cheopis*, is known to transmit the virus of some of the typhus-like fevers in America, North and South Africa, and Europe. Further, we have shown that in the laboratory it unfailingly transmits the virus of the urban (or shop) typhus of Malaya, and that the virulence of the virus is thereby enhanced. For tsutsugamushi virus attempted transmission in the laboratory has shown that the part played by the rat flea (*X. cheopis*) is insignificant. Many series of experiments were made (10) on guinea pigs fed on a vitamin-deficient diet; on white rats fed from birth on a diet deficient in vitamin A and bred from parents similarly fed; and on rabbits (the most susceptible laboratory animals when inoculated by the intra-ocular route). In one series of experiments on guinea pigs the evidence suggested that the flea might have a feeble power to transmit the tsutsugamushi virus; but in another series and in the experiments on rabbits and white rats no evidence of transmission was forthcoming.

A larval mite, *Trombicula deliensis*, is almost certainly the vector of tsutsugamushi in Malaya. Fletcher, Lesslar, and Lewthwaite (16), in an investigation of the reservoir (the rat), trapped 130 rats in endemic and nonendemic foci and found this larval mite only in rats from endemic foci (with one exception). In one endemic focus the mite was found more often in a particular area from which most of the cases came. Gater

(14) examined 743 wild rats—half from this same endemic area and half from the town of Kuala Lumpur—month by month for a year. He found on the town rats only three trombidiid mites known to attack man. *T. deliensis* was found on 21.3 per cent of the rural rats. Further, he suggested that *T. alkamushi* and *T. deliensis* were merely forms of the same species. These two larval mites are respectively the vectors of tsutsugamushi in Japan and the closely allied (if not identical) mite fever of Sumatra. *T. alkamushi* was by far the commonest ectoparasite found by Gater on laborers in the endemic area.

The reservoir. This concentration of the probable vector on the rats of an endemic area strongly suggests the rat as a likely reservoir of the virus. Anigstein (17) examining rats from this same area, found microscopical evidence of a scrotal reaction and of rickettsia bodies in the tunica vaginalis.

Nicolle (18) drew attention to a distinction between the virus of old-world typhus (*le typhus historique*) and that of rat typhus (*le typhus murin*) founded on success or failure to propagate them in the white rat. Whereas the former could not be maintained by him beyond the thirteenth passage in three separate series of white rats, the rat typhus could be maintained thus indefinitely. We maintained, with no loss of virulence, a strain of tsutsugamushi, isolated from man, through twenty-one generations of white rats, at which point the investigation was arbitrarily terminated. By Nicolle's criterion tsutsugamushi was thus shown to be derived from rats. We sought additional evidence (19). In one investigation twenty-three attempts were made to isolate, in the guinea pig, strains of tsutsugamushi from wild rats trapped in particular houses or circumscribed areas from which human cases had recently come. Three succeeded, and two strains were studied exhaustively. Among other signs of infection were scrotal swelling and the abundance of intracellular rickettsia bodies (the causal agent of tsutsugamushi) in the tunica vaginalis. In rabbits inoculated with virus from infected guinea pigs agglutination of the OX-K type of *Proteus* X strains to titers as high as 1 in 1700 and 1 in 1925 was obtained. One strain was established and maintained without difficulty in rabbits by the intra-ocular injection of virus. Cross-immunity tests made in rabbits between this rat strain and five strains isolated from men showed a complete reciprocal cross-immunity with four strains and a partial cross-immunity with the fifth strain.

This evidence indicates conclusively that the rat is a reservoir of tsutsugamushi in Malaya.

Rickettsia Diseases of Malaya

Experimental Infection of Animals

The early attempts made in Malaya to establish and maintain strains of tsutsugamushi in laboratory animals were frustrated by the insusceptibility of the guinea pig, rat, and rabbit. So attempts by Fletcher and Lesslar (1), Anigstein (17), and Lewthwaite (20) to isolate strains from upwards of 250 patients met with meager success. Later we (Lewthwaite and Savoor [21]) used three modifications of procedure which overcame this insusceptibility sufficiently to permit study of strains: the use of vitamin-deficient guinea pigs, the inoculation of rabbits by the intraocular route, and the intradermal inoculation of monkeys.

Guinea pigs. These were fed for some days before and after inoculation on a diet of water, autoclaved skimmed milk, and rolled oats—a diet recommended by Zinnser *et al.* (22) for enhancing the virulence of experimental infections with the endemic Mexican-American typhus. Still we failed, save for one notable exception. From 1 patient, by inoculation of blood drawn early in the fever, a strain was established and maintained at first precariously by passage of infected tissues for the first few generations and then more easily, until eventually the vitamin-deficient diet became unnecessary. This strain has now been maintained in guinea pigs for eight years without loss of virulence. The inoculum is usually brain tissue, less often heart blood, splenic tissue, or ascitic fluid. Of guinea pigs injected thus intraperitoneally 90 per cent die; use of the subcutaneous route diminishes this mortality. The clinical signs are an incubation period of seven to twelve days, followed by continuous fever, which may persist for nine days but more often ends by sudden defervescence and death about the fifth day of fever. Constant post-mortem signs are ascites and enlargement of the spleen. Rickettsia bodies are abundant in the ascitic fluid, especially in the fibrinous deposit usually present on the surface of the spleen, and their numbers increase with each succeeding day of fever. Typhus nodes may rarely be found in sections of the brain. Guinea pigs that recover are immune for at least fifteen months. This strain came from a patient who had no visible lesion at the time of examination; we wish to emphasize the fact that strains isolated from patients with a dermal lesion, though they could not be long maintained, gave the same clinical and post-mortem signs of infection in reacting guinea pigs of the early passages.

Rabbits. Intraperitoneal injection of infected human blood or of passage virus into rabbits led to a positive Weil-Felix reaction in about

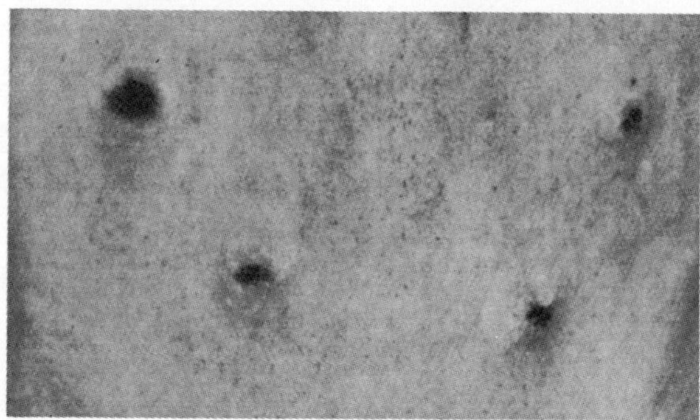

Fig. 3. Abdomen of macacus monkey inoculated intradermally with tsutsugamushi virus from a strain derived from a patient with an initial ulcer. Ulcers show well-marked central necrosis. Note the identical appearance of these dermal lesions and those shown in Fig. 4.

half the cases. The titers are lower than those given by human convalescent sera. Only the OX-K type of *Proteus* X strains are agglutinated. No other sign of infection is evident. Attempts to establish strains by intratesticular inoculation of virus failed. We then had recourse to the method of intra-ocular inoculation practised by Nagayo *et al.* (23) with the viruses of tsutsugamushi of Japan and typhus exanthematicus. Success was immediate. Injections of infected human blood from patients seen early in the disease yielded strains. The guinea pig strain can be transferred at will to rabbits by similar injection of infected blood or of ascitic fluid. A full account of the technique and results has been published elsewhere (21). After an incubation period an intense iridocyclitis develops in the inoculated eye, and agglutinins of the OX-K type appear in the serum of about half the rabbits. The causal rickettsia can readily be demonstrated at the height of ocular reaction in the cells of the endothelium covering Descemet's membrane at the back of the cornea. By successive inoculations of infected aqueous humor strains may be maintained with ease. Fever is fitful or absent, and the rabbits recover and are immune for at least twelve months. These signs and sequelae of infection are the same whether the strain has originated from a patient with a dermal lesion or from one in whom such a lesion has not been found.

White rats.   Infection of the white rat by our stock strain of tsutsugamushi is readily secured but is *inapparente* in type; fever is insignificant or absent, and scrotal swelling is never seen. At necropsy the only

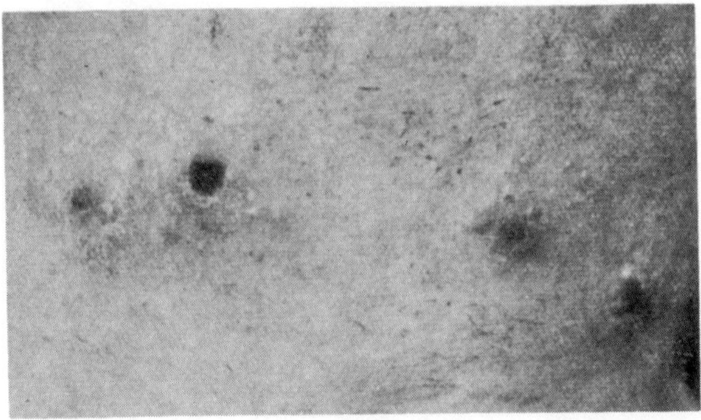

Fig. 4. Abdomen of macacus monkey inoculated intradermally with virus of a "rural-typhus" strain derived from a patient in whom an initial ulcer was not found. Ulcers show well-marked central necrosis (cf. Fig. 3).

constant finding is enlargement of the spleen; but ascites and a fibrinous exudate on the spleen are often present, and smears of these yield a few rickettsia bodies. Most of the infected rats die about the end of the second week.

Monkeys. In the first part of this paper we noted that a patient infected with tsutsugamushi might have a small ulcer, typical in its black necrotic center and surrounding red areola, that marked the site of inoculation by the insect vector. We noted also that until recently the presence of this ulcer differentiated tsutsugamushi from the rural form of tropical typhus. As our experimental work progressed, however, we were impressed by the identity of these supposed clinical entities in all other features, and to obtain experimental evidence about this apparent difference we inoculated monkeys and rabbits intracutaneously with strains derived from human cases of each clinical group.

One gibbon and three macacus monkeys were inoculated thus on either side of the abdomen with infected material from the eyes of rabbits; the strain was derived from a patient with an initial ulcer. Infection resulted in all, being shown by fever, leukopenia, a positive Weil-Felix reaction, and dermal lesions at the sites of inoculation. These lesions passed through macular and papular stages, and in the macacus monkeys, but not in the gibbon, progressed further to end as small circumscribed ulcers, with black necrotic centers and surrounding hyperemic areolae (Fig. 3). Swelling of the inguinal glands coincided with the development of necrosis in one monkey only.

One gibbon and six macacus monkeys were inoculated similarly

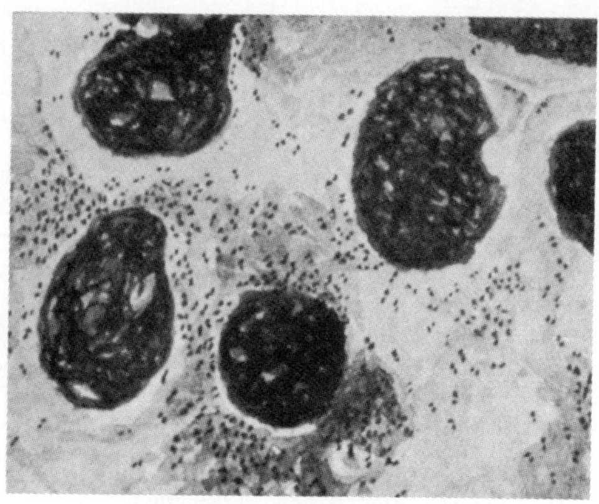

Fig. 5. Smear of scraping from the endothelium covering Descemet's membrane in the reacting eye, taken from a passage rabbit inoculated intraocularly with tsutsugamushi virus from a strain derived from a patient with an initial ulcer. A group of endothelial cells is seen, together with abundant rickettsia bodies, mostly intracellular, some extracellular. Note the identical appearance of these bodies and of those shown in Fig. 6. × 1300.

with infected material from strains derived from a patient in whom no initial ulcer was present when seen by us after the onset of the illness. The inoculum consisted of ascitic fluid from an infected passage guinea pig in five cases, and of infected material from the eyes of passage rabbits in two cases. All seven monkeys developed an infection manifested by precisely the same signs as those described above; the dermal lesions in the gibbon and in four of the macacus monkeys progressed beyond the papular stage to end as necrotic ulcers (Fig. 4); swelling of the inguinal glands developed in three.

Thus the experimental infections in gibbons and monkeys infected with virus from either clinical type were identical.

Rickettsial Nature of the Virus

Anigstein (17) reported the finding of rickettsia bodies in the tunica vaginalis of a guinea pig that had reacted to inoculation with the passage virus of a strain derived from a human patient with tsutsugamushi; since the patient had no primary ulcer, the case was at that time classified as scrub typhus. Subsequently we demonstrated rickettsia bodies constantly in laboratory strains derived from human patients with and without the primary ulcer, and less frequently in the brains

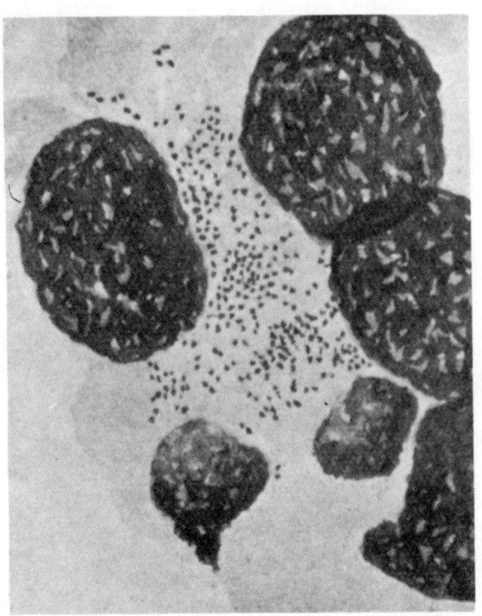

Fig. 6. Smear of fibrin covering spleen, taken from a passage guinea pig inoculated intraperitoneally with virus of a "rural-typhus" strain derived from a patient in whom an initial ulcer was not found. A group of endothelial cells is seen, with abundant intracellular rickettsia bodies (cf. Fig. 5). × 1700.

of fatal cases of tsutsugamushi in man. Ascitic fluid, especially scrapings of the peritoneum, from passage guinea pigs contains abundant rickettsia bodies, as also do scrapings of the endothelium lining Descemet's membrane from the reacting eye of passage rabbits (Figs. 5–7). In smears stained by Giemsa's method rickettsia bodies are seen lying within the cytoplasm of endothelial cells, mostly grouped as one or more clusters near the nucleus; rarely, extracellular forms are seen, apparently shed from ruptured cells. They are short rod-shaped bacilli showing bipolar staining. The polar granules are coccoid, purple, and connected by a narrow rod that stains blue. Average dimensions are 0.8–2.0 μ × 0.3–0.5 μ. In morphology, distribution, and staining characteristics they are identical with the *R. orientalis* described by Nagayo *et al.* (23) as the causal organism of tsutsugamushi of Japan.

Cross-Immunity Tests

In an investigation in laboratory animals of the identity or otherwise of two strains of a disease the most convincing test is that of cross-immunity. We (24) therefore paid particular attention to this test,

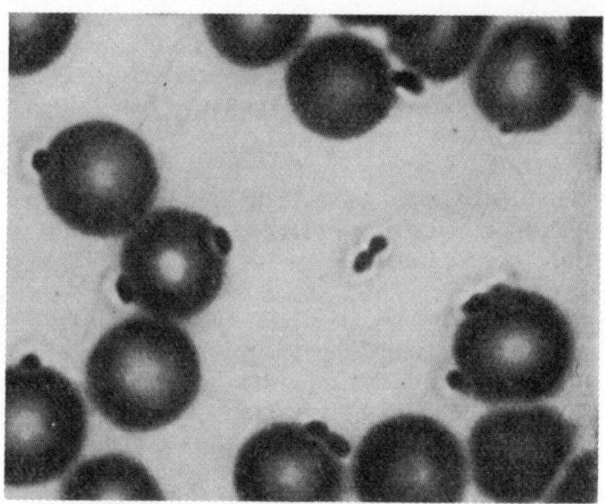

Fig. 7. Photomicrograph of pneumococci in the blood of a mouse, for comparison of the dimensions of pneumococci with those of the rickettsia bodies of tsutsuga-mushi. × *1700.*

using guinea pigs, rabbits, and monkeys. In each test reported below, one or more control animals were inoculated and reacted typically.

Guinea pigs. One strain derived from a patient in whom no initial ulcer was seen and two strains from patients with such an ulcer were used. The first of these has been firmly fixed for many years; the second and third strains became attenuated and were lost, but they furnished a sufficient number of reacting and immune animals to enable cross-protection tests to be done. The criterion applied was failure of a convalescent guinea pig to react with fever when inoculated with the virus of another strain. Eleven tests were made and showed cross-immunity between the strains to be complete and reciprocal.

Rabbits. The strains used were of the same two types as above. Three criteria were relief on: iridocyclitis, a positive Weil-Felix reaction, and, in a few cases, a dermal lesion at the site of inoculation.

Twenty-four rabbits that had developed a complete and identical iridocyclitis after intra-ocular injection, some with the first type of strain and others with the second type, were reinoculated in the other eye, a month or more later, with an inoculum of the other type of strain. Cross-protection was complete and reciprocal. Five rabbits that had given a positive Weil-Felix reaction after intraperitoneal inoculation with one type of strain proved to be immune when reinoculated intra-ocularly with the other type of strain.

Weil and Felix (25) showed that, in louse-borne typhus of East

European origin, when rabbits that have acquired an immunity to typhus are reinoculated with a homologous strain, the X-19 agglutinins produced as a result of the primary infection are not restimulated. Felix (26) emphasized the value of this test in the comparison of two strains of typhus virus; we applied it in our investigation. Eighteen rabbits that had developed a positive Weil-Felix reaction after inoculation with the virus of either the first or the second type were reinoculated, some with the homologous virus and others with the heterologous virus, some intra-ocularly and others intraperitoneally. A rabbit was presumed to be immune if there was no significant rise of agglutinins during sixty days after inoculation. In seventeen there was no significant rise of agglutinins; in one OX-K agglutinins developed to a degree slightly higher than the initial one.

Six rabbits that had previously reacted to intra-ocular inoculation of a strain derived originally from a patient with a primary ulcer were reinoculated intracutaneously with a strain derived from a patient in whom no ulcer had been found. In none did a dermal lesion develop, whereas typical dermal lesions developed in control rabbits. The immunity acquired lasted for at least a year.

Thus in the rabbit cross-protection is complete and reciprocal, between strains of either clinical type, whether inoculation is by the intra-ocular, intraperitoneal, or intradermal route, and whether the criteria are clinical (iridocyclitis and dermal lesion) or serological.

Monkeys. A gibbon was inoculated intracutaneously with a strain derived from a patient with a primary ulcer; it reacted typically developing the four cardinal signs of infection in the monkey: febrile reaction, dermal lesion, leukopenia, and agglutinins for the OX-K strain of *Proteus*. Three months later it was reinoculated, together with a control macacus, by the same route with a strain derived from a patient in whom no primary ulcer had been found. There was no reaction other than a mild leukopenia in the reinoculated animal; but in the control all four criteria of infection developed.

Thus the foregoing cross-protection tests in the guinea pig, rabbit, and monkey are in entire accord. They indicate that cross-immunity is complete and reciprocal between strains derived from human patients with an ulcer and from those in whom an ulcer has not been found.

Discussion

All the known features of etiology, epidemiology, serology, experimental pathology, and immunology point to the identity of strains derived from human cases of either clinical type; apart from the primary ulcer, the clinical syndrome of the two types in man is also identical. In the face of such evidence we think that an initial ulcer with attendant bubo is not enough to justify the separation of these cases from those in which no ulcer is found (hitherto termed rural or scrub typhus). We are convinced that the two clinical types are not separate entities but one and the same disease, in which the dermal lesion varies in duration and degree of evolution, being conspicuous, necrotic, and persistent in some cases; whereas in others it is inconspicuous, papular only, and fleeting, usually escaping recognition by completing its evolution before the onset of other symptoms and signs. As noted earlier, Schüffner suggested this possibility many years ago in tsutsugamushi in Sumatra.

In support of our conviction we wish to draw attention to certain of our observations on the dermal lesion. Earlier in this paper we described a fatal case in a European, unique in our experience, in that the dermal lesion was a tiny abraded papule which disappeared as early as the eighth day of illness. On the darker skin of an Asiatic it would almost certainly have been overlooked. Had the patient not been seen until the eighth day of illness, the case would have been classified as one without initial lesion and therefore as rural typhus. Yet the lesion was entirely comparable to the dermal lesion obtained experimentally in rabbits and monkeys—i.e., a papule which often does not progress to necrosis.

Consideration of the incidence of cases with an initial ulcer and of cases in which no ulcer was found in the labor force of an estate affords cogent evidence for the identity of the two clinical types. Thus Fletcher *et al.* (16) reported both types from the same endemic area of an estate. Wolff and Kouwenaar (27) reported from Sumatra that rural typhus and Sumatran mite fever (in which there is an initial ulcer) occurred in the same population group of estate laborers.

In our experience there have been among Europeans 10 cases with an ulcer for 1 without; among Asiatics 1 case with an ulcer for at least 40 without. The record of cases on a certain estate where both clinical types have appeared regularly for the past twelve years yields decisive evidence, in our view, on this problem of the initial lesion. Of the 7 European managers 5 have been infected, and an ulcer was found in 4 of them, whereas among the Tamil laborers supervised in the field by these Europeans more than 200 have been infected, yet in 2 only was an ulcer found. It is inconceivable that two viruses that were separate entities should show such a sharp racial discrimination between Europeans and Asiatics working together in the same area. Every line of investigation has converged to the conclusion that one and the same virus causes both clinical syndromes.

The disparity in the incidence of the ulcer according to race remains to be explained. In part it may be due to difficulty in finding an inconspicuous lesion on the dark skin of the Tamil. In part it is bound up with the greater sensitivity of the European to slight injury of the skin. The Tamil laborer wears scanty clothing while working, and constant exposure causes him to be less sensitive than the European to abrasions and bites. The European, unaccustomed to such exposure because he wears more clothing, is prone to scratch the site of an insect bite and thereby enlarge it and introduce secondary infection. Friction of clothes may also contribute to this local trauma.

Some observers, including ourselves, have in the past suggested that the uncertain incidence of an initial ulcer may be due to different modes of inoculation: that an insect vector with a short proboscis may inject the virus intradermally, and that another insect vector with a longer proboscis may penetrate the dermis and deposit the virus subcutaneously. With intradermal injection an ulcer would develop at the site of inoculation; with subcutaneous injection no lesion would develop, as we and others have shown experimentally in rabbits and monkeys for the OX-K type of virus. The tick has been suggested as a vector which might inoculate subcutaneously. It is known, however, that in India, South Africa, and the Mediterranean littoral, endemic typhus fevers, in the clinical picture of which necrotic primary ulcers frequently develop, are transmitted by a tick. It is no longer necessary to postulate two insect vectors and two routes of inoculation; our conception, based on human and experimental infections, of gradations of damage ranging from an ephemeral insignificant papule to a persistent well-defined necrotic ulcer, after intradermal inoculation, explains the presence or absence of a dermal lesion when the patient is first examined.

The same uncertain incidence of an initial ulcer is found in other fevers of the typhus group. Morishita has personally informed us that the initial ulcer is not always found in tsutsugamushi in Formosa. Kawamura *et al.* (28) have reported similarly. Such cases without an ulcer have hitherto been classed in Malaya as rural typhus, but in Formosa they are regarded as tsutsugamushi. Lépine (29), discussing a paper by Lewthwaite and Savoor (30), said that in *fièvre boutonneuse* the initial ulcer might be present or absent. Megaw (31), in the same discussion, said that in a case of tick typhus in India he had seen an initial ulcer (with attendant bubo) at the site from which a tick had been removed, although in most cases of this typhus-like fever no ulcer could be found. Unwin (4), reporting his 1500 cases of endemic tropical typhus (coastal fever) from North Queensland, wrote: "On close examination of many cases I have been able in several instances to find definite signs of an insect-bite, with its black central eschar and surrounding red areola." Thus the uncertain incidence of the initial ulcer in the endemic typhus fevers is not peculiar to tsutsugamushi of Malaya.

Summary

(1) Hitherto tsutsugamushi and the rural form of tropical (scrub typhus) have been thought to be separate diseases in virtue of the presence of a primary dermal lesion and attendant bubo in tsutsugamushi and their supposed absence in rural typhus.

(2) Their clinical picture, pathology, etiology, and epidemiology are described, and the results of experiments are recorded. From consideration of these, especially of cross-immunity tests between strains of the two clinical types, the conclusion is drawn that one and the same virus may cause various gradations of dermal lesion, and that tsutsugamushi and rural typhus are identical. Rural typhus not being a disease *sui generis*, this term should be discarded and the older term "tsutsugamushi" retained.

Acknowledgments

For permission to reproduce the various figures we wish to thank Dr. A. Neave Kingsbury, director of the Institute for Medical Research, F.M.S., and Dr. J. W. Field for Fig. 1, taken from *Bulletin* No. 1 of 1927 from that institute; the editor of the *Journal of Pathology and Bacteriology* for Fig. 2; and the editor of the *British Journal of Experimental Pathology* for Figs. 3–7.

For the more recent Weil-Felix reactions our thanks are due to Dr. R. Green, bacteriologist to this institute.

E. Gildemeister and E. Haagen

Typhus Fever Studies: I. Toxin in Rickettsia Egg Cultures (Rickettsia mooseri)

The first demonstration of toxic activity associated with living rickettsiae was reported by Gildemeister and Haagen in 1940. As occasionally happens in scientific research, this important discovery was serendipitous. Their original purpose, based on an erroneous premise, was to explore the value of a killed murine typhus vaccine for protection against epidemic typhus fever. In the course of testing the pathogenicity of murine typhus rickettsiae (*R. mooseri*), grown in the yolk sac of the developing chick embryo for the production of vaccine, they noted that mice inoculated intraperitoneally with heavy suspensions of the rickettsiae died within 4 to 20 hours. In the same report they showed further that the toxic property was neutralized by convalescent serum from either epidemic or murine typhus cases. Later, toxic activity was discovered in yolk sac tissue infected with *R. prowazeki*, the agent of epidemic typhus (1); *R. orientalis*, the agent of scrub typhus (2); *R. rickettsii*, the agent of Rocky Mountain spotted fever; and *R. conorii*, the agent of boutonneuse fever, South African tick bite fever, and Indian tick typhus (3).

Although rickettsial toxic activity has not been utilized extensively for diagnostic purposes, a toxin neutralization test was devised which played a vital role in the development and standardization of epidemic typhus vaccines (1, 4). In addition, the test has been successfully employed to demonstrate antigenic differences between the rickettsiae of epidemic typhus and of murine typhus (5) and in studies on the serological relations among the spotted fever group of rickettsiae (6). The mechanism of rickettsial toxicity and its mode of action have been studied by a number of workers (7, 8, 9, 10). The biochemical composition of rickettsial toxins and their precise functioning in the pathogenesis of rickettsial infections, however, has not been completely established. These are challenging areas for future research.

In the fight against typhus fever, elimination of lice is and will continue to be the most important factor. Only where the populace is infested with lice can typhus fever occur either endemically or epidemically. As a result eradication of the louse is synonymous with suppression of typhus fever. If typhus fever is introduced in a populace free of lice, the sickness generally is limited to a few cases if defensive measures are taken promptly.

Even immunization against typhus fever, which has made great advances during the past two years, cannot substitute for elimination of the louse in the fight against this disease. First of all, immunization does not provide absolute protection, and secondly, the production of vaccine for millions of people is not yet possible. We must therefore limit immunization to those persons who are especially endangered by virtue of their occupations, e.g., doctors, medical assistant personnel, police personnel, etc.

When we were faced with the necessity of producing typhus fever vaccine, it was clear to us that the method of Weigl—from the intestines of infected lice—could not be considered because of its complicated nature. The Weigl vaccine is the best available at this time, but numerous people who are immune to typhus fever are required for feeding of the infected lice, and they are not available in Berlin. We therefore decided on a process which has been employed in Germany for a long time by Otto and Wohlrab and has been tested under practical conditions. The causative agent of the classic typhus fever, *Rickettsia prowazeki*, is not used in this method but rather that of murine typhus fever, *R. mooseri*. Because of the close relation of the two types of rickettsia, one can perhaps expect a vaccine made with *R. mooseri* to be effective against the classic typhus fever.

Such vaccines can be obtained in three different ways: 1) from rickettsia which have multiplied in the peritoneums of mice, 2) from rickettsia which have been bred in cell cultures according to the method of Nigg and Landsteiner, and 3) from rickettsia obtained from incubated chicken eggs via the yolk sac method of Cox. Otto and Wohlrab have used the last method, for the most part, for some time. It is relatively easy to carry out and generally yields an ample result. We therefore decided to use this process ourselves. Otto and Wohlrab donated a strain of *R. mooseri*, which had been held in mice, to our efforts, for which we are grateful.

The continuous breeding of *R. mooseri* in white mice is very easy. The brains of typically ill mice are well ground in a mortar and mixed with 10 cc Ringer's solution. 0.25–0.5 cc of this brain suspension are injected into new animals intraperitoneally. The infected animals usually become sick on the fourth or fifth day and die about the sixth or seventh day. Rickettsiae can then be found in more or less large amounts in peritoneal smear slides.

The brains of mice thus infected and made sick are then used to breed rickettsiae in eggs which have been incubated for seven days. 0.2 cc of the above-described brain suspension is injected into the blunt end of the egg by means of a syringe. The shell of the egg is first sterilized with iodine, and a hole is made with a sterile needle. The hollow needle of the syringe is then inserted horizontally through this hole as far as possible and the contents of the syringe injected.

The eggs infected in this way are then incubated six more days and then opened by cutting off the blunt end with a shears. The embryo is thereupon removed and the remainder of the contents of the egg is poured into a sterile double dish. The yolk sac is then separated from the yolk by twisting around two sterile needles and placed into a sterile dish. Smear slides are then made from the yolk sac for examination for rickettsiae, and aerobic and anaerobic sterilization measures are taken, that is to say, it is checked for the presence of bacteria. Only those yolk sacs which contain rickettsiae and are free of bacteria are processed further.

The production of vaccine takes place in the following manner: put each yolk sac into a sterile glass bottle with glass balls; add 25 cc Ringer's solution; and shake the bottle for one hour on the vibrator machine. After material for further egg passage is removed, add 0.5 per cent Formol. Then shake for two to three days with the vibrator, filter through gauze in order to take out the remnants of the yolk sac, thicken to one half volume in the exsiccator with suction pump, and fill to make the original volume with Ringer's solution. The vaccine is now filled into tubes and placed in water bath at 60°C. for one hour on two successive days. This completes the production of the vaccine. It is best stored under refrigeration at 2–4°C.

In the course of this work we made observations which seem to us to be of basic importance and which will be reported below.*

As a means of determining whether the rickettsia egg cultures which we had started retained their pathogenicity for the white mice, a yolk sac which had been shown to have rickettsiae in the microscopic examination of a smear slide was shaken with Ringer's solution and amounts of 0.5 cc and 1 cc were injected into white mice intraperitoneally. To our surprise, all of the animals died within 4–20 hours, some of them with cramps. Since the yolk sacs were definitely determined to be free of bacteria, a bacterial effect could be discounted. Now, one possibility was that the yolk sac of incubated chickens egg was poisonous for mice. To clarify this point, chicken eggs which had been incubated for seven days were injected with 0.2 cc Ringer's solution instead of

---

* In our work with typhus fever, we were helped by our technical assistants, Miss Irmgard Ahlfelt and Miss Brigitte Crodel.

with rickettsiae and incubated for six days more. The yolk sac was removed in the usual way and shaken for one hour with 25 cc Ringer's solution, then injected intraperitoneally in amounts of 0.5–1 cc into white mice, but it showed itself to be completely free of poison; the animals remained alive and showed no signs of sickness.

Further experimentation showed that every rickettsia-positive yolk sac suspension from an incubated chicken egg killed mice which had intraperitoneal injections within 24, or at most 48, hours. Since it was injected intraperitoneally in amounts of up to 0.25 cc or less, less often 0.1 cc, the poison contained in these yolk sacs can be considered to be highly effective. The suspension kills only in exceptional cases when injected subcutaneously. The intracerebral method is likewise not dependable.

Guinea pigs given intraperitoneal injections of 1 cc of the rickettsia yolk sac suspension show no ill effects.

Yolk sac suspensions from eggs which have been infected with rickettsiae and incubated, but which show no rickettsiae under microscopic examination—in which, therefore, the infection did not take—also do not contain poison.

As regards the time when the poison developed in infected eggs, our experiments showed that after two days following the infection the yolk sacs of the incubated eggs did not contain the poison, but from the fourth day on they regularly did contain poison. Rickettsiae were also not to be found after two days, but after four days they were always found in amounts equal to those found after six days.

It is emphasized once more that there is no possibility that the poison came from any type of bacteria which happened to be in the eggs, since only those yolk sacs which were free of bacteria were used in the tests for poison. Furthermore, the mice killed by the poison were free of bacteria in their heart blood.

At this point it was necessary to determine other characteristics of this rickettsia poison. The experiments made in this connection showed that it is exceptionally labile. The effectiveness of the poison was destroyed by nothing more than keeping the rickettsia yolk sac suspension under refrigeration of 2°C. for seven days. The poison is also rapidly made ineffective through addition of Formol or by heating to 60°C. Thus the possibility of working with a poison which contains no rickettsiae is eliminated.

In order to clearly establish the specifity of the rickettsiae which we had demonstrated, neutralization tests were conducted with serums of

Table 1

Type and origin of serum	Amount of serum	Ringer's solution	Amount of rickettsia-yolk sac-Ringer's solution in cc	Number of mice	Number which died within 24–48 hours	later	Still living after ten days
Miss C, following labora-tory infection with	0.5	—	0.5	3	—	1	2
Rickettsia mooseri	0.2	0.3	0.5	3	—	3	—
Miss A, immunized with	0.5	—	0.5	3	1	2	—
Otto-Wohlrab vaccine	0.2	0.3	0.5	3	2	1	—
Miss H, immunized with	0.5	—	0.5	3	2	—	1
Weigl vaccine	0.2	0.3	0.5	3	1	2	—
Serum from retroplacen-tal blood (Homoseran)	0.5	—	0.5	3	2	1	—
	0.2	0.3	0.5	3	3	—	—
Normal human serum 1	0.5	—	0.5	3	2	1	—
	0.2	0.3	0.5	3	3	—	—
Normal human serum 2	0.5	—	0.5	3	2	1	—
	0.2	0.3	0.5	3	3	—	—

varying extraction. Serums from persons who had been immunized with Otto-Wohlrab vaccine and others with Weigl vaccine were tried. In addition, serum from one of our colleagues who had become infected during her work with egg cultures and suffered a mild illness was available (Weil-Felix after immunization with Otto-Wohlrab vaccine 1:50+, after the illness 1:1600). Further, there were three serums from persons who had recently survived the classic typhus fever (*Rickettsia prowazeki*), for which we have Dr. Kunert from the Hygienic Institute in Litzmannstadt to thank. Serums from coworkers who had not been immunized served as control serums, as did normal rabbit serums. For general interest we also used serum from retroplacental blood in the form of Homoseran (Anhal Serum Institute), which has shown a richness in protective material of various types (measles and poliomyelitis, for instance).

The tests were designed as follows:

To 1 cc of the rickettsia-yolk sac-Ringer's solution, equal or lesser amounts of the serum were added. If a lesser amount of serum was used, Ringer's solution was added in order to bring the volume up to 2 cc.

Table 2

Type and origin of serum	Amount of serum	Ringer's solution	Amount of rickettsia-yolk sac-Ringer's solution, in cc	Number of mice	Number which died within 24–48 hours	later	Still living after ten days
Miss C, following laboratory infection with	0.5	—	0.5	2	—	—	2
Rickettsia mooseri	0.25	0.25	0.5	2	—	—	2
Typhus fever serum Sl.	0.5	—	0.5	2	—	—	2
	0.25	0.25	0.5	2	—	—	2
Typhus fever serum Sk.	0.5	—	0.5	2	—	—	2
	0.25	0.25	0.5	2	—	—	2
G, immunized with Otto-Wohlrab vaccine	0.5	—	0.5	2	—	2	—
	0.25	0.25	0.5	2	—	2	—
Serum from retroplacental blood (Homoseran)	0.5	—	0.5	2	—	—	2
	0.25	0.25	0.5	2	—	—	2
Normal rabbit serum 1	0.5	—	0.5	2	2	—	—
	0.25	0.25	0.5	2	1	1	—
Normal rabbit serum 2	0.5	—	0.5	2	2	—	—
	0.25	0.25	0.5	2	2	—	—
Normal human serum 3	0.5	—	0.5	2	1	1	—
	0.25	0.25	0.5	2	1	1	—
Typhus fever serum R	0.5	—	0.5	2	1	—	1
	0.25	0.25	0.5	2	—	1	1
Control	—	0.5	0.5	2	2	—	—
	—	0.5	0.5	2	2	—	—

The mixture was left at room temperature for four to five hours, then refrigerated until the next day at 2°C. Then 1 cc of the mixture, which contained 0.5 cc of the rickettsia-yolk sac-Ringer's solution, was injected intraperitoneally into each of two mice.

The questions which these tests were intended to answer were the following: 1) Does immunity serum neutralize the rickettsia poison? 2) Can the rickettsiae also be rendered harmless by the serum? The answers to these two questions are given in Tables 1 and 2.

From Tables 1 and 2 we see the following:

1. *Effect upon the poison:* The typhus fever serum from Miss C.

(infection with *Rickettsia mooseri*) and the typhus fever serums (*Rickettsia prowazeki*) Sl. and Sk. neutralized the rickettsia poison very definitely when given in large enough doses; the typhus fever serum R did so with only one exception. The serum of the immunized persons makes the poison ineffective for the wide majority of the animals, while normal human serum and normal rabbit serum have the opposite effect for the most part. The serum obtained from retroplacental blood showed itself to be particularly effective: the poison was made ineffective in almost all cases.

2. *Effect upon the rickettsiae:* Here, too, the typhus fever serums proved to be effective. In a dose of 0.5 cc they usually prevented the taking of the infection. The serum of immunized humans was not able to do this except in one case. Similarly, the few mice which were not protected from the poison effect did not die. Especially noteworthy is the fact that Homoseran protected the mice against typhus fever in the same way (with sufficiently large dosage) as did the typhus fever serums.

We do not want to fail to mention the fact that the yolk sacs with the greatest concentration of rickettsiae are not best suited for passage breeding of rickettsiae in incubated eggs, because the chicken embryos injected with such material almost all die prematurely. Therefore the continuation of the experiment succeeds best when the medium rickettsia-content sacs are used. This fact, which we discovered shortly after the start of our tests, found its explanation in the demonstration of rickettsia poison. It was shown that the poisonous effect was greater when the yolk sac was rich in rickettsiae. It can then be assumed that the chicken embryo can withstand a certain dosage of rickettsia poison, but as soon as this is exceeded, the embryo dies.

Our experiments clearly proved the existence of a rickettsia poison. Here we cannot state definitely what type of poison it is, whether an exotoxin or an endotoxin. On the basis of our tests we are of the opinion that it may well be an endotoxin. Further tests are necessary to decide this question. In any event, it can now be stated that the main symptoms of a clinical case of typhus fever—the exanthema of the skin and the disturbance of the circulatory organs and the central nervous system—are based upon the effect of poison formed by the rickettsiae.

Our studies are of course not yet finished, but rather will be extended, especially in an effort to determine whether what we learned about *Rickettsia mooseri* also applies to *Rickettsia prowazeki*. This appears very likely. Another area to be checked is whether rickettsia poison can be found in tissue cultures in the same way as in egg cultures. Such tests have already been started.

Because the poison of the *Rickettsia mooseri*, as was shown, is very unstable, any attempt to kill the rickettsiae also makes the poison ineffective. For this reason it is not now possible to inoculate animals with pure poison without the presence of live rickettsiae. Nevertheless, such immunizations should be conducted—with poison and with living rickettsiae—in order to determine any difference between such immunity serums and those produced from killed rickettsiae.

Summary

1. Confirming the statements of Cox and of Otto and Wohlrab, it was found that *Rickettsia mooseri*, the causative agent of murine typhus fever, could be bred without difficulty in incubated chicken eggs.

2. A poison was demonstrated to be in the rickettsia-containing yolk sacs of such egg cultures, which, according to the above authors, are used in the production of typhus fever vaccines. This poison kills mice within 24, or at most 48, hours following intraperitoneal injection. This is the first demonstration of a toxin in rickettsia cultures.

3. The facility with which the rickettsia toxin in the yolk sacs can be demonstrated increases in direct proportion to the increase in the amount of rickettsiae present.

4. This toxin is very easily destroyed; it becomes ineffective through the addition of Formalin or by heating to 60°C. or after being stored for seven days. The resistance of the toxin, therefore, is no greater than that of the rickettsiae.

5. Typhus fever serums of the murine as well as of the classic typhus fever neutralize the poison. This can also sometimes be done with serums from persons who have been immunized with vaccines made from *Rickettsia mooseri* or *Rickettsia prowazeki*. Serum from normal human beings or rabbits does not neutralize the poison. It is noteworthy that serum obtained from retroplacental blood (Homoseran) promptly neutralizes the poison.

6. Typhus fever serums and Homoseran almost always protect mice from sickness following infection with *Rickettsia mooseri*. Serums from immunized persons do this only rarely.

7. The demonstrated rickettsia toxin is apparently an endotoxin.

8. The characteristic symptoms of a clinical case of typhus fever—exanthema, disturbance of the circulatory organs and the central nervous system—may be due to a toxin effect.

1943

Harry Plotz, Joseph E. Smadel, Thomas F. Anderson, and

Leslie A. Chambers

Morphological Structure of Rickettsiae

The earliest electron micrographs of rickettsiae were published in 1943 by Plotz and his associates in the brief paper reprinted here. The similarity in morphological appearance of the four strains of rickettsiae examined was of interest, and the discovery that an internal structure exists within these micro-organisms and that a limiting membrane surrounds the cytoplasm was an important finding. The presence of a limiting membrane in rickettsiae was confirmed in air-dried preparations (1) and in ultrathin sections (2).

Numerous studies were carried out later to determine the biochemical nature of this membrane, since it was considered to be analogous to the cell wall of bacteria. Schaechter and others (3), analyzing cell walls prepared from *R. mooseri,* found that their chemical composition was similar to that of bacteria cell walls in being composed mainly of amino acids and polysaccharides. Both type and group specific antigens were demonstrated in cell wall preparations. The detection in 1960 of muramic acid in cell walls of *C. burnetii* by Allison and Perkins (4) is of considerable taxonomic significance because muramic acid has been found only in bacteria and blue-green algae. Investigations on the biochemical components of rickettsiae are vitally important because they not only contribute to our understanding of the components' role in patho-genicity but may also aid in elucidating the evolutionary development of these infectious agents and of other microorganisms.

Rickettsiae are regarded by most workers in the field of infectious diseases as agents which occupy a position in the biological scale inter-mediate between the filterable viruses and the bacteria (1). Thus, the rickettsiae like the viruses are intracellular parasites but their size and staining characteristics emphasize their resemblance to bacteria. That the bacillary rickettsial forms do indeed represent the infectious agents is generally accepted. Information about the internal morphological structure of rickettsiae has been obtained during the course of other studies, and since it contributes to our understanding of the nature of this group of agents, it is presented at this time.

Materials and Methods

Four rickettsial agents were employed in the present studies: these were the Breinl strain of epidemic typhus, the Wilmington strain of

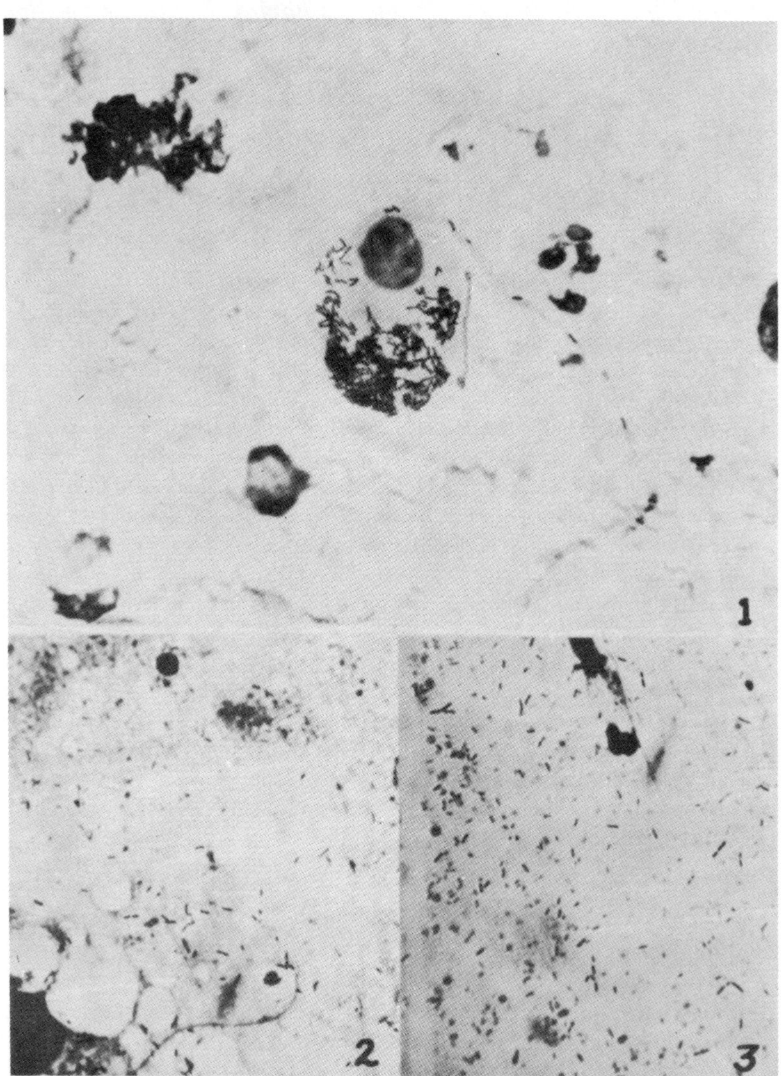

Fig. 1. A typical Neill-Mooser body is illustrated. This endothelial cell from the tunica of a guinea pig infected with endemic typhus contains many rickettsiae in its cytoplasm. The diplobacillary forms and short chains are also present in the streamer of cytoplasm seen to the right of the large cell. Macchiavello's stain. × 1000. Figs. 2 and 3. These represent photomicrographs of smears from emulsions of yolk sacs infected with epidemic and endemic typhus, respectively. Macchiavello's stain. × 1000.

endemic typhus, the Bitterroot strain of Rocky Mountain spotted fever, and the American strain of Q fever. These agents had been maintained by serial animal and cultural passages in the Virus Laboratory of the Army Medical School for some time, and their identities were checked at frequent intervals by means of cross-immunity and serological tests.

Most of the observations recorded in this report were made with the aid of a type B RCA electron microscope (2) on partially purified suspensions of Formolized rickettsiae which were obtained from egg yolk sacs inoculated by the technique of Cox (3); the method of purification of the rickettsial material will be described at a future date. In addition, suspensions of infectious rickettsiae of spotted fever were obtained from the scrapings of inoculated agar slant tissue cultures (4); these were washed by a process of differential centrifugation and used in the studies. Rickettsiae for examination in the electron miscrocope were placed on collodion films and washed by the method previously used for elementary bodies of vaccinia (5). In the case of the infectious rickettsiae of spotted fever such preparations were made at the Virus Laboratory and inactivated by one of two procedures, i.e., by exposure to Formalin vapor overnight, or by irradiation with ultraviolet light.

In order to illustrate the structure of rickettsiae as visualized by ordinary microscopy, impression smears of tunica tissue of guinea pigs infected with endemic typhus, and smears of crude emulsions of yolk sacs rich in rickettsiae were stained by Macchiavello's technique (6) and photographed by the usual methods.

Experimental Results

The bacteria-like rickettsial structures found in infected tissues are readily seen in smears and sections stained with aniline dyes and examined by ordinary microscopic techniques. The appearance of certain rickettsiae examined under these conditions is illustrated in Figs. 1 to 3. The cytoplasmic distribution of rickettsiae of endemic typhus in an endothelial cell from the tunica of an inoculated guinea pig is seen in Fig. 1. Wolbach (7) and Pinkerton and Hass (8) have emphasized the occurrence of rickettsiae of the spotted fever group in the nucleus as well as in the cytoplasm of diseased cells; this is in contrast to the distribution of the organisms of typhus fever which are found only in the cytoplasm. Figures 2 and 3 illustrate the pleomorphic rod-shaped structures which are found in stained smears of yolk sacs infected with the rickettsiae of epidemic and endemic typhus, respectively.

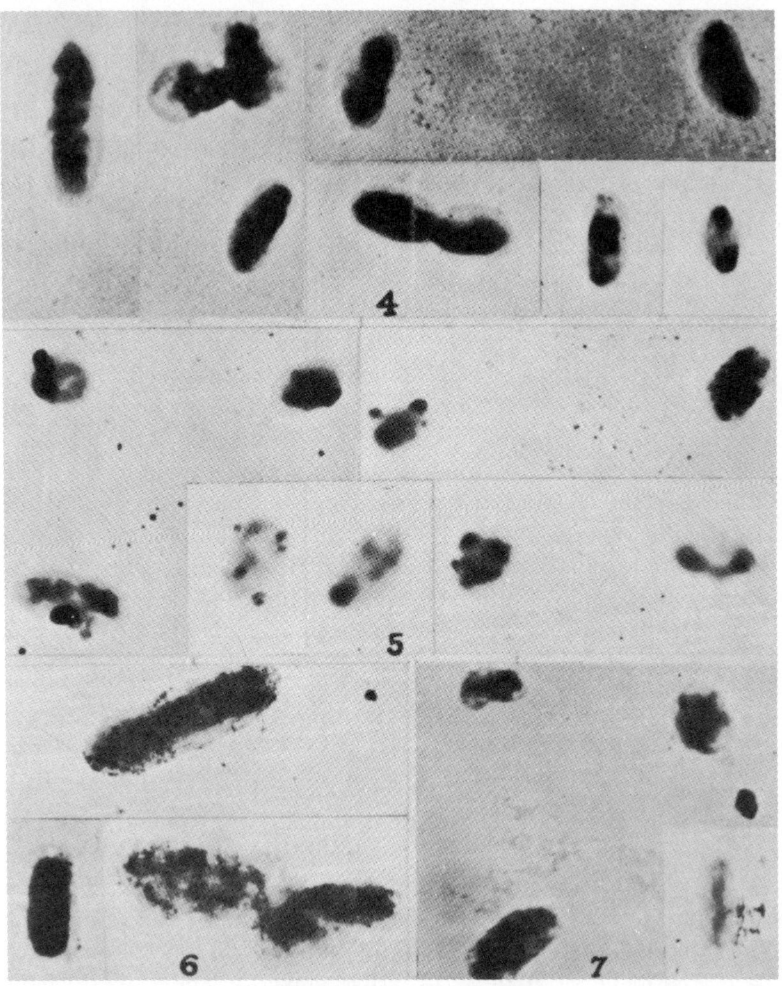

Figs. 4 to 7. *A series of electron micrographs of rickettsiae are reproduced; Fig. 4 portrays organisms of epidemic typhus, Fig. 5 those of endemic typhus, Fig. 6 those of Rocky Mountain spotted fever, and Fig. 7 those of Q fever. See text for descriptions of these figures. Original magnification 8000, enlarged twice for reproduction.*

The granule at the edge of the rickettsiae illustrated in Fig. 5c seems to have internal structure.

Morphological Structure of Rickettsiae

Examination by electron microscopy of the rickettsiae of epidemic and endemic typhus fever, of Rocky Mountain spotted fever, and of Q fever reveals a striking similarity in the morphological structure of these four agents. A number of representative examples of the four rickettsiae are illustrated in Figs. 4 to 7; organisms of epidemic typhus are portrayed in Figs. 4*a* to *f*, of endemic typhus in Figs. 5*a* to *e*, of Rocky Mountain spotted fever in Figs. 6*a* to *c*, and of Q fever in Figs. 7*a* to *c*. Suspensions of each type of rickettsiae contain many large bacillary forms that possess a limiting membrane which encloses a substance of moderate opacity to electrons. The membrane as well as the semiopaque substance suggests a structure comparable to that of bacteria as seen in the electron microscope (9). Rickettsiae are analogous to certain bacteria (9) in another important respect, namely, they contain granules which lie within the protoplasm. In most instances in which individual granules can be clearly recognized the bodies appear as comparatively large spherical structures. Sometimes they are joined together by a thread of material and present a picture suggestive of a string of beads, Figs. 4*b* and 5*a*. In other instances the granules seem unattached to the main irregular dense masses, Figs. 4*e*, 4*f*, or they push against the limiting membrane and produce a knobby external surface, Fig. 5.

The morphological structures observed in electron micrographs of all four rickettsial agents have not yet been studied sufficiently to enable one to distinguish one variety from another. Differences in the average sizes of rickettsiae of the four strains are apparent in Figs. 4 to 7. However, microscopy by ordinary light is also capable of bringing out gross differences in size, which indeed depend almost as much on the factors of nutrition and environment as on the type of the organism studied (1).

Particular stress is laid in this report on the structure of the large bacillary forms of rickettsiae because these are most readily identified as definite entities and they have been studied most extensively by the older techniques. Slightly smaller coccoidal forms of rickettsiae are easily recognized in the electron microscope for they too show evidence of a limiting membrane and of internal structure, Fig. 5. These small oval rickettsiae are of considerable interest since they cannot be differentiated with certainty from tissue particles by ordinary microscopy. The occurrence of such organisms may throw light on the concept of "invisible forms" of rickettsiae which has been brought forward to explain certain experiments in which rickettsiae have not been demonstrated in material of known infectivity (1, 10).

Small and medium-sized dense granules without surrounding semi-transparent substance or membranes are also found on examination of preparations of rickettsiae, Figs. 5*a*, 5*b*, and 7*a*; these seem unrelated to recognizable rickettsiae. They are well below the limit of resolution of the light microscope and may represent noninfectious cellular debris, salt crystals, or portions of disintegrated rickettsiae. The latter possibility would seem to account for at least part of the larger granules since similar structures are not found in suspensions of normal yolk sacs prepared by the same techniques used for obtaining the rickettsial suspensions and, since some of the organisms undergo destruction during treatment on the collodion film, Fig. 4*b*.

Suspensions of rickettsiae of epidemic typhus and of Rocky Mountain spotted fever were prepared by several other techniques and these suspensions in turn were treated with a number of materials after being placed on collodion films preparatory to examination in the electron microscope. Observations made on the various preparations indicated that the basic morphological structure of these rickettsiae is of the type illustrated in Figs. 4 and 6.

This great variation in the morphology of rickettsial bodies of the same strain may be contrasted with the relatively high degree of uniformity of structure observed in viruses. The elementary bodies of vaccinia virus which, in common with bacteria and the rickettsia, have an external membrane surrounding a differentiated internal structure, are brick-like in shape and the majority have five symmetrically arranged internal granules (5).

Summary

The morphological structures of the rickettsiae of epidemic and endemic typhus fever, Rocky Mountain spotted fever, and Q fever are similar to one another and to certain bacteria. The rickettsial organisms in common with the elementary bodies of vaccinia virus and all bacteria would appear to have a limiting membrane which surrounds a substance that seems to be protoplasmic in nature; numbers of dense granules are embedded in the inner protoplasm.

1944

Donald Greiff, Henry Pinkerton, and Vicente Moragues

Effect of Enzyme Inhibitors and Activators on the Multiplication of Typhus Rickettsiae: I. Penicillin, Para-aminobenzoic Acid, Sodium Fluoride, and Vitamins of the B Group

The successful development of specific chemotherapy of rickettsial infections may be traced to the concept of metabolite antagonism. The idea was based on the premise that the activating effect of the antagonism between para-aminobenzoic acid (PABA) and the sulfonamide drugs on bacterial growth might operate in a reversed manner on rickettsiae. The inhibitory action of PABA on the growth of rickettsiae was first demonstrated experimentally against murine typhus in 1942 by Snyder, Maier, and Anderson (1). Publication of this important finding was delayed, however, for reasons of wartime security.

Using an approach that may be considered unique in its time, Greiff, Pinkerton, and Moragues investigated both inhibitors and activators of the intracellular multiplication of rickettsiae in an effort to learn something of the specific enzyme systems involved in rickettsial metabolism. Independently, in the 1944 paper presented here, they established the rickettsiostatic activity of PABA against murine typhus, and in subsequent studies Greiff and his associates shed further light on the metabolic action of PABA on the general growth of rickettsiae (2). In experimental infections PABA was shown also to arrest the multiplication of the rickettsiae of Epidemic typhus, Rocky Mountain spotted fever, and scrub typhus (3, 4).

It was a remarkable demonstration of the inhibition of intracellular parasites by a compound generally regarded as a vitamin. In the first clinical trial of PABA a beneficial effect of the drug on the clinical course of epidemic typhus fever was reported by Yeomans, Snyder, Murray, Zarafonetis, and Ecke (5).

The exact mode of action of PABA has not been completely defined. Studies with PABA have continued to emphasize, however, its usefulness in investigations of rickettsial growth factors and in revealing clues to certain metabolic processes, e.g., the reversal of the rickettsiostatic action of PABA by para-hydroxybenzoic acid, indicating that the latter may be essential for rickettsia propagation (6, 7).

The importance of PABA in the management of rickettsioses was supplanted by the postwar development of broad-spectrum antibiotics. Chloramphenicol (8), Aureomycin (9), and Terramycin (10) were shown to possess potent anti-rickettsial properties. The action of these antibiotics is rickettsiostatic and not rickettsiocidal. The advent of antibiotic therapy in the treatment of rickettsial diseases has dramatically transformed the prognosis of tsutsugamushi disease (scrub typhus). The disease in Japan, formerly carrying a case mortality as high as 46 per cent, has been reduced to a benign illness of short duration carrying no mortality in treated patients (1). The effectiveness of antibiotics has been demonstrated in no other diseases as well as it has been in the rickett-sioses. Our general understanding of intracellular parasitism and our specific knowledge of the biological activities of rickettsiae were markedly enhanced during the ensuing search for chemotherapeutic compounds.

Introduction

Typhus rickettsiae, like the viruses, are obligate intracellular parasites, multiplying freely within their host cells when conditions exist which are favorable for their growth. It has been recognized for many years that favorable conditions for rickettsial growth are associated with a low rate of metabolic activity in the host cells (1, 2). Many viruses, on the other hand, particularly those of relatively small size, grow most freely in cells which are metabolizing actively (2). Riboflavin deficiency, which slows down cell metabolism by interfering with respiration, has been shown to be effective in bringing about conditions favorable for rickettsial growth in rats (3). On the other hand, riboflavin deficiency (4) and thiamin deficiency (5) protect mice to some extent against poliomyelitis (a small virus), significantly reducing the mortality from this infection.

By studying the effect of various enzyme inhibitors and activators on the intracellular multiplication of rickettsiae, it seems possible that information can be obtained concerning the specific enzyme systems involved in rickettsial metabolism. The enzyme activators to be employed will include many agents classed as vitamins as well as a variety of endocrine products. Enzyme inhibitors include chemotherapeutic agents, and many organic and inorganic chemicals which are known to interrupt or modify cellular metabolism.

In some instances the precise mode of action of the agent is known, while in other instances exact information is lacking. Although the intimate metabolism of living cells is in general incompletely understood, many specific facts have been established which, it is believed, can be applied advantageously to the solution of the problems of intracellular parasitism. It also seems reasonable to expect that knowledge of the enzyme systems themselves will be advanced by studies of this type.

In this report, the positive results obtained thus far will be presented in detail. Those agents which have shown no definite effect on the multiplication of rickettsiae will be mentioned briefly, since negative results are of some interest in this type of study.

Material and Methods

A murine strain of typhus, in its 30th passage in fertile eggs was used. This strain was originally isolated in Mexico. Its virulence for guinea pigs has remained unchanged in spite of 35 passages through eggs. In its earlier passages, this strain was used for testing the chemotherapeutic effectiveness of penicillin in the yolk sac (6) and in mice (9).

The technic of egg injection was essentially that used in previous experiments (6), with certain modifications which have been found to save much time and almost to eliminate bacterial contamination. When the control eggs in a previous series begin to die with heavy rickettsial infection (usually between the 6th and 8th days after injection), an egg in this series, preferably one with its embryo still active, is chosen as the source of inoculum. The end of the egg containing the air sac is swabbed with a 4 per cent alcoholic solution of iodine and the shell is removed piecemeal with sterile forceps. When the opening is sufficiently large, the inner air sac membrane is stripped away and the entire contents of the egg shell are allowed to slide out into a pyrex dish 5 cm. in height and 9 cm. in diameter across the top (the commercial pyrex custard dish). The dish previously has been sterilized with alcohol and flame and covered with the top half of a sterile petri dish.

The yolk sac membrane is grasped with sterile forceps and a segment estimated to weigh about 1 gm. is snipped off with curved scissors, and placed in the chamber of a Waring blender in which 100 cc of sterile physiological solution of sodium chloride has been placed previously. Blending is carried out for 4 minutes. The chamber of the Waring blender was provided by the manufacturer, at our request, with an outlet near the bottom, in which a rubber vaccine bottle stopper is fitted. The chamber is connected with a Cornwall pipetting unit (Becton, Dickinson, and Co., No. 1251), by means of rubber tubing and a 20 gauge needle. This pipetting unit, which is equipped with a two-way valve for continuous injection, is provided with a 21 gauge 2 inch needle and mounted on a metal stand at a convenient height. By means of specially constructed apparatus, injections are made with a foot treadle. The assembly of apparatus is shown in Fig. 1.

The fertile eggs to be injected, after preliminary incubation at

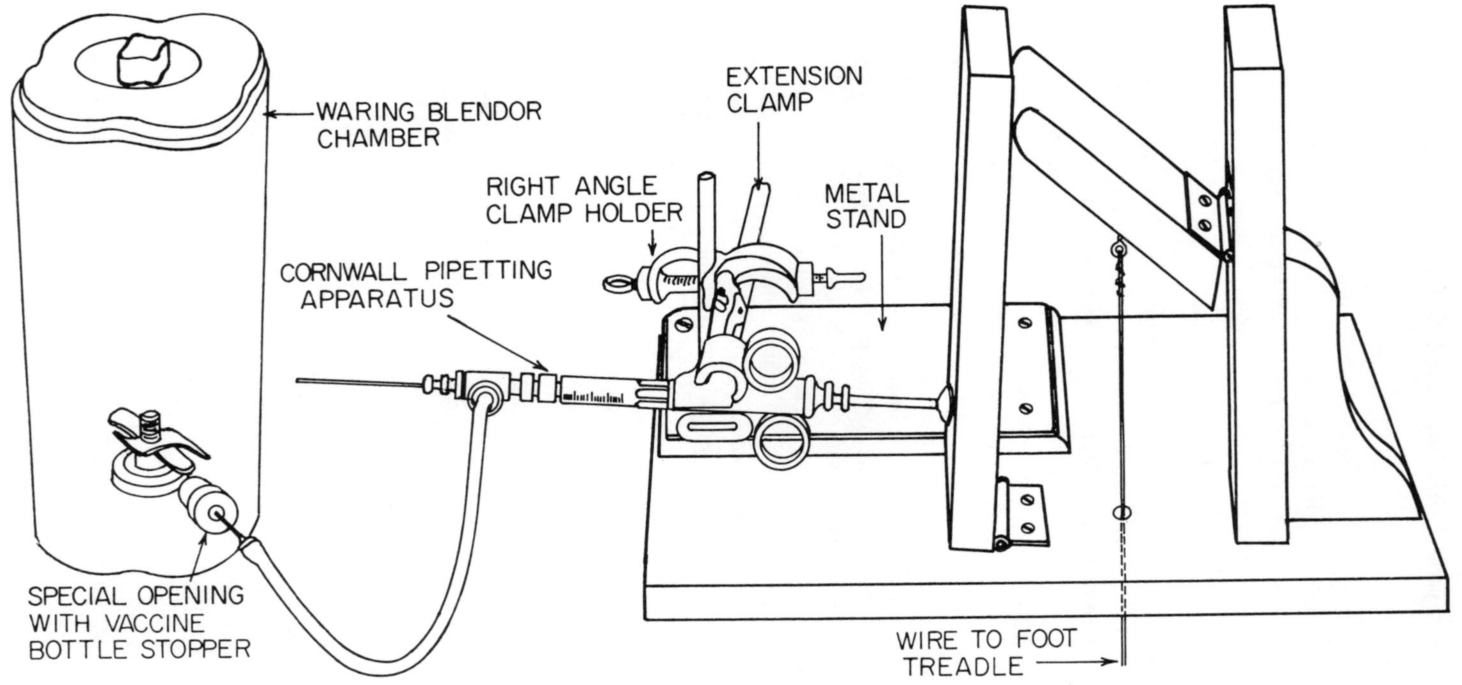

Fig. 1. *Apparatus designed for rapid injection of inoculum into the yolk sacs of fertile eggs. Depressing the foot treadle injects the desired amount of inoculum (governed by the adjustment of the pipetting apparatus) after the egg is in position. When the foot treadle is released, the spring in the barrel of the syringe automatically refills the syringe and restores the levers to their original positions. The levers and the base of the main stand are constructed of soft pine. The main stand is clamped onto a laboratory table through the top of which a hole is drilled to allow passage of the wire to the foot treadle.*

37.5°C. for 5 days, and after discarding those showing embryo death in the process of candling, are swabbed with iodine at the ends containing the air sacs. A minute hole is then punched in each (at the air sac end) by means of an automatically released blood lancet mounted on a metal stand. The point of the lancet is ground to a conical shape. With a little practice, by adjusting the depth of penetration, and by not holding the egg too firmly against the guard, small round holes may be punched with great speed, and without cracking the shell. The end of the shell is again swabbed with iodine after punching.

The actual injection of each egg is carried out by bringing the minute orifice in the shell in contact with the end of the fixed needle of the pipetting unit, pushing it in a straight line until the end of the needle in the yolk sac is approximately under the embryo, the position of which has been marked in lead pencil at the last candling, and injecting 0.1 cc of the emulsion containing the rickettsiae. (The presence of many rickettsiae and the absence of bacteria has been ascertained previously by the examination of Giemsa-stained film preparations.) After injection of the rickettsiae the orifice is sealed with a solution of parlodion in absolute acetone. The syringe refills automatically in preparation for the next egg.

By this method, 150 eggs can be injected in 30 minutes, and the entire process, including removal from the incubator, punching holes, injection, and replacing in the incubator, takes only about 2 hours. In order to eliminate the possibility of contamination, the needle of the pipetting apparatus is heated to dull redness after the injection of each of 12 eggs, and then washed and cooled by passing 1 cc of the inoculum through it. (This is caught in a beaker containing Formalin, in order to protect the operator.)

Subsequent introduction of the agents to be tested has been carried out by again swabbing with iodine, injecting the solution, and resealing with parlodion. For the injection, 1 cc tuberculin syringes provided with 24 gauge 1 inch needles are used. A separate syringe is used for each egg to avoid contamination. The solutions are made up separately and stored in sterile rubber-capped vaccine bottles. It has not been found necessary to work under a glass frame in order to avoid contamination.

Twelve to eighteen eggs served as controls for each experiment, while other groups of 8 to 12 eggs were injected with various concentrations of the substances to be tested, at varying intervals before or after the introduction of the rickettsiae. Estimates of the degree of infection were made from smear preparations of the yolk sac membrane of each egg, either after the death of the embryo or at other suitably chosen times. Such estimates were made independently by two different observers. In those rare instances where there was marked discrepancy in the results of the estimate, a careful restudy was carried out.

For testing chemotherapeutic effectiveness in laboratory animals, a method previously described, involving the use of mice of the dba strain (7, 8) was employed.

Penicillin and Para-aminobenzoic Acid

A brief report on the rickettsiostatic action of penicillin in the yolk sac has been made previously (6), and a corresponding positive chemotherapeutic effect in typhus infection in mice has been observed (9) when large doses of penicillin were given early in the course of the disease.

Because of the synergistic effect of PABA on the bacteriostatic action of penicillin reported by Ungar (10), it seemed desirable to find out whether the rickettsiostatic activity of penicillin would be similarly enhanced by this agent. The following experiment was carried out for the purpose of answering this question.

Experiment 1. The yolk sacs of 70 eggs were injected with typhus rickettsiae as described above. Fourteen eggs served as controls for the experiment as a whole; 48 hours after the injection of rickettsiae, 6.6 mg. of para-aminobenzoic acid dissolved in 0.4 cc of distilled water was introduced into the yolk sacs of 8 eggs. Eight eggs received 1000 units of penicillin, 8 received 100 units, and 8 received 10 units. The penicillin was dissolved in distilled water and injected in three divided doses of 0.4 cc each on the 2nd, 4th, and 6th days after injection with rickettsiae. Three additional groups of 8 eggs each were given penicillin as described above, and in addition to the penicillin each egg received 6.6 mg. of para-aminobenzoic acid in 0.4 cc of distilled water 48 hours after injection with rickettsiae. Assuming uniform solution in the entire fertile egg, this would represent a concentration of para-aminobenzoic acid of about 1:6000. Actually the concentration was probably greater, since the compound is presumably not soluble in the fat globules of the yolk. Another unknown factor is the distribution of the compound between the cells and the extracellular fluid.

Results. The results of this experiment are shown in Table 1, in which each symbol represents an observation on an individual egg. It is seen that 1000 units of penicillin exerted a definite inhibitory action, confirming previous experiments (6). A slight inhibitory action by 100 units and 10 units of penicillin is suggested, but the differences between these two groups and the control group are probably not significant. Survival of embryos beyond the 12th day is seen only in eggs receiving 1000 units of penicillin alone, para-aminobenzoic acid alone, or smaller amounts of penicillin in combination with para-aminobenzoic acid. Para-aminobenzoic acid in the concentration used is seen to have an inhibitory action on rickettsial growth about equal to that of penicillin. This result was quite unexpected. The strongly rickettsiostatic action of para-aminobenzoic acid by itself made the experiment inadequate for its original purpose of discovering a possible synergistic effect of this substance with penicillin, although the complete absence of rickettsiae in the group of eggs treated with 1000 units of penicillin plus PABA may be significant.

Experiment 2. This experiment was carried out for the purpose of determining the minimum concentration of para-aminobenzoic acid which would be effective, and also to compare the effect of neutralized para-aminobenzoic acid with the acid itself. Eighteen control eggs were injected with rickettsiae in the usual way. Twelve eggs received 6.6 mg. of PABA dissolved in 0.4 cc of distilled water, 8 eggs received 3.3 mg., 8 eggs 0.82 mg., and 8 eggs 0.20 mg. Twelve eggs received 6.6 mg. of PABA in a solution which had been made neutral to litmus by the addition of sodium hydroxide. All treatments were given 48 hours after the injection of rickettsiae.

Results. The results of this experiment (Table 2) indicate that 3.3 mg. of PABA had approximately the same rickettsiostatic activity as 6.6 mg., while 0.82 mg. and 0.20 mg. had no apparent effect. The action of neutralized PABA did not differ significantly from that of the acid itself. The inhibition of rickettsial growth is less striking in this experiment than in experiment 1, probably because the organisms began to multiply earlier, and had attained a relatively higher concentration before treatment was begun. It is to be noted that survival of embryos beyond the 8th day occurred only in eggs receiving 3.3 mg. or more of PABA.

Experiment 3. In this experiment, meta-aminobenzoic acid and ortho-aminobenzoic acid were compared with para-aminobenzoic acid from the point of view of rickettsiostatic activity. The chemicals to be tested were introduced into the yolk sacs 24 hours before the injection of rickettsiae.

Results. Inhibition of rickettsial growth by para-aminobenzoic acid is seen (Table 3) while the ortho and meta forms, in similar concentration,

Table 1. Growth of Typhus Rickettsiae in Eggs Treated with Combinations of Penicillin and PABA

Day following inocula-tion	Control	6.6 mg. PABA	1000 units penicillin	1000 units penicillin + 6.6 mg. PABA	100 units penicillin	100 units penicillin + 6.6 mg. PABA	10 units penicillin	10 units penicillin + 6.6 mg. PABA
	Degree of infection	Degree of infection	Degree of infection	Degree of infection	Degree of infection	Degree of infection	Degree of infection	Degree of infection
3		−	−	− −	−	(+)	−	− − −
4	−				−	−		− −
6	++							
7	++ +++	(+) −	−		+ ++	− −	++ +++	(+)
8	++++++ ++++ ++++++			−			++++	

9	+ + + + + + + + + + + + + + + + + + + +	+ +			+ + + + + + + + + + + + +		+ +	
10	+ + + + +	+ +				(+)	+ + + + + + + +	
11		−					+ + + +	
12	+ + + + + + + +	−[a]	(+)	−[a]	+ + + +	(+)[a]	+ + + +	−[a]
13		(+)[a]	− + −	−[a]		−[a]		
15			−[a] −[a]	− −[a] −[a]		−[a]		

− No rickettsiae recognizable with certainty.
(+) Less than one rickettsia per oil immersion field.
+ 1–10 rickettsiae per oil immersion field.
++ 10–100 rickettsiae per oil immersion field.
+++ 100–1000 rickettsiae per oil immersion field.
++++ 1000–5000 rickettsiae per oil immersion field.
+++++ 5000–8000 rickettsiae per oil immersion field.
++++++ 8000–12,000 rickettsiae per oil immersion field.
[a] Embryo alive at time of examination.

Table 2. Growth of Typhus Rickettsiae in Eggs Treated with Different Concentrations of PABA and with Neutralized PABA[a]

Day following inoculation	Control	1/3000 (6.6 mg.) PABA	1/6000 (3.3 mg.) PABA	1/24,000 (0.82 mg.) PABA	1/96,000 (0.20 mg.) PABA	1/3000 (6.6 mg.) PABA (neutralized)
	Degree of infection	Degree of infection	Degree of infection	Degree of infection	Degree of infection	Degree of infection
4	+ + + + + +		(+) + +	(+)	(+)	(+)
5	+ + + + +	+ + + + + + + + + + + + +	+ +	+ + + + + + + + + + + +	+ +	+ + + +
6	+ +	+ + + + + + + +		+ + + +	+ + + +	+ + +
7	+ + + + + + + + + +		+	+ + + + + + + +	+ +	+ + + + (+)
8	+ + + + + + + + + + + + + + + +	−[b]	+ + +[b]			(+) +
9		+[b] + +[b]	+ +			+ + +[b]
10		+ + +[b]				+ +[b]
11			+ +[b] + + +			+ +[b]

[a] For explanation of symbols, see Table 1.
[b] Embryo alive at time of examination.

Table 3. Growth of Typhus Rickettsiae in Eggs Treated with Para-, Ortho-, and Meta-aminobenzoic Acid[a]

Day following inoculation	Control	6.6 mg. PABA	6.6 mg. MABA	6.6 mg. OABA
	Degree of infection	Degree of infection	Degree of infection	Degree of infection
2		—	—	—
		—	—	+
4	+ +	+	+	
	—	—	+	+ +
	+ + +	—		+ +
	+			+ + +
	+ +			
	+			
	+ +			
	+ +			
	+			
	+ +			
5	+ + +	—	+ +	+ + +
	+ +		+ + + +	+ + + + +
			+	+ + +
			+ + +	+ + + +
6	+ + + + + +	+	+ + + + + +	+ + + + + +
	+ + + + + +	+ +	+ + + + +	+ + + + + +
	+ + + + + +	+ +	+ + + +	+ + + + + +
		—[b]	+ + + + + +	
			+ +	
			+ +	
7	+ + + + + +	(+)[b]	+ + + + + +	+ + + + + +
	+ + + +	+[b]	+ + + + + +	+ + + + + +
	+ + + + + +		+ + + + + +	+ + + + +
	+ + + +		+ + + + + +	
8		—[b]		
10		—[b]		
		—[b]		
		(+)[b]		
		(+)[b]		

[a] For explanation of symbols, see Table 1.
[b] Embryo alive at time of examination.

Table 4. Therapeutic Effect of PABA in Food on Murine Typhus Infection in Mice

Mice injected	Diet	Illness	Death	Time of death	Survived
8	Dog chow plus PABA	3	2	One on 4th day One on 7th day	6
8	Dog chow alone	8	8	All on 7th day	0

are without demonstrable action. Survival of embryos beyond the 7th day is noted only in eggs receiving para-aminobenzoic acid.

In another experiment, sodium benzoate, in a concentration of 6.6 mg. per egg, was found to have no demonstrable rickettsiostatic action.

Experiment 4. This experiment was planned to test the therapeutic effectiveness of para-aminobenzoic acid in murine typhus infection in mice. The experimental conditions were identical with those used in previous work (9) in which the therapeutic action of penicillin was demonstrated. The usual death rate in the control group under these conditions was 100 per cent. Sixteen mice of the dba strain were injected intraperitoneally with 0.5 cc each of a 10 per cent emulsion of brain tissue from a mouse dying of murine typhus after intraperitoneal injection of rickettsiae. These mice were kept at a room temperature ranging from 65–73°F. Eight of the mice were fed Purina dog chow in its original biscuit form. The other 8 mice were fed Purina dog chow, ground to a fine powder, with which 3 per cent of para-aminobenzoic acid was thoroughly mixed. All mice were given water *ad lib*. The treated mice were started on their diet containing PABA immediately after injection with rickettsiae.

Experiment 5. This was a duplication of experiment 4, except that 30 mice were used, fifteen of which had PABA added to their food. One mouse in the PABA series was killed on the 6th day for information.

Results. The mice apparently ate the powdered dog chow containing the PABA quite freely after the first 12 to 24 hours. One mouse in experiment 4 is believed to have died of starvation on the 4th day, however. The second mouse dying in experiment 4 on the 7th day probably died of typhus, although unfortunately smears were not made from the peritoneal cavity. This was the only mouse on the PABA diet which died from typhus infection presumably.

Table 5. Therapeutic Effect of PABA in Food on Murine Typhus Infection in Mice

Mice injected	Diet	Illness	Death	Time of death	Survived
15	Dog chow plus PABA	0	One killed for study		14
15	Dog chow alone	15	15	6th and 7th days	0

The results of experiments 4 and 5 are shown in Tables 4 and 5. A survival rate approaching 100 per cent is seen in the mice fed dog chow with PABA, as contrasted with a survival rate of zero in the mice fed dog chow alone.

Smears were made from the peritoneal cavities of all control mice shortly after death, and large numbers of rickettsiae were present in all instances. No evidence of secondary bacterial infection was found postmortem in any of the mice. A smear from the peritoneal cavity of the mouse in the PABA series, killed on the 6th day with no sign of illness, showed rare extracellular rickettsiae, and an occasional cell containing 15 to 20 organisms.

Sodium Fluoride

Sodium fluoride was chosen as a test substance because of its well-known effect of inhibiting glycolysis by interfering with phosphorylation. Preliminary experiments showed that the injection of 5 mg. of this substance into the yolk sac caused death of the embryos in 12 to 24 hours, while injections of 1 mg. or less were well tolerated.

In two experiments which will not be published in detail, series of eggs treated with 1 mg. and 0.1 mg. of sodium fluoride developed heavy rickettsial infection 24 hours earlier than the controls, and embryonic death occurred sooner than in the controls. In a repetition of this experiment, however, using 1 mg. of the substance, no significant differences were noted between the control and the treated groups.

Experiment 6. Sixteen eggs were injected with rickettsiae in the usual way. Forty-eight hours later 0.5 mg. of sodium fluoride in 0.5 cc of distilled water was introduced into the yolk sacs of 8 of these eggs.

Results. Only one of the control eggs showed an occasional rickettsia, and guinea pig inoculation from the yolk sac of this egg gave entirely negative results. Seven of the 8 eggs receiving sodium fluoride developed

Table 6. Effect of Sodium Fluoride on Rickettsial Multiplication in the Yolk Sac[a]

Day following inoculation	Control	0.5 mg. sodium fluoride
	Degree of infection	Degree of infection
3		—
4	—	+
7		+
8	—[b]	+++
9		++
11	—[b]	++[b]
12	(+)[b]	++++[b]
13	—[b]	+[b]
14	—[b]	
	—[b]	
	—[b]	

[a] For explanation of symbols, see Table 1.
[b] Embryo alive at time of examination.

visible rickettsiae, and in several eggs rickettsiae were numerous. The results are seen in Table 6. A guinea pig inoculated from one of the heavily infected eggs developed typical murine typhus after an incubation period of 3 days.

The failure of the control eggs to develop the usual picture of heavy infection is a phenomenon which has occurred in about one-fourth of our experiments. Whether it is due to insusceptibility of the eggs to infection, or to injection of material containing nonviable rickettsiae is not clear. The sodium fluoride injection, however, apparently produced conditions favorable for rickettsial growth in this experiment.

Penicillin and Para-aminobenzoic Acid with Sodium Fluoride

Experiment 7. The purpose of this experiment was to determine whether or not sodium fluoride would interfere with the rickettsiostatic action of penicillin and para-aminobenzoic acid. Forty-two eggs were injected with rickettsiae in the usual way. Forty-eight hours later, 12 eggs received injections of 6.6 mg. of para-aminobenzoic acid and 0.1 mg. of sodium fluoride. Similarly, 12 eggs received injections of 666 units of penicillin and 0.1 mg. of sodium fluoride.

Results. From the results as shown in Table 7 it is clear that the suppression of rickettsial growth by PABA and by penicillin was not markedly influenced by sodium fluoride in the concentration used.

Negative Results

Using the technic described above, the following agents have been tested for their ability to alter the multiplication of murine typhus rickettsiae in the yolk sac, when introduced in single doses 24 to 48 hours after the injection of rickettsiae. The figures following each agent indicate the amount injected into each egg. Riboflavin, 6 and 15 mg.; thiamin chloride, 3 and 15 mg.; choline chloride, 4 and 24 mg.; Bc, 0.0375 gamma; biotin, 0.1 mg.; physostigmine, 0.05 mg.; iodoacetic acid, 0.1 mg.

Discussion

Agents injected into the yolk sac in the above experiments were in intimate contact with the entodermal cells in which the rickettsiae grow. The observed inhibition or stimulation of rickettsial growth may have been brought about by direct action on the enzymes concerned with the metabolism of the rickettsiae themselves or by modifying the metabolism of the entodermal cells in such a way as to upset the delicate state of symbiotic equilibrium which exists between the rickettsiae and their host cells.

It has not been possible in any instance to determine with certainty which of these mechanisms is involved. In the case of penicillin, direct action on the metabolic enzymes of the rickettsiae themselves seems likely, since this strongly bacteriostatic substance has not been shown to modify the metabolism of animal tissues, and is probably an enzyme inhibitor rather than an enzyme activator. PABA, on the other hand, is believed to be a member of the B group of vitamins, and its effect may, like that of riboflavin (3), be due to stimulation of the metabolism of the host cells.

The increased survival rate in typhus-infected mice fed toluidine blue, reported by Peterson (11), is of particular interest in this connection. This dye has been shown (12) to increase the oxygen uptake of tissues, an effect which is neutralized by KCN. Assuming that the action of toluidine blue in mice is the result of this increased oxygen uptake, Peterson's work may be taken as confirmatory evidence that a high metabolic activity is unfavorable for the multiplication of rickettsiae in cells.

The resistance of cells to rickettsial infection may depend on a variety of factors which include temperature (8), presence in the cells of intact mechanisms for their own respiration and probably for other metabolic processes, absence from the cells of metabolic enzymes essential for

Table 7. Effect of Sodium Fluoride in Combination with Para-aminobenzoic Acid and Penicillin[a]

Day following inoculation	Control	6.6 mg. PABA and 0.1 mg. NaF	666 units penicillin and 0.1 mg. NaF
	Degree of infection	Degree of infection	Degree of infection
4	+ +	(+)	−
	+ +	(+)	(+)
	+ +	−	(+)
		−	
		+	
5	+ + +	+ +	(+)
	+ +	+ +	(+)
		−	(+)
			+ +
6	+ + + +		+ +
	+ + + + +		+ +
	+ + + +		+ +
	+ + + +		
	+ + + +		
	+ + + +		
	+ + + + +		
	+ + + +		
7	+ + + + + +	−	+ +
	+ + + +		
8	+ + + + + +	(+)[b]	(+)
	+ + + + +		
	+ + + + +		
9		+ + + +	
11		+ +	

[a] For explanation of symbols, see Table I.
[b] Embryo alive at time of examination.

rickettsial growth, and presence in the cells of enzyme systems antagonistic to rickettsial growth. The last two factors may determine absolute "natural" immunity, while variations in the first two factors may determine the severity of infection in the case of naturally susceptible cells. The peritoneal lining cells of rats may be made abnormally susceptible to rickettsial infection by partial riboflavin deficiency (3), and the administration of riboflavin has an immediate and striking rickettsiostatic action under these conditions (13). In normal mice the administration of large amounts of riboflavin is therepeutically ineffective (14).

On the basis of this hypothesis, an agent which is therapeutically effective in typhus infection in animals of one species might be ineffective in animals of another species, because of existing differences in metabolism. Murine typhus rickettsiae multiply in the peritoneal cavity of the normal rat, but produce little or no obvious evidence of illness. In the normal mouse, under the conditions used in the above experiments, murine typhus is a fatal disease. The addition of para-aminobenzoic acid to the food makes the disease in mice inapparent, as it is in the normal rat. It is to be noted that a few rickettsiae were found in the peritoneal cells of the mouse of the PABA series which was killed for information.

The stimulating effect of sodium fluoride, under certain conditions, on rickettsial growth in the yolk sac may be due to its interference with carbohydrate metabolism. By the use of this agent or of other similar agents, it may be possible to render the entodermal cells of the yolk sac susceptible to infection by rickettsia-like organisms to which they are normally resistant.

The extension of the type of investigation described above to the study of the metabolism of viruses seems to offer interesting possibilities for future exploitation.

Summary

By injection into typhus-infected yolk sacs, a number of agents were tested for possible inhibition or acceleration of rickettsial growth. The previously reported rickettsiostatic activity of penicillin was further confirmed.

Para-aminobenzoic acid, in single injections of 6.6 mg. and 3.3 mg. giving initial concentrations of approximately 1:6000 and 1:12,000 was found to have rickettsiostatic activity approximately equal to that of penicillin. No conclusion could be drawn regarding the possibility of a synergistic action of para-aminobenzoic acid and penicillin. Para-aminobenzoic acid neutralized with sodium hydroxide was found to be as effective as the acid itself, when given in single injections of 6.6 mg. Sodium benzoate, as well as the ortho and meta forms of aminobenzoic acid were found to be ineffective when given in similar amounts.

Para-aminobenzoic acid, when added to the food in a concentration of 3 per cent, was shown to have a remarkably effective chemotherapeutic action on murine typhus infection in mice.

Sodium fluoride was found at times to accelerate the growth of rickettsiae in the yolk sac, and to cause heavy infection under conditions such that the controls showed practically no multiplication of the organism. When rickettsiostatic substances (penicillin and para-aminobenzoic acid) were combined with sodium fluoride, their rickettsiostatic activity was not demonstrably changed. Other agents studied and found not to affect rickettsial multiplication are listed. The possible mechanisms involved in the observed inhibition and stimulation of rickettsial growth under these conditions are discussed.

Note: As this paper was going to press, it was learned that favorable therapeutic effects from para-aminobenzoic acid in experimental typhus infection had been described previously in unpublished confidential reports in the files of the United States of America Typhus Commission. The authors therefore wish to disclaim priority in the above observations, insofar as they deal with this chemical substance. Our observations were made independently, and without knowledge of this unpublished work.

Acknowledgment

This study was aided by a generous grant from the C. V. Mosby Company, St. Louis.

1945

Norman H. Topping and M. J. Shear

Studies of Typhus Fever Vaccines: III. Studies of Antigens in Infected Yolk Sacs

The discovery that rickettsiae possess soluble antigens as part of their intrinsic structure was an important one, leading to the further elucidation of their complex antigenic constitution and to the development of specific serological techniques for the diagnoses of rickettsial infections. Soluble antigens are serologically active, highly specific, noninfectious substances that are elaborated during the course of infection and are separable from the infectious agent. The association of soluble antigens with rickettsiae was demonstrated in 1942 by Topping and Shear, but for security reasons publication was withheld until 1945. At about the same time Plotz (1) independently obtained evidence of the existence of a soluble antigen in washings of rickettsial suspensions. Subsequently soluble antigens were demonstrated from the rickettsiae of epidemic typhus, murine typhus, Rocky Mountain spotted fever, rickettsialpox, boutonneuse fever, and Q fever (2).

Several practical applications resulted from studies on the nature of the soluble antigens of rickettsiae. Since immunization with soluble antigens was found to evoke complement-fixing antibodies and induce immunity to subsequent challenge with virulent rickettsiae, potent rickettsial vaccines were produced by combining soluble antigens with the infectious agent. Soluble group-specific antigens were obtained and employed in serological tests for the diagnosis of epidemic and murine typhus fevers and spotted fever and rickettsialpox complexes. Type-specific rickettsial suspensions, prepared by removing soluble antigens from the infectious agents, were used successfully in complement fixation reactions for routine differential diagnosis of epidemic and murine typhus (3). These developments have had obvious clinical and epidemiological significance.

The material for these studies was derived from yolk sacs infected with the Breinl strain of epidemic typhus fever after the method described by Cox. This strain has been carried in developing eggs for some time and is well adapted. It has become less virulent for guinea pigs but does produce, on occasion, large numbers of rickettsiae in the yolk sacs.

Clark, Rasmussen, and White have reported the use of ether in the separation of poliomyelitis virus from extraneous material, and Craigie has applied the use of ether to rickettsiae.* Craigie's technic gives a

* Personal communication from Dr. Craigie.

clean vaccine containing relatively large numbers of rickettsiae and is perhaps an improvement on the technic as described by Cox. We have employed certain modifications of the ether technic and have found an additional antigenic material in the developing yolk sac which is being discarded in the technic as described by Craigie. This substance can be found in the supernatant fluid after the first centrifugation. This immunizing substance has many of the characteristics usually found in soluble antigens in that some of it passes a Berkefeld N filter and the major portion remains in solution after centrifugation for 15 minutes at about 15,000 rpm. It has not been determined whether this substance is a true "soluble antigen" or whether it consists of minute rickettsiae or other bodies so small as to pass a filter and not be precipitated by centrifugation as described. Other academic questions regarding its chemical nature and properties are being pursued; however, some of its immunological properties have been briefly studied to date.

For purposes of discussion, we shall designate the substance present in the supernatant fluid after centrifugation as the soluble antigen, while the antigen present in the precipitate will be designated as rickettsiae because they are demonstrable there in large numbers. Three separate immunological procedures have been studied in comparing these two antigens. The first of these technics was complement fixation as described previously by Bengtson; the second was the ability of these two antigens to produce the Weil-Felix reaction in rabbits; and the third was a comparison of these two antigens in immunizing guinea pigs against a challenging dose of a passage strain of epidemic typhus fever virus.

Our technic for the preparation of the antigens is briefly as follows: 1) infected yolk sacs are harvested; 2) ground with alundum; 3) diluted to a 10 per cent suspension with saline containing 0.5 per cent Formalin; 4) shaken with one volume of ether, and sufficient time allowed to elapse for the phases to separate well (about 1 to $1\frac{1}{2}$ hours); 5) repeated extraction of the aqueous phase (either once or twice) until the excess ether is colorless; 6) removal of the ether at room temperature under reduced pressure.

After centrifugation, the sediment containing large numbers of demonstrable rickettsiae was resuspended in saline to the original volume; this suspension and the clear supernatant containing the "soluble antigen" were tested for their ability to fix complement in the presence of specific immune guinea pig serums. Two of these titrations are presented in Table 1.

Table 1

Primary manipulation				
Number	Manipulation	Designation	Material	Complement fixation reaction
ET34	Centrifuged 4000 rpm 1 hour	a	Sediment (contains rickettsiae)	Pos. 1:8[a]
		b	Supernatant (soluble antigen)	Pos. 1:128
ET5	Centrifuged 4000 rpm 1 hour	a	Sediment (contains rickettsiae)	Pos. 1:32
		b	Supernatant (soluble antigen)	Pos. 1:64

Secondary manipulation				
Number	Manipulation	Designation	Material	Complement fixation reaction
ET34		—	—	—
	Centrifuged 15,000 rpm 15 min	c	Supernatant	Pos 1:128
		d	Sediment	Negative
ET5	Washed and recentrifuged at 4000 rpm	d	Sediment	Pos. 1:32
		e	Supernatant	Negative
	Filtered Berkefeld N	c	Filtrate	Pos 1:16

[a] Only 3+ and 4+ reactions were considered positive.

It will be noted in Table 1 that there were two separate lots, ET 34 and ET 5; these lots were composed of three pooled yolk sacs each. It is known that there is usually a considerable variation in the numbers of rickettsiae to be found in the harvested yolk sacs and that the amount of antigen present is roughly proportionate to the numbers of rickettsiae present in the preliminary smear, preparation direct from the yolk sac. In both lots in Table 1 the supernatant fluid fixed complement to a higher dilution than did the sediment, and further, this antigen in the supernatant was not sedimented at 15,000 rpm for 15 minutes, nor was it completely removed by filtration through a Berkefeld N filter. It will also be seen that one washing of the rickettsiae of the sediment No. 5a did not remove the complement-fixing antibody.

A control experiment was done using a supernatant solution and a sediment prepared in an identical manner but from eggs not inoculated

Table 2

Rabbit num-ber	Original Weil-Felix			Inoculated with	Date	Weil-Felix						
						Date						
	1:10	1:20	1:40			Feb. 18	Feb. 20	Feb. 23	Feb. 26	Mar. 2	Mar. 5	Mar. 10
29304	2[a]	1	0	ET 5d (sediment table 1)	Feb. 11, 1942	Pos.[a] 1:40	Pos. 1:320	Pos. 1:160	Pos. 1:320	Pos. 1:80	Pos. 1:40	Pos. 1:40
29305	3	0	0	ET 5b (supernatant table 1)	do	Pos. 1:160	Pos. 1:320	Pos. 1:160	Pos. 1:80	Pos. 1:40	Pos. 1:40	Pos. 1:20

[a] Only 3+ and 4+ reactions were considered positive.

Table 3

Guinea pig number	Immunizing material 1 cc each of	Dates	Date bled	Complement fixation	Date of challenge with 10-per cent Breinl strain	Days of fever	Comment
29314	ET 5b, ET 34b (Supernatants)[a]	Feb. 11, 19	Feb. 26	1:64	Feb. 28, 1942	2	Abscess palpable in abdomen
29315	do.	do.	do.	1:256	do.	0	Immune
29316	do.	do.	do.	1:512	do.	0	Do.
29317	do.	do.	do.	1:512	do.	0	Do.
29318	ET 5d, ET 34a (Sediments)[a]	do.	do.	1:16	do.	3	Abscess palpable in abdomen
29319	do.	do.	do.	1:512	do.	0	Immune
29320	do.	do.	do.	1:128	do.	0	Do.
29321	do.	do.	do.	1:256	do.	0	Do.
29468	Controls					8+	No immunity
29469						6+	Do.
29470						8+	Do.
29471						8+	Do.

[a] See table 1.

with epidemic typhus virus. The results were entirely negative with both fractions. Further, these two fractions were each inoculated into four guinea pigs; two inoculations of 1 cc each were given at weekly intervals. Both fractions failed to produce complement-fixing antibodies in their serums.

Several of the fractions containing antigenic properties, as tested by the complement fixation test, have been injected intravenously into rabbits and observations made of the Weil-Felix reaction. Two of these are presented in Table 2.

Table 2 shows that both the sediment ET 5d and the supernatant solution, ET 5b, are about equally effective in producing the Weil-Felix reaction in rabbits.

These fractions have been inoculated into guinea pigs for the purpose of observing their ability to produce complement-fixing antibodies, as well as to immunize them against a challenge inoculation of living epidemic typhus virus. The results of these tests are presented in Table 3.

In Table 3 it will be noted that the four guinea pigs vaccinated with the soluble fraction produced complement-fixing antibodies in their serums at least as well as did the four guinea pigs vaccinated with the sediment containing the rickettsiae. This same statement can be made concerning their immunity. It is interesting further to note that in each group of four guinea pigs there was one (29314 and 29318) that did not produce as high a titer in the complement fixation test as the others, and that each of these guinea pigs developed fever during the immunity test. In both of these male guinea pigs a large abdominal abscess could be palpated easily, perhaps due to a perforation of the rectum while temperatures were being taken. Any attempted explanation of these results would only be conjecture.

From the foregoing evidence it would appear that there is a soluble substance present in the supernatant fluid after ether extraction and centrifugation that has the same immunological properties (as far as we have gone) as does the sediment containing the rickettsiae. This substance is antigenic in the complement fixation test, produces a Weil-Felix reaction when inoculated into rabbits, produces complement-fixing antibodies in the serums of vaccinated guinea pigs, and finally immunizes those guinea pigs against a subsequent inoculation of virulent epidemic typhus virus.

Robert J. Huebner, Peggy Stamps, and Charles Armstrong

Rickettsialpox—A Newly Recognized Rickettsial Disease: I. Isolation of the Etiological Agent

In sharp contrast to the usual outbreaks of rickettsial infections, which have occurred primarily among residents of urban slum areas and primitive rural regions, a rickettsial disease was discovered in 1946 among the inhabitants of modern luxury apartments. The occurrence of this disease in such lofty surroundings exemplifies one of the many facets of rickettsial agents—their ecological adaptability. Cases of the disease appearing in the New York metropolitan area were described independently by Sussman (1) and by Greenberg, Pellitteri, Klein, and Huebner (2). The investigative efforts of Robert J. Huebner and his associates in unraveling the identity of the mysterious malady were outstanding. Whereas, in the past, decades often elapsed before some new rickettsioses were thoroughly characterized, this etiological agent was isolated and classified, and the transmission, ecology, and epidemiology of the disease outlined, approximately seven months after the first case was recognized.

A series of papers was published that described the successful characterization of the new disease entity. In the paper reprinted here, Huebner and his collaborators reported on the first isolation of the etiological agent from a human patient and noted that the agent possessed the morphological and cultural features of rickettsiae. The disease was aptly named rickettsialpox to denote that it is caused by a member of the genus *Rickettsiae* and that a spotty rash is a noticeable clinical manifestation. The name *Rickettsia akari* (Greek-mite) was proposed for the causative agent (3). From the tissues of mites (*Allodermanyssus sanguineus*), ectoparasites of house mice, rickettsiae were recovered that were indistinguishable from earlier isolates of the infectious agent. The recovery of *R. akari* from the tissues of a naturally infected house mouse (*Mus musculus*), trapped at the site of an outbreak of the disease, indicated that this host was the reservoir for the disease (4). This finding, together with the accumulated evidence, strongly implicated the mite as the vector for the transmission of the disease to humans. In subsequent studies the epidemiology of the disease in man was outlined (5) and the histopathology of the cutaneous lesions was described (6).

Since the original outbreak of rickettsialpox was described in the New York area, cases have been reported from many of the large cities on the Eastern seaboard of the United States and from as far west as Utah. A rickettsial agent, similar if not identical with *R. akari*, has been found in French Equatorial Africa, South Africa, and the Soviet Union. In addition to being isolated from the mite and house mouse, *R. akari* has been culled from the domestic rat and the Korean vole (7). The recovery of the infectious agent from these last two hosts, and the demonstration that the infectious agent can be transmitted by the tropical rat mite, suggest the existence of other ecological cycles and relations and implies that the epidemiology of rickettsialpox may be more involved than previously realized.

During July 1946, a peculiar febrile disease characterized by an initial lesion and an eruption of a vesiculo-papular type was reported to the National Institute of Health. The outbreak occurred in a housing development in New York City and cooperative studies were undertaken—members of the city health department* and the authors participating in various phases of the work. An investigation of 80 cases during the succeeding 10 weeks disclosed a strikingly uniform clinical entity.

Because of a clinical resemblance to chickenpox and because the organism isolated from one patient has the morphological and cultural characteristics of rickettsiae, the name "rickettsialpox" is proposed. Sussman (1) recently reported three cases resembling those observed by us.

In the course of these etiological studies, 15 blood specimens, 1 bone marrow specimen, 1 skin lesion washing, and 1 lymph node washing were inoculated into animals. An organism possessing the morphological, cultural, and staining characteristics of a rickettsia was recovered from the tissues of a single mouse, which had been inoculated with blood drawn on the second day of fever from one of the patients (M. K.).

It is the purpose of this paper to describe the isolation of the M. K. organism, and to record observations on the illness produced by it in certain laboratory animals. Antigens prepared from yolk sac cultures of the M. K. organism and serums from 19 ill or convalescent patients were studied in the complement fixation test. The results of this study are also presented.

Isolation of the M. K. Organism

Whole blood drawn from the patient M. K. on July 26, 1946, 2 days after onset of fever was immediately placed in a dry ice container. Approximately 2 hours later the specimen was thawed rapidly and inoculated intraperitoneally into five mice and two guinea pigs. Nine days later (August 4, 1946) two of the five mice appeared ill. Inactivity,

* Dr. Morris Greenberg, Dr. Ottavio Pellitteri.

rapid breathing, and ruffled fur characterized the general appearance of both mice. Central nervous system symptoms were absent. The three other mice, which were observed for 30 days, at no time presented signs of illness. One of the sick mice became moribund and was sacrificed. The second sick mouse died during the night and was unfit for further study. Autopsy of the first mouse revealed a small amount of blood-tinged peritoneal fluid, large lymph nodes, an enlarged edematous liver, and a dark engorged spleen which was enlarged 8 to 10 times. The respiratory and intestinal tract appeared normal. The liver and spleen, the brain, and the pooled lymph nodes were suspended in saline and inoculated intraperitoneally into three groups of white mice (Swiss strain). In addition, the liver and spleen suspension was inoculated intraperitoneally into two guinea pigs.

The three suspensions used for inoculation produced objective signs of illness in each group of inoculated mice and in the two guinea pigs—the latter responding with 3 and 4 days of fever and marked scrotal reactions. The signs of disease in the mice were immobility, rapid breathing, and ruffled fur. Two of the mice in the liver and spleen passage died on the seventh day after inoculation. A second liver and spleen passage was made on the ninth day, and autopsy of the donor mouse revealed the same gross pathology as the original mouse. The liver and spleen line of passage at the time of writing is in its fourth subpassage in mice. It still produces objective illness but deaths are rare.

In the brain passage deaths did not occur, although ruffled fur and immobility were observed on the ninth day. On the twelfth day after inoculation the brain was removed from one of the mice which still appeared quite ill; a suspension was made in saline and this was inoculated into the yolk sacs of fertile eggs that had been incubated 7 days. The suspension produced no growth on blood agar. Seven days later all the embryos were moribund or dead. Films made from the yolk sacs revealed large numbers of minute intracellular and extracellular diplobacilli staining well by Machiavello's method but poorly with methylene blue. Embryonic fluid of all the eggs produced no growth when placed on plain and blood agar.

The mice inoculated with lymph node passage material developed ruffled fur but no other apparent signs of illness. On the ninth day one of the mice was sacrificed, and typical post-mortem findings were observed. Since there was considerable blood-tinged peritoneal fluid, this was aspirated, placed on blood agar, and inoculated into the yolk sacs of fertile eggs.

Table 1. Titrations of Crude and Ether-extracted M. K. Antigens against Five Serums in the Complement Fixation Test

Antigens	Serums used in fixed dilution	Serum dilution	Results with various antigen dilutions						Results with antigen control dilutions	
			Un-diluted	1:2	1:4	1:8	1:16	1:32	1:1	1:2
M. K. No. 1—10 per cent crude antigen	Endemic typhus	1:16	0	0	0	0	0	0	0	0
	Rocky Mt. spot-ted fever	1:16	4	4	4	4	4	4		
	Q fever	1:16	0	0	0	0	0	0		
	H. B.[a]	1:10	4	4	1	1	0	0		
	J. M.[a]	1:10	4	4	3	2	1	0		
M. K. No. 2—10 per cent ether-extrac-ted antigen	Endemic typhus	1:16	0	0	0	0	0	0	0	0
	Rocky Mt. spot-ted fever	1:16	4	4	4	4	4	4		
	Q fever	1:16	0	0	0	0	0	0		
	H. B.	1:10	4	4	4	3	1	1		
	J. M.	1:10	4	4	4	4	1	(b)		
R161—30 per cent ether-extracted Rocky Mt. spot-ted fever antigen	Endemic typhus	1:16	0	0	0	0	0	0	0	0
	Rocky Mt. spot-ted fever	1:16	4	4	4	4	3	2		
	Q fever	1:16	0	0	0	0	0	0		
	H. B.	1:10	4	4	4	3	1	(b)		
	J. M.	1:10	4	4	4	4	1	0		
NYS—10 per cent crude normal yolk sac antigen	Endemic typhus	1:16	0	0	0	0	0	0	0	0
	Rocky Mt. spot-ted fever	1:16	0	0	0	0	0	0		
	Q fever	1:16	0	0	0	0	0	0		
	H.B.	1:10	0	0	0	0	0	0		
	J. M.	1:10	0	0	0	0	0	0		

[a] Serums of rickettsialpox patients taken 30 days after onset.
[b] Transient.

Seven days later there was no growth on the blood agar slant but all the chick embryos were dead or moribund. Again the yolk sacs showed a profuse growth of bipolar rods resembling rickettsiae. Subcultures on blood agar again were negative.

A third yolk sac isolation of what proved to be the same organism was made from the blood of one of the two guinea pigs inoculated with the liver and spleen suspension from the original mouse. The organism was not apparent in the yolk sacs until 13 days after inoculation, suggesting a relative paucity of M. K. organisms in guinea pig blood.

These three isolations from the original mouse appear to be identical. Reinoculation of yolk sac suspensions of the M. K. organism into mice and guinea pigs results in a disease similar to that produced by animal passage material. All attempts to cultivate the M. K. organism on acellular media have failed; in addition to ordinary media, special media such as tryptose agar, Casman's blood agar, chocolate blood agar, and glucose cystine agar were employed in aerobic, anaerobic, and 20 per cent carbon dioxide atmospheres.

The M. K. Organism as a Complement-Fixing Antigen

A 10 per cent suspension of first-passage yolk sacs containing many visible M. K. organisms was prepared and titrated as an antigen in the complement fixation test† against convalescent serums of two patients, H. B. and J. M. Serum pools collected from guinea pigs which had recovered from endemic typhus, Rocky Mountain spotted fever, and Q fever were also employed. A portion of the 10 per cent suspension was extracted with ether and the aqueous layer tested as an antigen against the same serums. The results (shown in Table 1) reveal a complement-fixing reaction between the M. K. antigens and three of the serums—the Rocky Mountain spotted fever, the H. B., and the J. M. serums.

The M. K. antigen achieved its highest titer with the Rocky Mountain spotted fever serum. This is in contrast to the lower titers given against the same serums by R161, an ether-treated Rocky Mountain spotted fever antigen. It should be noted that ether treatment increased the titer of the M. K. antigen in the presence of the serums of both patients.

More potent M. K. antigens were subsequently prepared, ether extraction by method No. 1 and method No. 2 of Topping and Shepard (2) being the methods of choice. As with antigens prepared from *Rickettsia prowazeki, R. mooseri,* and *R. rickettsi,* a soluble antigen which could not be precipitated by high-speed centrifugation (4000 rpm.) for 1 hour was found to be present in the M. K. antigens. Except for cross-reaction with Rocky Mountain spotted fever, the antigens possessed a high degree of specificity in the complement-fixation test (Table 2). Generally, the titer of human Rocky Mountain spotted fever serums has been lower when tested with the M. K. antigens than with homologous antigens.

† The Bengtson technique was used throughout.

Table 2. Specificity of M. K. Antigens in the Complement Fixation Test, showing the Results given by the Various Types of Serums Tested To Date against the M. K. Antigens

Type of serums tested	Total number of serums	Number of serums negative	Number of serums positive	Titer or range of titers of positive serums
Human serums				
Normal	18	17	1	1:4 (3+)
Endemic typhus	6	6	0	—
Tsutsugamushi	3	3	0	—
Q fever	6	4	2	1:4 each
Syphilis	4	4	0	—
Rocky Mountain spotted fever	11	1	10	1:8 to 1:512
Do	19	0	19	1:32 to 1:640
Guinea pig serums				
Normal	7	7	0	—
Endemic typhus	1	1	0	—
Q fever pool	1	1	0	—
Rocky Mountain spotted fever	7	0	7	1:16 to 1:512
Do	23	0	23	1:8 to 1:512

Serological Reactions of Serums from Typical Cases, Including Serums from M. K.

Serums from patients with typical symptomatology were tested against M. K. antigens and a Rocky Mountain spotted fever antigen in the complement fixation test. M. K. No. 2 and M. K. No. 3 as well as R161, a Rocky Mountain spotted fever antigen, were used. Proteus OX-19, and OX-2 and OX-K agglutinations were also done.

In Table 3, it will first of all be noted that the serum of each patient tested reacted in the convalescent stage with the M. K. antigen, one of the highest titers being afforded by the convalescent serum of M. K. Significant but lower reactions occurred in the presence of the Rocky Mountain spotted fever antigen in 15 cases, which represent 79 per cent of the total. Most significant, however, is the rise in titer against M. K. antigen shown by the serums of 4 cases, M. S., Mr. S., L. A., and D. G. Convalescent serum from a guinea pig which had shown a typical response to the M. K. mouse liver and mouse spleen passage was strongly positive when tested with the M. K. antigen but was completely negative in the presence of R161. Many of the convalescent serums have been tested with typhus and Q fever yolk sac antigens. In every instance they have been negative.

Table 3. Complement Fixation Results on Serums of Patients Tested with M. K.[a]
and Rocky Mountain Spotted Fever[b] Antigens

Patient	Date of onset	Date of specimens	M. K. titer	Rocky Mountain spotted fever titer
	1946	1946		
J. R.	Mar. 7	July 24	1:32	Negative
Mrs. C.	Mar. 15	July 24	1:16	1:4
Mr. C.	Mar. 29	July 24	1:256	Negative
B. B.	June 9	July 11	Not done	1:128 (AC[c] 1:16)
		Aug. 29	1:256	1:128
M. B.	June 23	July 11	1:32	Negative
		Aug. 21	1:16	Negative
C. F.	July 11	July 12	Not done	Negative
		Sept. 13	1:64	1:16
Mr. S.	July 7	July 26	1:32	Negative
		Aug. 8	1:64	1:4
M. S.	July 14	July 24	Negative	Negative
		Aug. 18	1:256	1:64
C. B.	July 17	Aug. 29	1:64	1:8
L. A.	July 18	July 24	1:8	Negative
		Aug. 18	1:128	1:128
J. M.	July 18	Aug. 18	1:640	1:320
A. G.	July 20	Aug. 4	1:320	1:80
Mrs. S.	July 25	Aug. 18	1:64	1:64
H. B.	July 27	Aug. 18	1:320	1:80
M. K.	July 22	Aug. 29	1:512	1:256
W. N.	July 22	Sept. 11	1:64	1:8
M. M.	Aug. 10	Aug. 29	1:64	Negative
A. A.	Aug. 18	Aug. 29	1:128	1:8
		Sept. 11	1:128	1:32
D. G.	Aug. 31	Sept. 7	1:4	Negative
		Sept. 11	1:32	1:16

[a] M. K. No. 2 and No. 3.
[b] R 161.
[c] Anticomplementary.

Proteus reactions were without significance in every case except two:
J. M. who had a convalescent titer of 1:200 against *Proteus* OX-19, and
J. R. with a titer of 1:100 also against *Proteus* OX-19. Since only one
serum specimen was available for examination in both instances a rise
in agglutinin titer was not demonstrated.

Negative results were obtained in agglutination tests for tularemia, brucellosis, leptospirosis, and the typhoid group. Heterophile agglutinations were also negative. Repeated blood cultures taken during acute stages of the disease were in every instance sterile.

Behavior of the M. K. Organism in the Yolk Sacs of Fertile Eggs and in Certain Laboratory Animals

The M. K. organism at the time of writing has been carried through four yolk sac passages. Yolk sac seed materials diluted 1:10 to 1:10,000 produce death of the embryos 4 to 7 days after inoculation. Yolk sac films stained by Machiavello's technique show red-staining diplobacillary and diplococcal forms which resemble *R. prowazeki* and *R. mooseri* in morphology. Many M. K. organisms appear on smear to be located within the nuclei of yolk sac cells.

The staining characteristics of the M. K. organism in yolk sac films are quite similar to those of *R. prowazeki*. Machiavello's method provides the best results, Geimsa's stain is adequate, but methylene blue and Gram's method give poor results. Apparently the organisms are decolorized by the acetone of the Gram method but take the counterstain only with indifferent success.

Behavior in Mice

In white mice (Swiss strain) the M. K. organism has been carried through four passages of both brain and spleen suspensions. Intraperitoneal inoculation results in definite objective signs of illness, but few deaths occur. Ruffled fur is noticed as early as the sixth day after inoculation. Immobility and rapid breathing associated with no apparent interest in food and water mark the peak of the disease which is reached between the ninth and thirteenth days. Deaths may occur any time during this period. Intracerebral inoculation of infected brain produces signs of illness earlier and results in a larger percentage of deaths than with intraperitoneal inoculation.

One cubic centimeter of heart blood taken from a sick mouse failed in one attempt to cause visible signs of illness when inoculated into the peritoneum of three fresh mice. The brain from this same mouse produced typical signs of illness when inoculated intraperitoneally into four fresh mice.

Heavily infected yolk sacs diluted 1:10 in 50 per cent skim milk produced death in mice within 5 to 7 days after intraperitoneal inoculation. Less potent suspensions resulted in typical signs of illness, but death was not uniformly produced. Intravenous inoculation into mice of a potent suspension has thus far provided no evidence of a toxic substance. However, in one experiment a yolk-sac dilution as high as 1:320 was lethal within 7 days for the four mice inoculated. In lower dilutions, death occurred as early as the fourth day, and signs of illness appeared within 3 days.

Tissues of M. K. mice placed repeatedly on ordinary culture media have failed to lead to the cultivation of an organism of any significance. Occasional colonies of staphylococci and salmonella were obtained but these are occasionally encountered in work with mice at the National Institute of Health.

Behavior in Guinea Pigs

The M. K. organism has been maintained without difficulty through four passages in guinea pigs by means of intraperitoneal inoculation of tunica washings. Redness and swelling of the scrotum and irreducible testes, often the first signs of the disease, occur usually on the fifth day after inoculation. The onset of fever may occur anywhere from the fourth to the sixth day. A short febrile course (3 to 5 days) is marked by remissions. It is not uncommon for a guinea pig to show marked redness and swelling of the scrotum and a temperature of 40.5°C. on the fifth morning after inoculation, a normal temperature on the sixth morning, and a temperature of 40.0°C. on the seventh morning.

Temperatures taken twice daily, in the morning and in the afternoon, give a more accurate picture of the thermal reaction to the disease, often revealing a fever later in the day after a normal morning temperature has been recorded.

Effect in Guinea Pigs of Various Inocula

When tunica washings are used as passage material, redness and swelling of the scrotum are a constant pathological finding although the temperature curve may often show only a single insignificant elevation.

We have been unable to reproduce signs of disease with any degree of regularity in guinea pigs when heart blood is used as passage material. On the few occasions when intraperitoneal inoculation of guinea pig blood produced any reaction, the very mild objective signs of the disease were delayed until 10 to 15 days after inoculation.

Ten per cent yolk sac suspensions inoculated intraperitoneally produce a more acute and severe febrile reaction. An abbreviated incubation period (1 or 2 days) is followed by a sudden onset of high fever (41°C. and higher) which is sustained without remissions for 4 or 5 days.

The onset of the scrotal reaction is usually delaye duntil the fourth day.

Gross pathology in the infected guinea pig is characterized by: (a) periorchitis with adherence of the testes to the tunica vaginalis which is thickened and markedly injected; (b) moderately enlarged spleen and lymph nodes; (c) occasional small areas of pneumonic consolidation; and (d) frequent indurated cutaneous and subcutaneous nodules at the site of inoculation.

No systematic attempt has been made as yet to examine animal tissues for visible organisms. However, a few small red-staining diplobacilli have been seen in films made of the peritoneum and tunica vaginalis stained by Machiavello's method.

Discussion

Despite the fact that only one isolation of an organism (a rickettsia) has thus far been made, the evidence presented in the foregoing account we believe to be sufficient to establish it as the causative agent of the disease under study.

Classification of the M. K. organism as a rickettsia, we believe is justified. The arthropod vector will be described in a subsequent communication.

The characteristics of the M. K. organism on yolk sac cultivation and its behavior in guinea pigs coupled with a serologic relationship to Rocky Mountain spotted fever are suggestive of *Rickettsia conori*, the causative agent of fièvre boutonneuse.

Certain differences between the reported behavior of *R. conori* in the laboratory and the M. K. organism have, however, been observed. We have been unable to produce any signs of illness in monkeys even with large doses of potent yolk sac suspensions (4). The ability to produce objective illness in white mice apparently is not shared by *R. conori*, although this point seems not to have been extensively pursued by the Mediterranean investigators.

The failure of the disease under study to stimulate agglutinins for Proteus OX-19 and OX-2 in the serums of most of the New York patients would seem to differentiate it in this respect from fièvre boutonneuse which is reported to produce such agglutinins regularly (3).

Preliminary tests (4) suggest a partial but incomplete cross-protection of guinea pigs convalescent from infection with the M. K. organism against challenge with the Bitter Root strain of *R. rickettsi*. Complete reciprocal cross-immunity has been reported (5) as characterizing the immunological relationship of fièvre boutonneuse and Rocky Mountain spotted fever.

Summary

An organism having the morphologic and cultural characteristics of a rickettsia has been isolated from a patient during the course of an unusual outbreak of disease occurring in New York. This organism produces illness in mice and guinea pigs and grows well in the yolk sacs of fertile eggs.

Ether-extracted yolk sac antigens have been prepared which fix complement with convalescent serums drawn from typical cases. This reaction is apparently specific insofar as it has been tested, except for cross-reactions with Rocky Mountain spotted fever.

The behavior of the M. K. organism in fertile eggs, mice, and guinea pigs has been described. Certain similarities to R. *conori* have been pointed out, but further work will be necessary before any conclusion as to further similarities is possible.

Note: Since this paper was submitted for publication, a second strain of rickettsialpox has been isolated from the blood of a patient, M. S. The M. S. strain is culturally and immunologically indistinguishable from the M. K. strain.

More recently, a report of cases by Dr. Benjamin Shankman has appeared in the New York State Journal of Medicine (6).

Acknowledgments

The aid given by Commissioner Israel Weinstein, Dr. Samuel Frant, Dr. Morris Greenberg, and Dr. Ottavio Pellitteri, of the New York City Health Department, facilitated this work immeasurably.

Dr. Ralph Muckenfuss, director, and Miss Annabel W. Walter, bacteriologist, of the New York City Bureau of Laboratories, helped with the early laboratory work in addition to providing laboratory animals, space, and equipment.

We wish also to acknowledge the cooperation offered by the physicians in charge of the patients included in this study. We are particularly grateful for the help of Dr. Benjamin Shankman and Dr. Harry N. Zeller of Kew Gardens, Dr. Leon N. Sussman of Manhattan, and Dr. Irving S. Klein, assistant medical superintendent of the Willard Parker Hospital, New York.

1949

Marianna R. Bovarnick and John C. Snyder

Respiration of Typhus Rickettsiae

This classic report by Bovarnick and Snyder, the first to demonstrate independent metabolic activity by rickettsiae, provided the impetus for extensive and fruitful studies on rickettsial metabolism. Their findings established a distinctive respiratory activity, glutamate oxidation, for purified suspensions of epidemic and murine typhus rickettsiae that was not exhibited by normal yolk sac suspensions prepared in the same manner. The rate of oxygen uptake in the presence of glutamate, the chief substrate, was directly proportional to the concentration of viable rickettsiae. That rickettsiae possess enzymes for the aerobic oxidation of glutamate was confirmed with murine typhus microorganisms by Wisseman, Jackson, Hahn, Ley, and Smadel (1), and conclusively established by the studies of Karp (2). The latter showed that the rate of glutamate oxidation remained unchanged, although other enzymatic activities were abolished, when purified rickettsia suspensions were treated with antiserum against normal yolk sac preparations. Evidence obtained from studies of the oxidation pathways suggested that the utilization of glutamate proceeded through steps involved in the Krebs cycle (3). The presence of an operative Krebs cycle in *C. burnetii* has been reported by Ormsbee and Peacock (4).

Bovarnick and Miller (5) found evidence of the existence of a transaminase enzyme, glutamate-oxalacetate, and indications that phosphate was necessary to maintain an optimal glutamate oxidation rate. This led to the important discovery that rickettsiae are capable of converting oxidative energy into high energy phosphate bonds resulting in the formation of adenosine triphosphate (ATP) from diphosphopyridine nucleotide (DPN), Coenzyme A, adenosine diphosphate (ADP), and inorganic phosphate (6). The chief energy source of rickettsiae, therefore, results from oxidative phosphorylation.

Studies on the physiology of *C. burnetii* have revealed that these rickettsiae possess an ATPase and an ADPase (7). The presence of these enzymes is in accord with the phosphorylation activities in rickettsiae described previously by Bovarnick. Although rickettsiae are capable of performing some reactions necessary for their own proliferation, they are from a metabolic standpoint obligatory intracellular parasites that exhibit certain enzyme deficiencies and a concomitant dependence on the enzymes of the host system. Rickettsiae appear to rely on host cells for their source of energy and the necessary substrates and cofactors to function metabolically. Metabolic studies on the rickettsiae enlarge our general understanding of host-parasite relations and help define the mechanisms involved in the pathogenicity exhibited by these microorganisms since there is a close association of rickettsial virulence with metabolic activity (see paper by Gilford and Price, 1955).

Respiration of Typhus Rickettsiae

Studies yielding information concerning the growth or metabolism of obligate intracellular parasites should be of obvious theoretical and possibly practical importance. Rickettsiae, a group of intracellular parasites which appear to be physiological as well as morphological intermediates between the viruses and bacteria, seem to offer a favorable group for such studies. The experiments reported below indicate that this indeed may be the case.

Methods

Three strains of typhus rickettsiae were used in this study: the Breinl strain of epidemic typhus, the Madrid E strain of epidemic typhus (3, 5) and the Wilmington strain of murine typhus. The three strains were maintained by serial passage in embryonated eggs (4).

Preparation of Rickettsial Suspensions. Suspensions of typhus rickettsiae were prepared from infected yolk sac pools which were homogenized in a Waring blender with 1 volume of a buffered isotonic salt solution and quickly shell frozen in an alcohol-dry ice mixture. The composition of the salt solution is described below. A portion of the 50 per cent yolk sac suspension was thawed, diluted with $2\frac{1}{2}$ volumes of the same salt solution, and centrifuged at 5000 rpm in an angle centrifuge for 45 minutes. The supernatant was discarded; the precipitate was resuspended to the same volume, treated with 1 gm. of celite (6, 12) for each 6 gm. of yolk sac, and centrifuged at 1000 rpm for 30 minutes to remove cell fragments. The supernatant was again centrifuged at 5000 rpm and the precipitate resuspended to the desired volume, usually equal to one-half that of the original yolk sac. This suspension was centrifuged at 500 rpm for 10 minutes to remove any remaining particles; the supernatant turbid fluid constituted the final suspension which was used for measurements of respiration. It generally contained about 50 per cent of the rickettsiae originally present as estimated by its toxicity for mice. The protein nitrogen content was around 0.5 to 1 mg. N per ml., but varied somewhat with each preparation. All procedures were carried out at 0–5°C. and the suspensions were used immediately after preparation.

The salt solution for washing the rickettsiae consisted of 0.122 M KCl; 0.0074 M NaCl; 0.0041 M KH_2PO_4; and 0.0078 M Na_2HPO_4; pH 7.0. In many instances 0.04 per cent casein hydrolysate or 0.0045 M potassium glutamate was also present, except in the solution used for resuspension of the final precipitate. More recently respiration measurements have been carried out at pH 7.5 rather than at pH 7.0 as the oxygen uptake is greater at the higher pH. In such cases the final precipitate was resuspended in a solution of the following composition: 0.126 M KCl; 0.0018 M NaCl; 0.0012 M KH_2PO_4; 0.0106 M Na_2HPO_4; pH 7.5.

Oxygen Consumption Measurements. These were carried out by the conventional Warburg method at 34.3°C. The reaction mixture consisted of 1.5 ml. of a rickettsial suspension; 0.2 ml. of a solution of 0.012 M $MgCl_2$ and 0.004 M $MnCl_2$; substrate, neutralized with KOH, at the indicated concentration, and salt solution of the indicated pH to bring the total volume in the vessel to 2.4 ml. The center well contained 0.1 ml. of 10 per cent KOH. Readings were taken at intervals for 3 to 4 hours but the rates given in Table 1 were those observed for the first 2 hours.

Glucose concentration was determined by the method of Nelson (9), and pyruvate as described by Lardy (7). Toxicity of the rickettsial suspensions for white mice was estimated by the intravenous injection of 0.25 ml. of serial threefold dilutions of the rickettsial suspensions using 4 mice for each dilution (2). Deaths were counted after 24 hours and the dilution of the final rickettsial suspension required to kill 50 per cent of the mice was estimated by the method of Reed and Muench (11). The infectivity of the epidemic typhus preparations was estimated in cotton rats in the manner described in a previous report (8).

Results

Table 1 contains the data of the experiments which show that partially purified rickettsial preparations from yolk sac infected with *R. prowazeki*, strain E, had a definite oxygen consumption with casein hydrolysate as substrate. The product of similar preparations from normal yolk sac had an insignificant oxygen uptake under the same conditions indicating that the observed metabolic activity was a property of the rickettsiae themselves. This conclusion was further confirmed by the observation that the oxygen uptake of rickettsial preparations from various pools of strain E was directly related to the concentration of viable rickettsiae as determined by two accepted assays for rickettsiae, namely toxicity for white mice and immunization end-point in cotton rats. The direct proportionality which exists between the rate of oxygen uptake and toxicity for white mice is shown by the constancy of the ratio between these two values given in columns (*k*) and (*l*) of the table. Furthermore, this same correlation of oxygen uptake with the concentration of viable rickettsiae occurred with the Breinl strain of *R. prowazeki* and the Wilmington strain of *R. mooseri*.

Respiration of Typhus Rickettsiae

Table 1. Oxygen Uptake by Purified Preparations of Typhus Rickettsiae

| Rickettsiae | | | Rate of oxygen uptake | | | | | | | |
Strain	Pool no.	pH	No substrate	Casein hydrolysate 0.3 per cent	Glutamate 0.0125 M	Pyruvate 0.004 M	Succinate 0.0125 M	Toxicity for mice[a] LD_{50}	$k_C = e/j$[b]	$k_G = f/j$[b]
(a)	(b)	(c)	(d)	(e)	(f)	(g)	(h)	(j)	(k)	(l)
				microliters O_2/hr./ml. rickettsial suspension						
Madrid E	2958[c]	7.0		5.5			11.5	13	0.42	
Madrid E	2955	7.0	1.9	10.6		4.2	6.4	20	0.52	
Madrid E	2937	7.0		21.1		5.5	19.1	55	0.38	
Madrid E	2956[c]	7.0	2.3	24.1		8.9	8.9	50	0.48	
Madrid E	3006	7.0		10.4	10.8			17.2	0.60	0.63
Madrid E	3006	7.4		15.7	20.8					
Breinl	3040G	7.0		45.3	61.8	8.1		100	0.45	0.62
Breinl	3040E	7.0			96.4		20.4	172		0.56
Breinl	3040	7.4			107.0	14.1	18.1			
Breinl	3040, frozen[d]	7.4			10.0	5.6	39.2			
Wilmington	3096	7.4			28.0	2.9	3.5	55		0.51
Wilmington	3097	7.4			54.5	5.3	4.6	100		0.54
Wilmington	2676	7.4	0.7		87.7	6.8	6.9	172		0.51
Wilmington	2676, frozen[d]	7.4			5.5	0.0	23.1	19		0.29
Normal	1	7.0		0.4		0.0	3.1			
Normal	2	7.4			0.5	0.3	1.4			
Normal	2, frozen	7.4			0.4		1.3			

[a] The toxicity for mice is expressed as that dilution of the rickettsial suspension used for measurements of oxygen uptake, 0.25 ml. of which will kill 50 per cent of the mice.

[b] The constancy of k_C and k_G, the ratio of the rate of oxygen uptake with casein hydrolysate and glutamate respectively to the dilution required to kill 50 per cent of the mice, is a measure of the proportionality between rickettsial viability and respiratory activity.

[c] The 50 per cent immunization end-point in cotton rats for pool 2958 corresponded to a dilution of the original yolk sac pool of $10^{6.5}$, that for pool 2956 to a dilution of $10^{7.5}$, when 0.25 ml. amounts were inoculated into cotton rats.

[d] These were portions of the preceding rickettsial suspensions which had been frozen and thawed.

The chief constituent of casein hydrolysate responsible for the observed oxygen uptake is probably glutamic acid since this amino acid brings about an oxygen uptake equal to or, usually, greater than that in the presence of casein hydrolysate (see columns (*e*) and (*f*) in the table). Not all of the amino acids have yet been tried, but to date none has been found other than glutamic acid that leads to an increased oxygen uptake by rickettsiae. Carbon dioxide is also produced from glutamic acid, but the R.Q. of 0.85 indicates that the oxidation is incomplete.

No other substrate has been found that is oxidized as rapidly as glutamic acid. It was surprising to find that not only is there no oxygen uptake with glucose or lactate, but also no disappearance of glucose either aerobically or anaerobically, with or without addition of adenosine triphosphate, cozymase, hexosediphosphate, magnesium, and manganese. However, a very slow oxygen uptake, roughly proportional to the rickettsial activity, occurs with pyruvate. This oxygen uptake disappears after about 4 hours, in contrast to that with glutamate, which decreases only 10 to 20 per cent in this time. The significance of the small oxygen uptake with pyruvate was checked by measurements of the disappearance of pyruvate in the presence of normal and infected yolk sac preparations. With the former, there was no change in substrate concentration (0.001 M) in 5 hours; with the latter, in one instance 1.2 micromols, with a second more active preparation, 2.3 micromols disappeared in 5 hours.

Succinate increases the oxygen uptake of rickettsiae, but in this instance there is a small oxygen uptake with similar preparations from normal yolk sac. Furthermore, there was no parallelism between rickettsial toxicity and the rate of oxygen uptake in the presence of succinate. It is possible that live rickettsiae may be impermeable to succinate since on freezing in the absence of protein or other protective substances, the viability of rickettsiae as indicated by their toxicity for mice, and their activity toward glutamate and pyruvate are greatly reduced while their rate of oxygen uptake with succinate is doubled or trebled (see table, pools 3040 and 2676).

It is clear from these results that typhus rickettsiae which have been separated from the greater part of the tissue in which they were grown exhibit definite metabolic activity. This phenomenon is quite different in nature from the changes in metabolism observed in some virus-infected tissues. The latter appear to be due to changes in the tissue metabolism brought about by the presence of the virus rather than to activity of the virus itself (1, 10).

Respiration of Typhus Rickettsiae

Summary

Partially purified suspensions of typhus rickettsiae have been shown to exhibit metabolic activity as evidenced by consumption of oxygen and production of carbon dioxide in the presence of glutamate. Similar activity at a much lower rate occurs in the presence of pyruvate. The rate of oxygen uptake was directly proportional to the concentration of viable rickettsiae, as estimated by their toxicity for mice. Normal yolk sac suspensions prepared in the same manner showed only a very slight oxygen uptake under the same conditions. Glucose was not metabolized by the rickettsial suspensions.

Acknowledgments

This work was supported by a grant from the Division of Research Grants and Fellowships of the National Institute of Health, United States Public Health Service, and was conducted with the aid of the Commission on Virus and Rickettsial Diseases, Army Epidemiological Board, Office of The Surgeon General, United States Army, Washington, D.C.

1949

Hans Ris and John P. Fox

The Cytology of Rickettsiae

An important contribution that added to our comprehension of the biochemical nature of rickettsiae was this 1949 report by Ris and Fox on the nucleic acid content of these microorganisms. These investigators not only demonstrated deoxyribonucleic acid (DNA) in the internal (chromatin) bodies found in rickettsiae (see paper by Plotz *et al.* 1943) but detected the presence of ribonucleic acid (RNA) in the cytoplasm. Their findings were substantiated by Price (1), who reported both DNA and RNA in *R. rickettsii*. The failure of previous researchers to detect RNA in rickettsiae was attributed to the washing procedures employed during purification which resulted in the complete loss of RNA or low RNA to DNA ratios (1:3). Cohn, Hahn, Ceglowski, and Bozeman (2) demonstrated that RNA comprised 75 per cent of the nucleic acid components lost by rickettsial cells. They found that *R. mooseri* had an RNA-to-DNA ratio of 3.5:1, which was similar to that reported for many bacteria. The presence of both RNA and DNA as constituents of rickettsiae was added evidence that these microorganisms possess a cellular organization and biochemical composition similar to, and as complex as, that of bacteria.

In recent years it has been shown that all bacterial cells which have been adequately examined are essentially similar to the cells of higher organisms with the demonstration of deoxyribonucleic acid-containing, regularly dividing nuclear structures and the presence of ribonucleic acid in the cytoplasm (1, 2). It is not yet clear whether these Feulgen-positive bodies are similar to chromosomes in higher organisms or whether the genic material is organized in a different way. Since chromosomes exhibit a very special structure and behavior during cell division in addition to containing DNA and being self-reproducing, this name should not be applied to the Feulgen-positive bodies of bacteria. Instead the less specific terms *nuclear structure* and *chromatinic body* (Robinow [1]) will be used here.

Rickettsiae are usually considered to be essentially like bacteria in morphology though they resemble viruses in being obligate intracellular parasites (cf. reference 3). Photographs with the electron microscope have revealed some internal structures similar to those found in bacteria (4). Chemical analysis of isolated rickettsiae, however, has shown the presence of deoxyribonucleic acid only, no ribonucleic acid having been detected (5, 6). The present study was undertaken in order to investigate, first, whether RNA can be demonstrated in unwashed rickettsiae using cytochemical methods, and secondly, whether the DNA is present in nuclear structures as in the bacteria above mentioned, or is diffusely distributed through the rickettsial bodies.

Materials and Methods

The material used in this study came from chick embryo yolk sacs infected with the Breinl strain of epidemic typhus (*Rickettsia prowazeki*). Yolk sac smears were air-dried, heat-fixed, and then immersed in Carnoy or in 20 per cent Formalin. Concentrated suspensions of rickettsiae were obtained from yolk sac emulsions by repeated washing in saline.

Ultraviolet photographs (2537 Å) were obtained using a G.E. germicidal lamp (4 watt) with quartz-condensing lens, a Bäckström filter (20 per cent $NiSO_4$ plus 8.5 per cent $CoSO_4$ in distilled water), Zeiss 1.7 mm. quartz objective and Zeiss × 10 quartz ocular.

Rickettsiae for electron microscope photographs were extracted from yolk sacs, sulfate-precipitated, and inactivated with 1:5000 merthiolate. A drop of this suspension was dried on formvar film, washed in distilled water to remove salts, and dried again for examination in the RCA Universal electron microscope.

Unstained smears of rickettsiae were also photographed with the phase contrast microscope (Spencer 1.8 mm., medium dark contrast objective).

To determine the presence of RNA in unwashed rickettsiae they were fixed in 20 per cent Formalin and treated with ribonuclease (preparation of Dr. Kunitz, 0.2 mg. per ml. in distilled water, 45 minutes at 50°C.). Controls were treated the same way except for the enzyme. Buffer solutions were not used because they were found to extract the basophilic material from rickettsiae on the control slides. The slides were then stained together in methyl green pyronine for 20 minutes and differentiated in acetone.

Demonstration of Ribonucleic Acid in the Cytoplasm of Rickettsiae

Tovarnickij et al. (5) studied the chemical composition of rickettsiae isolated from mouse lungs and washed with physiological saline. Cohen (6) analyzed rickettsiae isolated from phenol-treated typhus vaccines. Both authors reported the presence of DNA, but no RNA was found. They concluded that rickettsiae were similar to viruses in containing only one type of nucleic acid, while bacteria and higher organisms

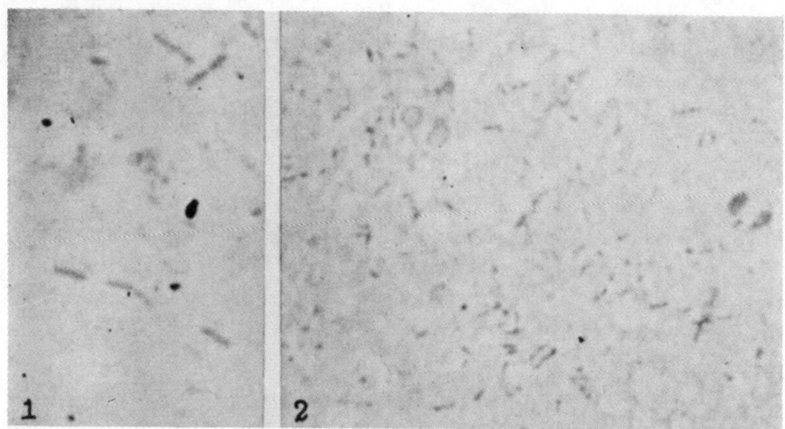

Figs. 1 and 2. Rickettsiae in yolk sac smears, stained with methyl green pyronine. Fig. 2 shows the rickettsiae after treatment with ribonuclease, Fig. 1 in the control slide. In the control the cytoplasm is stained intensively with pyronine. After ribonuclease treatment only the nuclear structures are stained. Zeiss 2 mm. NA 1.3 objective, × 2400.

always have both RNA and DNA. However, it has been shown that ribonucleoproteins are easily extracted from cells with physiological saline (7). It is therefore possible that no RNA was present in purified rickettsiae because it had been washed out during preparation. The presence of RNA in cells can be demonstrated cytochemically using ribonuclease and basic dyes (8). We therefore treated yolk sac smears fixed with 20 per cent Formalin with ribonuclease and stained with methyl green pyronine. On the control slide the rickettsiae stain more or less solidly red with pyronine (Fig. 1). The intensity of the staining varies somewhat from one cell to the other. After digestion with ribonuclease, however, the overall staining is always very much decreased (Fig. 2). Rickettsiae therefore contain RNA in variable amounts, probably depending on the physiological state as has been demonstrated for bacteria (9). Since it was not found in purified suspensions of rickettsiae it must have been lost during preparation. The effect of saline for instance on the staining with pyronine is marked. Fresh rickettsiae and rickettsiae washed with saline were smeared on the same slide and stained with pyronine. Unwashed rickettsiae stain uniformly red. Rickettsiae washed once stain very faintly and those washed more thoroughly do not stain at all with pyronine.

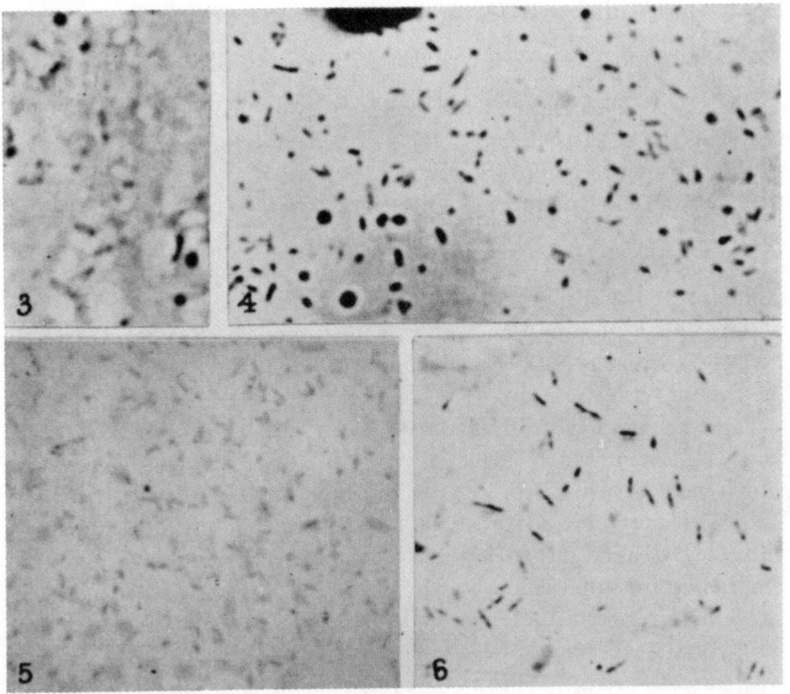

Fig. 3. Photograph of unwashed rickettsiae in yolk sac smear taken with the phase contrast microscope. Spencer 1.8 mm. dark medium, × 2700.

Fig. 4. Rickettsiae in yolk sac smear, hydrolyzed with N HCl 10 minutes, stained with Giemsa. Zeiss 2 mm. NA 1.3 objective, × 2400.

Fig. 5. Rickettsiae washed with saline, photographed in ultraviolet light (2537 Å), Zeiss 1.7 mm. quartz objective, ca. × 2500. The nuclear structures absorb more intensely than the cytoplasm.

Fig. 6. Rickettsiae in yolk sac smear, digested with ribonuclease, stained with methyl green pyronine, photographed with the phase contrast microscope. Spencer 1.8 mm. dark medium objective, × 2700. The chromatinic bodies stand out most sharply with this technique.

Recently Callot and Vendrely (10) studied the effect of deoxyribonuclease and ribonuclease on rickettsiae. They found that after deoxyribonuclease the staining with Giemsa was greatly reduced, but no marked decrease in staining was detected after digestion with ribonuclease. It is possible that the RNA was washed out during incubation in the control, or that they were dealing with rickettsiae in a physiological state with low RNA content in the cytoplasm.

Demonstration of Nuclear Structures in Rickettsiae

With the phase contrast microscope two or more dark bodies are visible in the rickettsial rods (Fig. 3). These structures are very similar to the chromatinic bodies in bacteria. In order to determine whether they are nuclear structures like those in bacteria it must be shown that they contain DNA.

Staining with Basic Dyes. In bacteria the nuclear structures can be demonstrated with basic dyes after removal of the RNA of the cytoplasm. This is accomplished either with ribonuclease (11) or through hydrolysis with 1 N HCl (12). Robinow (13) hydrolyzes in 1 N HCl and then stains with Giemsa.

Rickettsiae in fresh yolk sac smears stain solidly with basic dyes such as basic fuchsin (Macchiavello's procedure) and pyronine. Rickettsiae which have been washed with saline before fixation lose the ability to stain with these dyes. If washed rickettsiae, or rickettsiae hydrolyzed with 1 N HCl at 60° for 10 minutes are stained with Giemsa chromatinic bodies become apparent (Fig. 4).

Methyl green is a basic dye with high specificity for DNA. Washed rickettsiae were stained with methyl green pyronine. The nuclear structures stained purplish and the cytoplasm faintly pink. Photographed at 630 mμ near the absorption maximum of methyl green, the nuclear structures were clearly visible. The chromatinic bodies, however, appeared most distinct after treatment with ribonuclease and staining with basic dyes. Fig. 2 shows rickettsiae stained with methyl green pyronine after ribonuclease treatment. The nuclear structures stained purplish and stand out clearly in the practically colorless cytoplasm. Fig. 6 is a photograph from the same slide, but taken with the phase contrast microscope.

Ultraviolet Absorption. Photographs of washed rickettsiae at 2537 Å show strongly absorbing structures inside the rickettsial bodies (Fig. 5), corresponding to the structures staining with basic dyes. This is further evidence for the presence of nucleic acid in these structures.

Feulgen Reaction. Yolk sac smears were fixed in Carnoy and stained with the Feulgen reaction [modification of Rafalko (14)]. The nuclear structures stained very faintly red. With a green filter (Wratten 74) the small dots of the chromatinic bodies could be seen, but nothing else of the rickettsiae was visible. Though the stain was so weak that by itself

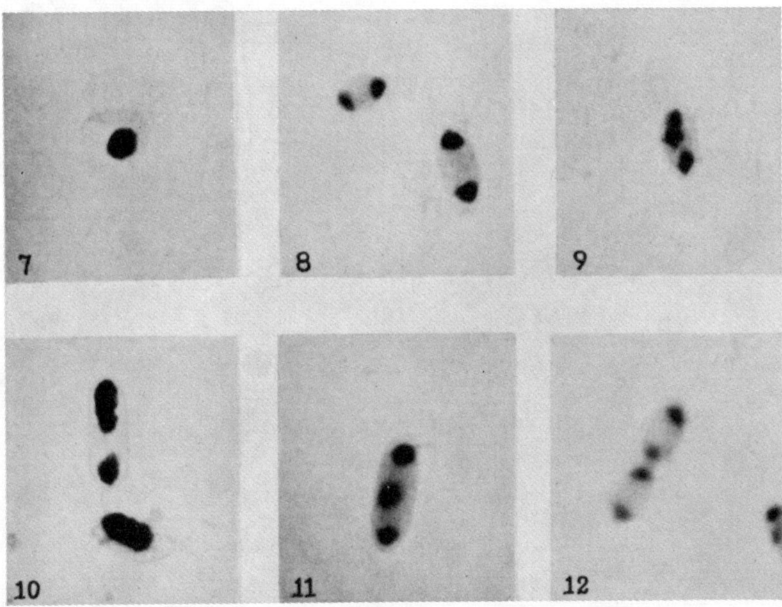

Figs. 7 to 12. Electron microscope photographs of rickettsiae extracted from yolk sacs, sulfate-precipitated, and inactivated with merthiolate. RCA Universal electron microscope, ca. × 15,000. Compare with Fig. 6.

it would be questionable as a demonstration of DNA, it indicated that the DNA found in purified rickettsiae must be concentrated in these small structures inside the rickettsial bodies. The absolute amount of DNA in one rickettsial organism was obviously extremely small.

The behavior of these chromatinic bodies toward basic dyes, especially after digestion with ribonuclease, the absorption at 2537 Å, and the Feulgen staining therefore leave little doubt that the DNA found in rickettsiae is localized in definite nuclear structures. Spherical rickettsiae contain one nuclear body. In rod-shaped rickettsiae one finds two bodies which are close together in short rods and farther separated in long rods. Sometimes long rods may contain three or four chromatinic bodies. These are usually spherical, but occasionally one sees dumbbell-shaped structures which suggest a chromatinic body in the process of division (Fig. 13 and Figs. 6 and 9).

Electron microscope photographs of rickettsiae washed with saline revealed internal structures which correspond to the chromatinic bodies

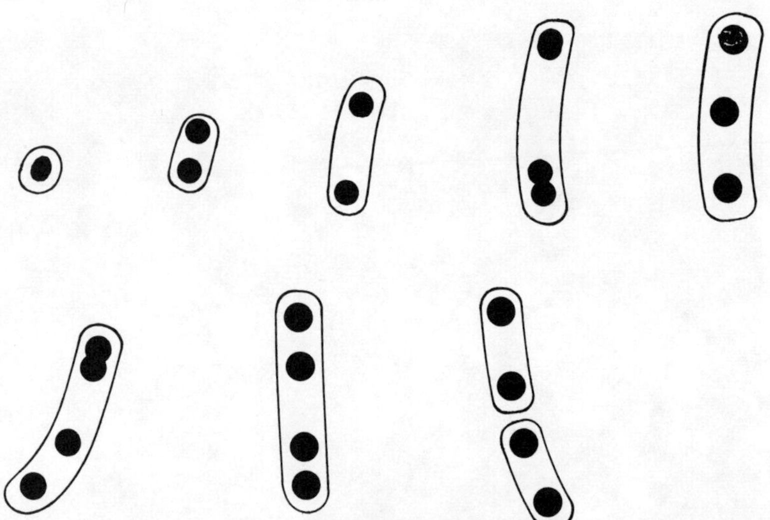

Fig. 13. Nuclear structures in various forms of Rickettsia prowazeki. Compare with Figs. 6 and 7 to 12.

described above.* Rickettsiae with one, two, or three chromatinic bodies were common (Figs. 7 to 12). Sometimes two nuclear structures were very close together, possibly representing the division of a chromatinic body (Figs. 9 and 10). Plotz et al. (4) described structures which seem to be identical with our chromatinic bodies.

Summary

Internal structures of rickettsiae seen with phase contrast microscopy and in the electron microscope contain deoxyribonucleic acid and are therefore nuclear structures similar to those found in bacteria. They are minute spherical bodies, either single as in spherical rickettsiae or varying in number from 2 to 4 in rod-shaped forms. Occasional dumbbell-shaped chromatinic bodies are thought to represent these structures in the process of division. The presence of ribonucleic acid in the cytoplasm of rickettsiae was demonstrated with the use of ribonuclease and basic dyes. Rickettsiae therefore have a cellular organization similar to that of certain bacteria, with a clear differentiation into nuclear structure and cytoplasm.

* The electron microscope photographs were prepared by Dr. E. G. Pickels, formerly of the Rockefeller Institute.

1952

*Herbert L. Ley, Jr., Joseph E. Smadel, Fred H. Diercks,
and Philip Y. Paterson*

Immunization against Scrub Typhus: V. The Infective Dose of Rickettsia tsutsugamushi *for Men and Mice*

The comparative susceptibility of laboratory animals to rickettsial infections and the minimum infective dose required to induce disease have been the subjects of several investigations. Fox (1) described the relative vulnerability of laboratory animals and chick embryos to new and established strain isolates of murine and epidemic typhus rickettsiae. Through intricate and carefully executed experiments, Fuller (2) established that the human body louse is as susceptible as the cotton rat to experimental infection with epidemic typhus rickettsiae. That the number of rickettsiae contained in an infective dose is remarkably low was revealed by Price, Emerson, Nagel, Blumberg, and Talmadge (3), who demonstrated that a dose of ten epidemic typhus rickettsiae was sufficient to infect 50 per cent of the cotton rats.

The following paper by Ley, Smadel, Diercks, and Paterson (1952) was the first to define the infective dose of a rickettsial agent for man. By correlating infection rates in human volunteers with intraperitoneal infectivity for mice, they found that the infecting doses of *R. tsutsugamushi* for man and for mice were equivalent. One infective unit was capable of inducing scrub typhus in either host. In another study involving volunteers but with a different rickettsial agent Tigertt and Benenson (4) found that the minimal infecting doses of *C. burnetii* administered by the respiratory route were of the same order of magnitude for man and guinea pig. Studies of this nature, revealing the comparative susceptibility of man and experimental animals to certain rickettsial infections, provide a basis for relating to the human being such data as are derived from animal experimentation on the efficacy of new vaccines and chemotherapeutic agents.

During the course of studies on the immunization of man by a combined procedure employing living vaccine and specific chemoprophylaxis, it was found that intradermal injection of a small number of *Rickettsia tsutsugamushi* was sufficient to induce scrub typhus (1, 2, 3). The use of this combined vaccine-chemoprophylactic procedure is founded upon the concept that a reproducible number of infectious doses of *R. tsutsugamushi* can be obtained in a given inoculum. The required uniformity and stability of a suspension of the organisms apparently had been achieved with properly lyophilized infected yolk sac materials used in the original investigation, for these suspensions contained approximately the predicted number of mouse infectious units and uniformly induced scrub typhus in volunteers injected with 10 to 25 such units. In recent studies on immunization of man, however, an unexpected drop in infectivity of the lyophilized vaccine occurred, and, as a result, a number of volunteers received less than an infective dose. Subsequent studies employed varying amounts of lyophilized vaccines which produced markedly different rates of infection in the volunteers.

The present report gathers together all the observations on infection rates in a number of groups of volunteers who received various scrub typhus vaccines and correlates these findings with the observed intra-peritoneal infectivity of each material for mice. We have been impressed with the equivalence of the infective doses of *R. tsutsugamushi* for man and for the mouse. Indeed, they appear to be of the same order of magnitude, e.g., one infectious unit is capable of inducing scrub typhus in either host. Because there are relatively few instances in which data of this general nature are available for other infectious diseases of man, the existing information on this subject has been reviewed and is summarized in this report.

Materials and Methods

General. The procedures employed in the selection and care of volunteers were those which have been employed over a period of years in similar studies carried on by our group in Malaya. These methods are mentioned in some detail in the previous paper (1), which also contains references to earlier reports where the subjects are presented more extensively.

When arrangements were completed for the vaccination of a given group of volunteers, a pool of living vaccine was prepared by rehydrating the lyophilized infective yolk sac material contained in 3 separate ampules of a given lot of vaccine. This pool was then divided into two portions. One was diluted in sucrose PG solution (4) containing 10 per cent inactivated human serum so that, on the basis of previous mouse titrations, 0.1 ml. of the final dilution contained approximately the desired number of mouse minimal infectious doses (mouse MID). This material was promptly injected intradermally in 0.1 ml. amounts over the left deltoid muscle of the volunteers. To provide an estimate of the current mouse infectivity of the vaccine, serial 10-fold dilutions of the second portion of the original pool were prepared over the range of 10^{-1} to 10^{-6} at the same time the volunteers were inoculated, and groups of 6 mice were injected intraperitoneally with 0.2 ml. of each dilution.

The lyophilized infectious yolk sac preparations of the Gilliam, Karp and CP-14 strains of *Rickettsia tsutsugamushi* used in the current work were from the same lots used in concurrent studies on the duration of immunity in persons recovered from scrub typhus infection (2). Two groups of volunteers who were vaccinated during the previous year received the lyophilized Gilliam vaccine described in the report concerned with the earlier studies on immunity (3).

Estimation of infectivity of rickettsial materials. Different methods were required for estimating the mouse infectivity of the 3 strains of *R. tsutsugamushi* employed because the lethal and infectious doses of Karp and CP-14 organisms are essentially identical, whereas the lethal dose of the Gilliam organism is generally several thousand times larger than the infectious dose. The procedures employed, which are described in detail elsewhere (4, 5), permitted expression of results as the number of mouse MID's of rickettsiae contained in a given volume and dilution of suspension.

The volunteers were considered to be infected with *R. tsutsugamushi* if they developed clinical disease and presented positive laboratory findings. Clinical illness was defined as beginning with the onset of sustained temperatures of 100°F. or over, headache, conjunctival injection, and tender, enlarged regional lymph nodes. Laboratory evidence of infection consisted of either demonstrable rickettsemia during the acute febrile period, or a 4-fold or greater rise in Weil-Felix OX-K agglutinins during convalescence. Both of these laboratory criteria of infection were fulfilled in the majority of patients. When a given inoculum caused clinical illness in volunteers, they were promptly hospitalized and were given specific antibiotic therapy within 48 hours of onset of sustained fever. Prompt therapeutic control of the disease invariably followed treatment.

Results

Minimal infectious dose of Rickettsia tsutsugamushi *for man.* The relationship between the number of mouse MID of 3 strains of *Rickettsia tsutsugamushi* inoculated into groups of volunteers and the incidence of infection in these volunteers is summarized in Table 1, which includes

Table 1. Human Susceptibility to Infection with Three Strains of *R. tsutsugamushi*

| Inoculum | | Number of volunteers | | Incubation periods (mean day of onset) | | Reference[c] |
| | | | | | | |
Strain	Mouse MID	Vaccinated	Hospitalized	Fever	Primary lesion	
Gilliam	1,000	8	8	10.6	8.5	2
Lot 6	100	4	4	10.5	6.0	
	100	3	3	11.7	7.6	2
	22[a]	8	8	9.0	4.7	3
	9[a]	6	6	8.3	4.2	3
	2.5	4	0			
Karp	150[b]	6	6	9.7	5.8	
Lot 14	125	7	7	10.1	5.8	2
	90	3	3	10.3	5.0	2
	60	12	12	10.6	5.1	1
	15[b]	6	6	12.3	7.2	
	1.5[b]	4	1	16	10	
CP-14	20	1	1	10	3	2
Lot 2	8[b]	2	2	11.0	5.0	
	0.8[b]	2	2	12.0	8.5	
	0.08[b]	2	0			
	0.008[b]	2	0			

[a] The inocula used in these 2 instances were diluted in sucrose salt solution without serum.

[b] These 7 groups furnish the basis for Table 2.

[c] References are to articles from which the data were extracted; undesignated data are from current studies.

data obtained from immunization studies conducted in Malaya during the past 2 years. The experience with the Gilliam, Karp, and CP-14 strains of this organism shows that a few mouse MID's of each are regularly capable of infecting man. Indeed, an estimated 0.8 mouse MID of the CP-14 strain, 9 of the Gilliam strain, and 15 of the Karp strain, induced disease in all volunteers who received these inocula. On the other hand, 3 of the 4 volunteers inoculated with 1.5 MID of the Karp strain and all of those who were vaccinated with 0.08 MID of the CP-14 strain and 2.5 MID of the Gilliam strain failed to develop disease.

Additional information on groups of volunteers inoculated at one time with different amounts of either Karp or CP-14 living vaccine is presented in Table 2 along with data obtained simultaneously by

Table 2. Comparative Susceptibilities of Men and Mice to *R. tsutsugamushi*

Titration host	*Rick.* strain	Volume inj. (ml.)	Inoculum						Host-specific MID_{50}/ml. yolk sac
			Dilution used						
			10^{-1}	10^{-2}	10^{-3}	10^{-4}	10^{-5}	10^{-6}	
Man	Karp	0.1 (I.D.)	6/6[a]	6/6	1/4				5×10^3
Mouse	(Lot 14)	0.2 (I.P.)		6/6	6/6	0/6	0/6		15×10^3
Man	CP-14	0.1(I.D.)	2/2	2/2	0/2	0/2			3×10^3
Mouse	(Lot 2)	0.2 (I.P.)	3/6	5/6	1/6	0/6	0/6	0/6	8×10^2

[a] Numerator = number of men hospitalized or mice dying; denominator = number of men or mice in group.

titration of the same preparations in mice. The units of the last column of this table, "Host-specific MID_{50}/ml. yolk sac," were selected to simplify comparison of the infectivity of the preparations for the two hosts. The results entered in this column were obtained by first determining from the data the host-specific MID_{50} titers for each suspension by the method of Reed and Muench (5). Then, with corrections for the different volumes of inocula used for mouse and man, the number of host-specific MID_{50} per ml. of undiluted yolk sac was computed and entered in the table. This method of expressing infectivity illustrates well the close correspondence between the infectious doses of either vaccine for mice and men. Indeed, this close correlation appears somewhat unusual, when the standard deviations of the titration end points are determined (6). To be significantly different, the host-specific LD_{50} titers of a given suspension, tested in groups of 6 mice and 2 men per dilution, would have to differ by at least 1.6 log units, i.e., one titer would have to be 40 times greater than the other. The observed host-specific infectivities of the two strains do differ, but only by a factor of 3 (15,000/5,000) for the Karp strain and 3.75 (3,000/800) for the CP-14 strain. In addition, these differences show no consistent bias, for man appears to be more susceptible to the Karp strain, and the mouse to the CP-14 strain. Therefore, the statistical treatment supports the observations that one infectious unit for the mouse approximates one infectious unit for man.

Relation between size of infecting dose and incubation period. Inspection of

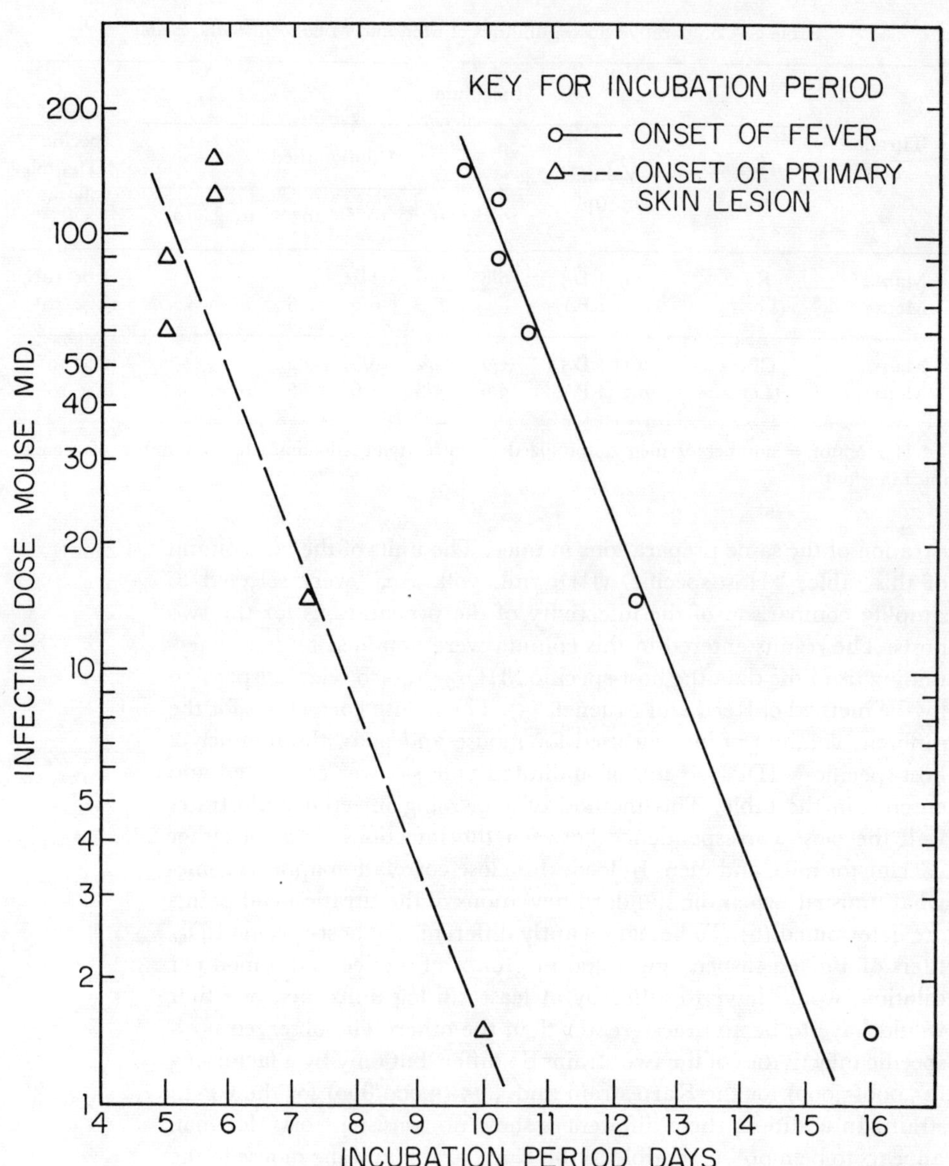

Fig. 1. *Incubation periods of fever and skin lesions in man as a function of infecting dose of* R. tsutsugamushi.

Table 1 reveals a reciprocal relationship between the number of mouse MID of the Karp strain administered to the volunteers and the incubation period of their disease as measured by the onsets of sustained fever or of primary skin lesion. This impression is confirmed when the data on the Karp strain are arranged graphically as in Fig. 1. A linear relationship appears to exist between the logarithm of the infecting dose of rickettsiae and the incubation period of both the febrile illness and the skin lesion. This relationship is more nearly exact for the onset of fever, which can be determined objectively with ease. The early definition of the skin lesion presented some difficulty since changes in environmental temperature apparently influenced the ease with which the early lesion could be discerned. Despite these uncertainties, it is apparent from the figures that the skin lesion usually appeared about 5 days before onset of sustained fever.

Information on the Gilliam and CP-14 strains in Table 1 is less reliable and does not provide a correlation of the type observed with the Karp strain. The numbers of volunteers who were injected with the CP-14 strain are inadequate for analysis. The main inconsistencies in the data on the Gilliam strain are found in groups injected with 9 and 22 mouse MID of rickettsiae, for the individuals in these groups had shorter incubation periods than those volunteers who received 100 or more mouse MID. It should be pointed out that the live vaccines administered to the aberrant groups were diluted in unmodified sucrose PG solution whereas the materials employed with the other groups were diluted in sucrose PG solution containing 10 per cent inactivated human serum. It is our opinion that the diluent used for the groups that received 9 and 22 mouse MID of the Gilliam strain influenced the results, but we have no information that indicates whether the effect was mediated through the animals or the volunteers.

Discussion

These observations suggest that under appropriate circumstances man develops scrub typhus when injected intradermally with the number of *Rickettsia tsutsugamushi* which constitute approximately one intraperitoneal infectious unit for the mouse. This fact prompted an examination of the literature for comparable studies dealing with other human pathogens which might be sufficiently detailed to permit determination of the human minimal infectious dose by 50 per cent end-point methods. A summary of the pertinent observations of others, analyzed in this fashion, is given in Table 3.

Table 3. Summary of Minimal Infective Dosages of Microbial Agents in Man

Infective agent	Number of microbial units required to infect man			Evidence of human infection	Laboratory method of quantitation of microbial units	Reference
	Number	Units	Route in man[a]			
R. tsutsugamushi	$\frac{1}{4}$ to 3	Mouse MID$_{50}$	I.D.		I.P. mouse titration	7
P. vivax	< 10	Trophozoites	I.V.		Microscopic count	8
S. meleagridis	40×10^6					8
S. anatum	4.7×10^6					9
S. newport	1.4×10^6			Clinical		9
S. derby	15×10^6	Organisms	Oral		Bacterial plate counts	9
S. bareilly	1.7×10^6					10
S. pullorum	1.3×10^9					11
Sh. paradysenteriae	2.5×10^9					
Poliomyelitis virus	$< 8.6 \times 10^2$	Mouse MLD$_{50}$	Oral	Laboratory[b]	I.C. mouse titration	12
West Nile virus	1.2×10^3	Mouse MLD$_{50}$	I.V. & I.M.	Laboratory	I.C. mouse titration	13

[a] I.D. = intradermal; I.V. = intravenous; I.M. = intramuscular.
[b] Infection demonstrated by isolation of virus or by development of neutralizing antibodies.

Among the agents listed in Table 3 other than *R. tsutsugamushi*, *Plasmodium vivax* required the lowest number of microbial units to induce disease in man. Boyd and Kitchen (7) demonstrated that 10 parasites, determined by direct microscopic examination, induced malaria in men when inoculated by the intravenous route. Of the pathogenic enteric organisms listed in Table 3, more than a million were required to induce illness in human beings according to the work of McCullough and Eisele (8, 9, 10) and of Shaughnessy and his coworkers (11). The only recorded instances available to us in which known numbers of microbial units of viral agents have consistently produced recognizable infection in man are those of Koprowski and his colleagues (12) with poliomyelitis virus and Southam and Moore (13) with West Nile virus. Clinical disease did not occur with either agent but evidence of infection was obtained either by isolation of virus or by demonstration of the development of specific neutralizing antibodies. It is of interest that less than 1,000 microbial units of poliomyelitis virus but more than 100,000,000 microbial units of West Nile virus were required to induce subclinical infection of man.

Although the literature abounds with much valuable information on accidental infection or purposeful inoculation of man with a variety of pathogenic agents, these reports do not provide definitive information on the minimal number of microbial units required to produce human infection. Because it is not feasible to review these observations at length, we hesitate to single out certain reports for specific mention. Nevertheless, the observations of Nicolle and Conseil on shigellosis in North Africa (14), Morales-Otero on brucellosis in Puerto Rico (15), Kawamura et al. on scrub typhus in Japan (16), Kreis on choriomeningitis in France (17), Smorodintsev on hemorrhagic nephroso-nephritis (epidemic hemorrhagic fever) in the U.S.S.R. (18), and Blanc et al. on Q fever in Morocco (19) are worthy of careful review by those interested in the problem.

Direct microscopic enumeration of plasmodia or plate counts of bacteria provide satisfactory methods for estimating the number of these organisms required to infect man by a given route. On the other hand, the microbial unit determined by titration in animals may, but probably does not, represent a single structural unit of the infectious agent. Examples known to virologists are legion in which the LD_{50} of a given virus suspension varies many fold when titered by different routes of inoculation in the same host, or when titered by the same route in different hosts. Moreover, the apparent infectivity of a preparation may be modified appreciably by the progressive adaptation of an agent to a new host. An example of this phenomenon occurred in the work of Sabin (20) on the dengue virus which originally produced striking clinical disease in man but no apparent illness in mice. After a number of passages in mice, it produced mild disease in this host but no clinically apparent illness in man although the latter became immune to unadapted virus. As a result, it is difficult to interpret the results of comparative studies on infectivity of different lines of dengue virus tested in human and rodent hosts.

The demonstration in this report of the equivalence of the infective dose of *R. tsutsugamushi* for man and for the mouse is perhaps subject to criticism since different routes of infection were used for the two hosts. Despite this objection, the work remains, to the best of our knowledge, the only study in the literature in which the infecting dose for man of a rickettsial agent has been defined with accuracy.

Summary

Data collected during the course of other studies have been assembled to yield an estimate of the minimal infective dose of *Rickettsia tsutsugamushi* for man. Despite the biological variations inherent in the methods employed, approximately a single mouse infectious dose of each of 3 different strains of this organism was capable of infecting man by intraderman inoculation.

Acknowledgments

The authors extend their thanks to the many volunteers who took part in the investigations from which this report is drawn and who cheerfully experienced the discomforts inherent in their service. To Dr. J. W. Field, Director of the Institute for Medical Research, Kuala Lumpur, to the entire staff of the Institute and to the Government of the Federation of Malaya, particularly the Medical Service, grateful acknowledgment is made for continued cooperation in making available the laboratory and clinical facilities required for these studies.

1955

James H. Gilford and Winston H. Price

Virulent-Avirulent Conversions of Rickettsia rickettsii in Vitro

In recent years studies on the factors influencing the stability of rickettsiae *in vitro* have found that the physiological state of these infectious agents markedly affects certain of their metabolic activities and biological properties. Bovarnick and Allen (1) discovered the phenomenon of reversible inactivation, in which the hemolytic and respiratory activities, infectivity, and toxicity of typhus rickettsiae were all lost as a consequence of freezing and thawing in isotonic saline; these activities were restored after incubation of rickettsiae for a short time in the presence of diphosphopyridine (DPN) and Coenzyme A. A similar but more complete type of reversible inactivation was obtained by Bovarnick and Allen (2) at 0°C. They later (3) described another form of the phenomenon, wherein typhus rickettsiae incubated at 36°C. in the absence of substrate exhibited loss of activities that could be prevented by the presence of adenosine triphosphate (ATP) or glutamate; only the latter was capable of restoring the lost activities, however. The cessation of rickettsial activities at 0°C. and 36°C. indicated that different metabolic patterns are involved, since different factors are required to prevent their loss or to restore them.

The findings of Gilford and Price reprinted here (1955) explain the mysterious fluctuations of virulence exhibited by the rickettsiae of Rocky Mountain spotted fever by correlating induced physiological changes in the infectious agent with pathogenicity. Several years previously Spencer and Parker (4) had noted that virulent *R. rickettsii* in the tick host became avirulent for guinea pigs after refrigeration but regained virulence if the ticks were warmed or fed on blood. The pertinent aspects of this phenomenon were reproduced *in vitro* by Gilford and Price. Virulent-to-avirulent conversion of *R. rickettsii* was accomplished in the presence of para-aminobenzoic acid (PABA), and reactivation to the virulent form by the addition of DPN or Coenzyme A. The loss and restoration of *R. rickettsii* virulence for the guinea pig closely resemble the reversible inactivation of typhus rickettsiae described by Bovarnick and Allen except that *R. rickettsii* remains virulent for chick embryos but the typhus rickettsiae, under similar conditions, do not. Gilford and Price also showed a correlation between rickettsial virulence for guinea pigs and adsorption of rickettsiae onto guinea pig tunica cells *in vitro*, and the role of certain organic metabolites in promoting attachment of the infectious agent to cells. These provocative and important findings, though they have been cited extensively in the scientific literature and have gained a measure of acceptance, still await independent confirmation.

Studies like these have enlarged our comprehension of the biology of rickettsiae. They have helped to elucidate some of the metabolic patterns operating in the rickettsial cell and confirmed the close relation between metabolic activities, rickettsial invasiveness, and varied manifestations of virulence. The accumulation of fundamental information on the biochemical reactivity of rickettsiae is applicable also to understanding the epidemiology of these infections and the mode of action of chemotherapeutic agents.

Earlier reports (1, 2) from this laboratory have demonstrated that virulent strains of *Rickettsia rickettsii*, the etiological agent of Rocky Mountain spotted fever (RMSF), exist under certain conditions in an avirulent phase in its arthropod vector, *Dermacentor andersoni*. This phase is virulent for chick embryos but avirulent for guinea pigs and many other laboratory animals (2). Previous experiments also showed that temperature (1, 3) and the molting process (2) of the arthropod were important in controlling the virulence of the rickettsiae in the arthropod vector. The correlation between the virulent-to-avirulent changes and the epidemiological behavior of *R. rickettsii* has been discussed previously (2).

In this paper is reported (a) the *in vitro* conversion of virulent *R. rickettsii* to an avirulent state by para-amino-benzoic acid (PABA); (b) the *in vitro* reactivation or conversion of the PABA-avirulent and arthropod-avirulent rickettsiae (1) to the virulent form by the addition of Coenzyme I (CoI) or Coenzyme A (CoA); and (c) the observation that the state of virulence for guinea pigs parallels the adsorptivity of *R. rickettsii* to minced guinea pig tunica.

Results

In Vitro Conversion of Virulent R. rickettsii *to an Avirulent State by PABA.* In Table 1 are given the results of a typical experiment in which a 10 per cent virulent yolk sac suspension of *R. rickettsii* (1) in sucrose-phosphate-glutamate (SPG) solution (4) was incubated at 25°C. for 60 hours with 5 mg./ml. of PABA. Although in the absence of PABA the egg infectivity of the agent was lost by the incubation, in the presence of PABA 4 of the 6 logs of egg infectivity survived but the material failed to produce RMSF in guinea pigs.* Parahydroxybenzoic acid (POB), CoI, and CoA mixed with PABA prevented this loss of virulence. POB is known (5) to reverse the rickettsiostatic effect of PABA. CoII could not replace CoI under the conditions shown in Table 1.

* One egg LD_{50} of the virulent phase is approximately equal to 1 guinea pig ID_{50} as determined by clinical symptoms [see reference (6)].

Virulent-Avirulent Conversions

Table 1. Effect of POB, CoI, and CoA on PABA-treated Ricksettsiae

Sample[a]	(Addition (mg./ml.)	Titer after 60-hour incubation (egg LD_{50})	Spotted fever in guinea pigs[a]	Adsorption to guinea pig tunica (egg LD_{50})[b]
1. Virulent phase	None	$< 10^{0.5}$	0/6	—
2. Virulent phase	5.0 PABA	$10^{4.3}$	0/6	$< 10^{0.5}$
3. Virulent phase	5.0 PABA + 2.0 POB	$10^{4.5}$	6/6	$10^{2.3}$
4. Virulent phase	2.0 POB	$10^{3.6}$	6/6	$10^{2.3}$
5. Virulent phase	5.0 PABA + 0.5 CoI	$10^{4.6}$	6/6	$10^{2.5}$
6. Virulent phase	5.0 PABA + 0.3 CoA	$10^{4.2}$	6/6	$10^{2.3}$

[a] Numerator shows number of guinea pigs developing spotted fever. All guinea pigs except those of sample 1 received approximately $10^{3.0}$ egg LD_{50} intraperitoneally [see reference (6)]. All samples were incubated 60 hours at room temperature before being inoculated into the animals. The initial titer was $10^{6.5}$ egg LD_{50} before incubation.

[b] Guinea pig tunica was minced into approximately 1.0-mm. pieces and washed 4 times with Hanks' solution. Samples weighing 0.5 gm. were put into 25-ml. Erlenmeyer flasks, and 2.0 ml. of inoculum containing the appropriate rickettsial suspensions after the 6-hour incubation period were pipetted into each flask and shaken gently at room temperature for 90 minutes. The titer of each inoculum was approximately $10^{4.0}$ egg LD_{50}. After a 90-minute adsorption period the tissues in the various flasks were washed 4 times with 10 ml. of SPG solution. No rickettsiae were detected in the final wash fluid as determined by egg titration (6). The various samples were then ground in a mortar in a total volume of 5 ml. of SPG solution, centrifuged at 800 × g for 5 minutes, and the supernatant fluid then titered in chick embryos (6). The addition of CoI to the avirulent phase results in as many rickettsiae being adsorbed to guinea pig tunica as are found when fully virulent rickettsiae are studied. When 100 egg LD_{50} of the virulent phase was injected intraperitoneally along with 5 mg. of PABA, the guinea pigs developed typical spotted fever. As a further control, 10 per cent normal yolk sac was incubated with 5 mg of PABA for 60 hours. At this time 10 egg LD_{50} of the virulent phase was added to the suspension, mixed well, and injected intraperitoneally. The guinea pigs developed typical spotted fever. It is clear that the avirulence of sample 2 cannot be due to PABA being carried over in the inoculating suspension.

After reactivation had taken place, the suspensions could be diluted 1000-fold and still cause RMSF when injected into guinea pigs. Since these conversions in virulence take place *in vitro* and occur under conditions which are unfavorable for rickettsial multiplication, it would appear that more than 99 per cent of the viable organisms are concerned in these transformations. If as little as 3 egg LD_{50} of the virulent rickettsiae are mixed with 100 egg LD_{50} of the PABA-treated avirulent suspensions, the injection of such suspensions into guinea pigs results in RMSF.

In Vitro Reactivation or Conversion of Tick Avirulent to Virulent R. rickettsii.

Table 2. Effect of CoI, CoA, and POB on the Virulence of the Tick Avirulent Phase

Sample	Additions (mg./ml.)	Titer after 6-hour incubation (egg LD_{50})	Spotted fever in guinea Pigs[a]	Adsorption to guinea pig tunica (egg LD_{50})[b]
1. Avirulent phase	None	$10^{3.5}$	0/6	$< 10^{0.5}$
2. Avirulent phase	0.500 CoI	$10^{4.3}$	6/6	$10^{2.3}$
3. Avirulent phase	0.300 CoA	$10^{3.7}$	6/6	$10^{1.6}$
4. Avirulent phase	2.0 POB	$10^{4.6}$	0/6	$< 10^{0.5}$
5. Virulent phase	None	$10^{3.5}$	6/6	$10^{2.1}$
6. Virulent phase	2.0 POB	$10^{4.5}$	6/6	$10^{2.4}$

[a] Numerator shows number of guinea pigs injected intraperitoneally with $10^{3.5}$ egg LD_{50} of the various samples which developed spotted fever. Samples 1–6 were incubated 6 hours at 30°C. before being injected into the animals. Similar results were obtained if the suspensions were diluted 100-fold and injected into guinea pigs. The initial titer before incubation was $10^{5.6}$ egg LD_{50} in all samples, 50 ticks being ground in 50.0 ml. of SPG solution. The incubation period is necessary for the conversion of the avirulent tick suspension to the virulent phase. If CoI is added to the avirulent tick preparation and this suspension immediately inoculated intraperitoneally into guinea pigs, the rickettsiae remain avirulent and the guinea pigs develop no clinical symptoms of RMSF.

[b] The adsorption experiments were carried out as described in Table 1.

Table 2 illustrates the results of experiments in which tick avirulent rickettsiae (1) were incubated 6 hours at 25°C. with CoI or CoA. With either coenzyme the rickettsial agent took on the properties of the virulent phase for guinea pigs. Incubation with POB did not produce virulent rickettsiae. Experiments not shown here, with various preparations of CoI, showed that their capacity to convert the avirulent to virulent rickettsiae paralleled the CoI activity.

In addition, destruction of the CoI with snake venom pyrophosphatase† also destroyed the material which changed the avirulent into the virulent form. All this is strong evidence that CoI (6) is the active component in the *in vitro* conversion mechanism. This is of interest in view of the stimulatory effect of this coenzyme on the respiratory of *R. rickettsii* (6). Bovarnick and Allen (7) reported that CoI and CoA increase the infectivity of the E strain of *R. prowazeki* for both eggs and animals under conditions of freezing and thawing which had destroyed its infectivity. This situation is different from the reactivation of *R.*

† Pyrophosphatase was kindly supplied by Dr. G. Rafter. The CoI in most experiments was 95 per cent pure and was obtained from the Nutritional Biochemicals Corporation, Cleveland, Ohio. The CoA was obtained from the same firm and was 75 per cent pure.

rickettsii in that the avirulent phase of *R. rickettsii* is virulent for chick embryos (1).

In Vitro Conversion with Normal Tick Extracts. When normal (un-infected) adult ticks are incubated at 35°C. for 24 hours and then ground up, the suspension will raise the virulence of *R. rickettsii* under the conditions described in Table 2. This same is true for normal nymphs that have received a blood meal. No such activity can be found in ticks kept at low temperatures. Thus, from those two phases of *D. andersoni* in which reactivation takes place naturally, it is possible to prepare extracts which will duplicate the reactivation *in vitro*. Since the various phases of the tick life-cycle are under the control of one or more molting hormones, it is suggested that this probably plays a direct or indirect role in the formation of the active metabolites which convert the rickettsiae from one form to another, since it has been shown that the virulence of *R. rickettsii* is decreased when a nymph of *D. andersoni* infected with a virulent strain of *R. rickettsii* molts to the adult stage (2), and this low virulent phase can be raised to a more virulent phase by the addition of tick extracts as described above.

Relationship of Virulence to Adsorption. Since the virulent strains of *R. rickettsii* grow very well in the tunica of guinea pigs, a suspension of minced guinea pig tunica was used to test the adsorption of the various rickettsial preparations. The results are shown in Tables 1 and 2. It may be seen that the avirulent phase showed very low adsorption to the minced tunica and that whenever the virulence increased, as shown by the production of disease in guinea pigs, the adsorption to tunica suspensions increased. This suggests that the avirulence is due to failure to adsorb, and apparently this requires CoI or CoA or perhaps other biological materials.

Conclusion

The above results suggest, first, that the changes in virulence of *R. rickettsii* can be produced *in vitro* and need not be due to selection, mutation (in the usual sense of the word), or a combination of these two factors, since they take place under conditions which are considered unfavorable for rickettsial multiplication. Furthermore, the results show that more than 99 per cent of the organisms are involved in these virulence changes. Second, the data also indicate that the organic metabolic compounds, CoI, CoA, PABA, and POB, affect the attachment of *R. rickettsii* to guinea pig tunica, and, if the rickettsiae cannot attach, they obviously cannot infect a host cell. Such information might prove useful in a search for chemotherapeutic agents against rickettsiae and large viruses. Third, the results show that the virulence of an arthropod-borne microparasite can be modified by specific metabolic substance(s) formed by the arthropod and that the formation of this substance(s) may be under the control of a hormone of the arthropod.

This work was supported by Contract No. Nonr-248(44) between the Office of Naval Research and Johns Hopkins University, under the direction of W. H. Price.

1956

M. G. P. Stoker and P. Fiset

Phase Variation of the Nine Mile and Other Strains
of Rickettsia burneti

Phase variation of *Coxiella burnetii* (i.e., *Rickettsia burneti*) probably constitutes the only present known example of a distinct, reproducible genetic variation among rickettsiae. The discovery of this phenomenon evolved gradually from observations of the wide variations exhibited by strains of *C. burnetii* in their complement-fixing activity. Stoker and Fiset were instrumental in clarifying and defining phase variation of *C. burnetii*—the term applies to the reversible adaptation of the rickettsial strains. Freshly isolated strains from man, animals, or ticks were considered to be in phase 1; strains passed in eggs were in phase 2. Strains in phase 1 did not react in the complement fixation test with early antibody but were able to evoke both early and late antibodies in animals, whereas egg-adapted phase 2 strains reacted with both antibodies in the complement fixation test. A reversal from an egg-adapted strain of phase 2 to phase 1 could be induced by one or more passages in adult animals. The interest stimulated by this phenomenon considerably advanced our knowledge of the surface antigens of *C. burnetii* and their range of reactivity (1).

The phase variation phenomenon assumed practical importance when it was related to the protective potency of Q fever vaccines. Ormsbee, Bell, Lackman, and Tallent (2) demonstrated that Q fever vaccines made from *C. burnetii* in phase 1 were immunologically superior to phase 2 vaccines. The former induced a 100- to 300-fold greater protective potency for guinea pigs than the latter. The data amassed from experimental studies helped to explain the significant differences in protective potencies of Q fever vaccines made from different strains on the basis of phase differences rather than strain differences. Studies on phase variation of strains of *C. burnetii* are fundamental to the preparation of an effective vaccine for protection against Q fever infection. The techniques for identifying and manipulating the phases may be relevant in the development of efficacious vaccines against other rickettsial diseases.

Introduction

Several authors have reported that strains of *Rickettsia burneti* from different sources vary in their serological behavior (1, 7, 12). Those which have been studied may be broadly divided into two groups according to their activity in complement fixation tests: group 1, strains such as Henzerling and Nine Mile, which although not identical (11) yield antigens which react well with guinea pig sera prepared against homologous and heterologous strains of *R. burneti* and with antisera from a wide range of naturally infected animals; group 2, strains such as the Panama (2) and Konitzer (1), which unless used in high concentration react poorly with all antisera, including those which show high titers with Henzerling or Nine Mile antigens.

Two strains of *R. burneti* isolated in Great Britain appeared at first to be in group 2 because antigens prepared from early yolk sac passages, although rich in rickettsiae, failed to react with homologous or heterologous antisera. After further egg adaptation, however, a change occurred and antigens made from the fifth and subsequent yolk sac passages resembled those made from the Henzerling and Nine Mile strains and reacted with a wide range of Q fever antisera (9, 10). This variation, which was not due to an increase in numbers of rickettsiae in the antigens, was confined to their behavior in fixation of complement with antibody. It did not extent to their agglutinability, either by Q fever antibody itself, or, after absorption of Q fever antibody, by anti-globulin serum (3).

A similar variation during egg adaptation was found by other workers [(6) and Berge, personal communication] and this raised the possibility that it might be of general application to *R. burneti*, and might account for some of the differences between strains in groups 1 and 2 described above, because the strains were not compared after an equal number of egg passages. If so, an admittedly good complement-fixing strain, such as the classical Nine Mile strain, would react poorly with antisera when the strain was in the early stages of egg adaptation.

The Nine Mile strain was isolated from ticks in Montana (5) and was later adapted to growth in yolk sacs (4). Since it yields antigens which react with antisera against many different strains of *R. burneti*, the Nine Mile strain is widely used for the routine diagnosis of Q fever. Most lines of this strain have already undergone numerous egg passages and are unsuitable for study of the early stages of egg adaptation; but one line of the Nine Mile strain has been maintained at the Rocky Mountain Laboratory, Montana, entirely by guinea pig passage.

We have studied the variability of this guinea pig adapted strain on passage in yolk sacs, and of other strains freshly isolated from ticks, sheep, and cows. We have also reversed the variation by passage of the egg-adapted strains in animals, and have investigated the antibody response of man and guinea pigs with antigens prepared from strains in different stages of the variation.

Phase Variation of Rickettsia burneti

For convenience we refer to strains as being in phase 1, when in the early stages of egg adaptation they react poorly with complement-fixing antibody; and in phase 2, when, after further passage in yolk sacs, they react well with such antibody. The phenomenon in general is referred to as phase variation.

Methods and Materials

For passage of strains in animals, fully grown guinea pigs, weighing 300 to 500 gm., were inoculated peritoneally with 2 ml. quantities of the appropriate suspensions of yolk sac, or of spleen from previously inoculated animals. Hamsters were similarly inoculated with 1 ml. and mice with 0.25 ml. of the suspensions. Ten per cent horse serum in tryptic digest broth was used as diluent throughout. The methods of yolk sac inoculation, passage in fertile hens' eggs, and preparation of antigens from yolk sac suspensions by ether extraction and differential centrifugation were those already described (10).

Serological Tests

Human antisera were obtained from patients, including the patient from whom the Christie strain had originally been isolated, at varying times after an attack of Q fever; guinea pig antisera were obtained by cardiac puncture. After separation from the clot, antisera were stored at $-20°C.$, and were heated to $60°C.$ before testing.

Complement fixation tests were carried out by the standard technique used in this laboratory (11). Most of the antigens were tested by titrating increasing doubling dilutions of the antigen with increasing doubling dilutions of homologous antiserum in the presence of two minimal hemolytic doses of complement. Such titrations with graded concentrations of antigen as well as of antiserum, are referred to as chessboard titrations. In Figs. 1, 2, and 3 these chessboard titrations are recorded pictorially. The four antigen dilutions on the vertical scales range from 1:10 to 1:80. The antiserum dilutions on the horizontal scales start at 1:10 and finish at 1:1280 for the Nine Mile antiserum and at 1:320 for the Christie antiserum.

Strains of R. burneti

The Christie strain was described in previous communications (9, 10). The Nine Mile strain, as used for routine preparation of diagnostic antigen, was received as lyophilized yolk sac suspension from Dr. Cox of the Lederle Laboratories in 1949, after 50 or more egg passages. This egg-adapted line, which reacts well with a variety of Q fever antisera, is referred to as the NM (Led) strain.

The guinea-pig-adapted line of the Nine Mile strain was received from Dr. Lackman of the Rocky Mountain Laboratory as lyophilized spleen suspension from the 307th guinea pig passage. This line, which had never been passaged in eggs, is referred to as the NM (Rocky) strain.

The source of other, freshly isolated, strains is given below.

Standardization of Rickettsial Concentration

When comparing the behavior of various rickettsial suspensions as antigens, it is obviously important that the concentration of organisms in each suspension should be approximately the same. Since the organisms do not obviously vary in size, and, judging by direct and electron microscopy, there is practically no extraneous material in the final preparation, the antigens were matched by opacity in a photo-electric densitometer with an NM (Led) strain antigen containing 31.3 mgm. of nitrogen per 100 ml. as a standard.

To find whether antigens matched by this method contained approximately equal numbers of rickettsiae, direct counts were made of the organisms in eight selected antigens using the electron microscope technique of Williams and Backus (13). The numbers of rickettsiae in the matched antigens were found to lie between 2×10^{13} and 3×10^{13} per ml.; differences of this order did not affect the significance of results obtained in the complement fixation tests.

Results

Variation of the Nine Mile Strain

The lyophilized material from the 307th guinea pig passage of the NM (Rocky) strain was inoculated into guinea pigs; spleens taken during the febrile period in this 308th guinea pig passage were then inoculated as 10 per cent suspensions into yolk sacs of fertile hens' eggs. The embryos died 11 days later and the smears from the yolk sacs showed a profuse growth of rickettsiae. Antigens prepared from these yolk sacs were tested for fixation of complement, in chessboard titrations with homologous guinea pig antiserum taken 21 days after inoculation with the NM (Rocky) strain in the form of infected guinea pig spleen suspension. Stock antigen prepared from the egg-adapted NM (Led) strain was also tested with the same antiserum.

Phase Variation of Rickettsia burneti

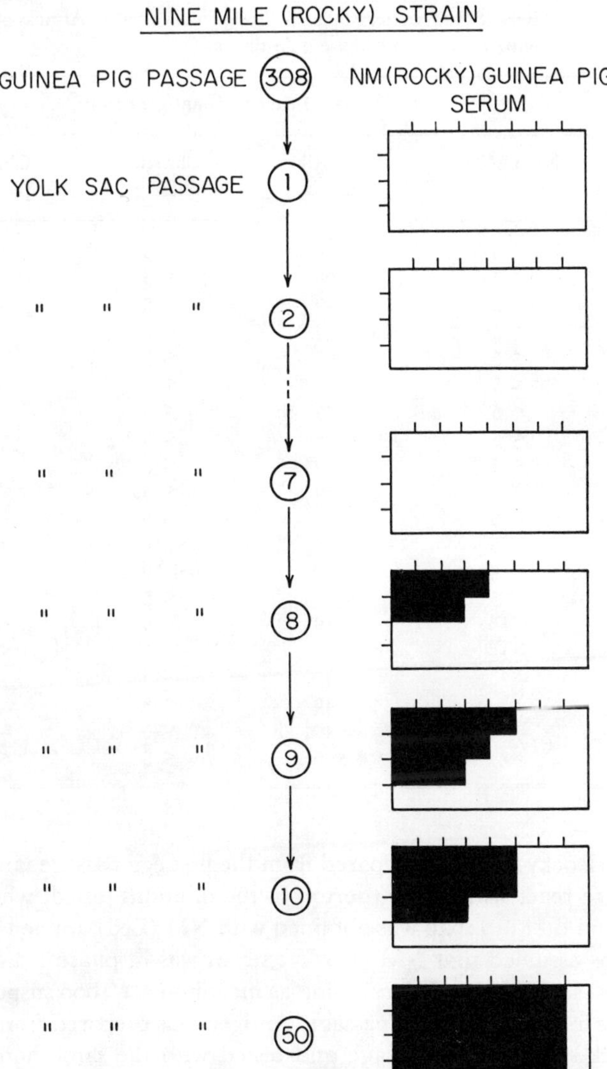

Fig. 1. *The effect of successive yolk sac passage on antigens from the Nine Mile (Rocky) guinea-pig-adapted strain of* R. burneti, *tested by complement fixation with homologous guinea pig antiserum. (For explanation of the diagrams, see Methods, Serological Tests.)*

Table 1. Complement Fixation Titers of Human Sera taken at Long Intervals after Attacks of Q Fever, with Phase 1 and Phase 2 Antigens

Serum obtained (years after illness)	Reciprocal of titer with antigens from			
	Nine Mile phase 1	Nine Mile phase 2	Christie phase 1	Christie phase 2
1	5	160	5	160
1	< 5	80	< 5	80
1	< 5	20	< 5	10
2	< 5	40	< 5	20
2	< 5	20	< 5	10
2	< 5	10	< 5	< 5
3	< 5	40	< 5	20
3	< 5	< 5	< 5	< 5
4	< 5	80	< 5	20
4	< 5	80	< 5	20
4	< 5	40	< 5	20
4	< 5	20	< 10	10
4	< 5	20	< 10	10
4	< 5	< 10	< 5	< 5
4	NT[a]	< 10	< 5	< 5
4	NT	< 5	< 5	< 5
12	NT	40	10	40
12	NT	40	< 5	20
14	NT	40	< 5	10
14	NT	< 5	< 5	< 5

[a] NT = Not tested.

NM (Rocky) antigen prepared from the first egg passage failed completely to react with the antiserum in the dilutions tested, whereas an antiserum titer of 1:640 was obtained with NM (Led) antigen (Fig. 1).

It was assumed that NM (Rocky) strain was in phase 1 and it was passaged serially in yolk sacs, using as inoculum a 1/1000 suspension of yolk sac from the previous passage. Antigen was prepared from four or five yolk sacs at each passage and tested with the same homologous guinea pig antiserum. At the eighth passage the antigen reacted with the antiserum and in subsequent passages the degree of complement fixation increased, but was not as marked as that shown by the NM (Led) antigen prepared from the 50th or greater yolk sac passage (Table 1). In a later experiment, however, yolk sac passages were carried out with a more concentrated inoculum, diluted 1 in 10 instead of 1 in 1000, starting at the sixth passage in the original series.

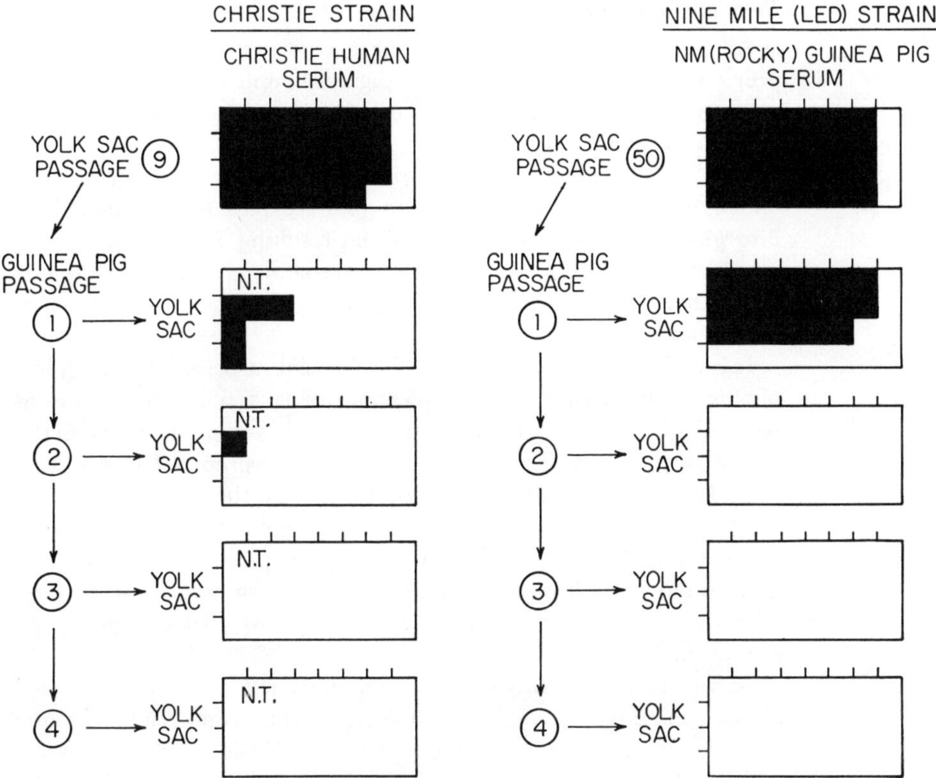

Fig. 2. The effect of successive guinea pig passage on antigens from the egg-adapted Christie strain of R. burneti, *tested by complement fixation with human convalescent serum; and from the egg-adapted Nine Mile (Led) strain, tested with homologous guinea pig antiserum. (For explanation of the diagrams, see Methods, Serological Tests.)*

This led, from the eighth passage, to the development of antigens closely resembling those prepared from the NM (Led) strain.

When the antigens were tested with other antisera, for example, from guinea pigs inoculated with NM (Led) strain, or with Christie strain human antiserum, similar results were obtained.

Thus it is clear that the Nine Mile strain, like the Christie strain, is subject to the variation and changes from phase 1 to phase 2 when passaged in yolk sacs.

Reversal of the Variation

All the strains found to be in phase 1 on first growth in eggs had previously been passaged in guinea pigs. Attempts were therefore made to reverse the variation by inoculation of egg-adapted phase 2 strains into guinea pigs.

Yolk sac suspensions of the Christie strain in its ninth egg passage, and of the NM (Led) strain in its 50th (or more) passage, were inoculated into guinea pigs. At the height of the resulting febrile response the guinea pigs were killed and 10 per cent suspensions of spleens were used for further passage. Five guinea pig passages of the two strains were carried out.

It is difficult to make satisfactory rickettsial suspensions from guinea pig tissues for testing the complement-fixing activity of the strains. Accordingly, some of the spleen suspension at each passage was used to inoculate yolk sacs, from which antigens were prepared in the usual way. The validity of this procedure depends on the assumption that if the strains had reverted to phase 1 in the guinea pigs, one yolk sac passage would not be sufficient for reversion to phase 2. These antigens, derived indirectly from each successive guinea pig passage, were tested with the corresponding Christie human or NM (Rocky) guinea pig antiserum (Fig. 2).

Before inoculation into guinea pigs both the egg-adapted strains were in phase 2 and reacted well with homologous antiserum. When reisolated from the first guinea pig passage at the acute febrile stage and grown in yolk sacs, they were still reacting partly as phase 2 strains. From the second guinea pig passage onwards, however, the Nine Mile strain had reverted completely to phase 1 and the Christie strain almost completely.

After five guinea pig passages the NM (Led) strain, now in phase 1, was readapted to yolk sacs, and seven passages were needed for reversion to phase 2. Thus the behavior in yolk sacs of the strain after five guinea pig passages was much the same as that found with the NM (Rocky) strain after 308 guinea pig passages.

When material for passage was taken early in the course of infection of the animals, at the height of the febrile response, the change from phase 2 to phase 1 occurred at the second or third guinea pig passage. Since *R. burneti* persists for long periods in the tissues of guinea pigs it seemed possible that the reversion might occur in the first passage if reisolation from the animals was delayed sufficiently. Accordingly Christie ninth-egg-passage material in phase 2 was inoculated into a

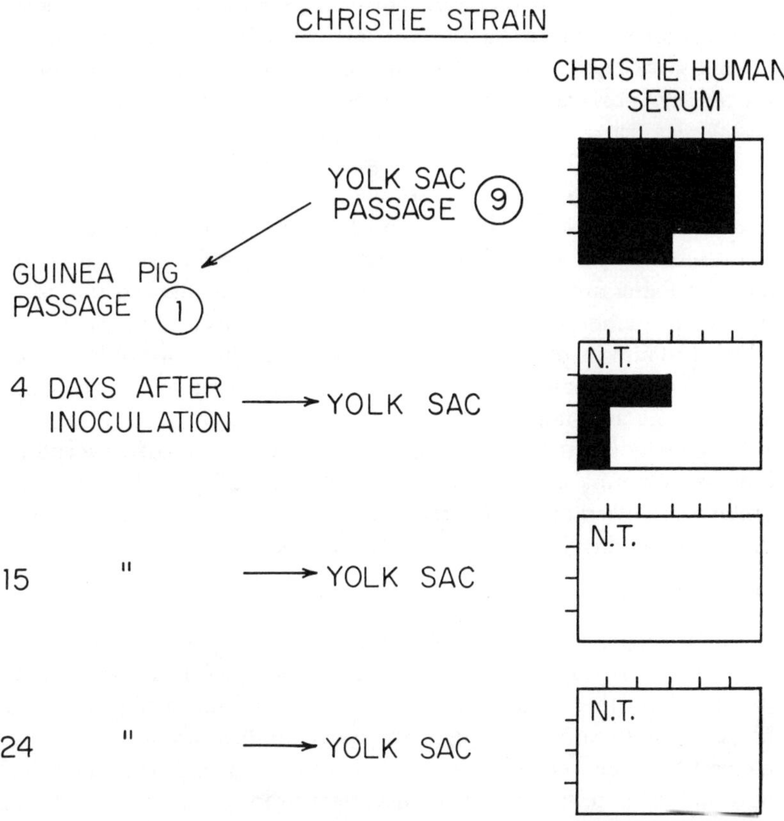

Fig. 3. The change in complement fixation with human convalescent serum by antigens from the egg-adapted strain of R. burneti, *reisolated at intervals during the course of infection in the guinea pig. (For explanation of the diagrams, see Methods, Serological Tests).*

number of guinea pigs. At successive intervals after inoculation, animals were killed, and spleen suspensions inoculated into yolk sacs for preparation of antigen. Reversion to phase 1 occurred in rickettsiae isolated from the guinea pigs 15 days or more after inoculation or 11 days after the acute febrile period (Fig. 3).

Since growth of the rickettsiae in the guinea pig led to reversion from phase 2 to phase 1, attempts were made to cause reversion in other animals. Hamsters and mice were inoculated with Christie strain in the ninth egg passage, in phase 2. Thirty days after inoculation pooled spleen suspensions from hamsters or mice were inoculated into batches of yolk sacs. There was insufficient growth for antigen preparation in the first egg passage from either species of animal, so a further yolk sac passage was carried out. Tests on antigens prepared from these second passage yolk sacs showed that, after growth for 30 days there had been complete reversion to phase 1 in mice and almost complete reversion to phase 1 in hamsters. Abinanti and Marmion (personal communication), who for other purposes devised a technique for preparing complement-fixing antigens direct from mouse spleens, showed that after mouse inoculation with a phase 1 strain the spleens contain rickettsiae which are also in phase 1, demonstrating that the phase 1 state does occur in the animals themselves and is not limited solely to the early stages of egg adaptation.

We conclude that *R. burneti* exists in phase 1 when grown in susceptible laboratory animals, and only alters to phase 2 after fairly prolonged growth in yolk sacs. In this state it reverts to phase 1 again almost immediately after inoculation into the animals.

State of Naturally Occurring Strains of R. burneti

The biological significance of phase variation depends on the phases in which the organisms exist in their natural hosts. Strains are usually isolated from these sources by inoculation into guinea pigs, mice, or hamsters, and passage in these laboratory animals would in any case convert them into phase 1. To determine the original state of the strain it would be necessary to make an antigen from the natural source of material, or to isolate the strain by direct yolk sac inoculation and to test the antigenic behavior at an early passage. Strains from ticks, cows, and sheep were tested by the latter method.

A suspension of 371 adult and nymphal ticks (*Haemaphysalis punctata*), collected in Kent and known to be infective for guinea pigs at a dilution of 10^{-4}, was mixed with 1000 units of penicillin per milliliter and inoculated directly into yolk sacs of fertile hens' eggs. Cows' milk known to be infective for guinea pigs was also mixed with penicillin and inoculated directly into yolk sacs. Both these strains grew sufficiently for the preparation of antigens from yolk sacs in the first passage.

A 20 per cent suspension of a placenta from a Kentish sheep, known to contain $10^{4.5}$ guinea pig infective doses of *R. burneti* per gram was filtered through a gradocol membrane with an average pore diameter of 0.7 μ, and the filtrate was inoculated into yolk sacs. There were not sufficient rickettsiae for an antigen preparation in the first yolk sac passage, but antigen was made from the second passage of this strain.

Antigens from first passage yolk sacs of the tick and milk strains and second passage yolk sacs of the sheep placenta strain, tested with high titer NM (Rocky) guinea pig antiserum, were all in phase 1.

Antibody Response in Man and Guinea Pigs

Smadel and his colleagues (8) showed that antibodies to the poorly complement-fixing strains of *R. burneti* eventually appeared in guinea pig sera two months or more after inoculation. Berge and Lennette (1) confirmed this, and found similar antibodies in pools of human sera taken 16 to 28 months, but not in the first six weeks, after natural infection.

Guinea pig and human sera were studied to find whether antigens from strains in phase 1, although not reacting with antisera taken at the usual time, three to five weeks, after infection, would nevertheless fix complement with antibody appearing much later in the immune response. Guinea pigs inoculated with the NM (Rocky) strain in phase 1 in the form of guinea pig spleen suspension were bled at frequent intervals during a five month period. The sera were tested with phase 1 antigens prepared from the second yolk sac passage of the NM (Rocky) strain, or the third yolk sac passage of the Christie strain, and phase 2 antigens from the 50th (or more) passage of the NM (Led) strain, or the 10th yolk sac passage of the Christie strain.

Instead of chessboard titrations the sera were tested with the optimum antigen dilution of the phase 2 antigens, as previously determined by chessboard titration with standard antisera (11), and with phase 1 antigens in an equivalent rickettsial concentration.

In all guinea pigs there was a rapid rise of phase 2 antibody, reaching a peak in the second week after inoculation and then declining, but persisting at a lower level at least until the end of the experiment. Phase 1 antibodies also appeared but were not detectable until five to six weeks after inoculation, increasing until the 10th week and then persisting at about the same level as the phase 2 antibodies. Figure 4 exemplifies the antibodies detected by the four antigens.

The only homologous human serum available was that obtained from the patient infected with the Christie strain. Specimens taken up to four months after the illness were tested; no antibody was detectable up to this time with phase 1 Christie antigen, even in sera with a titer of 1:320 with the phase 2 Christie antigen.

Serum from other patients collected after longer intervals, ranging

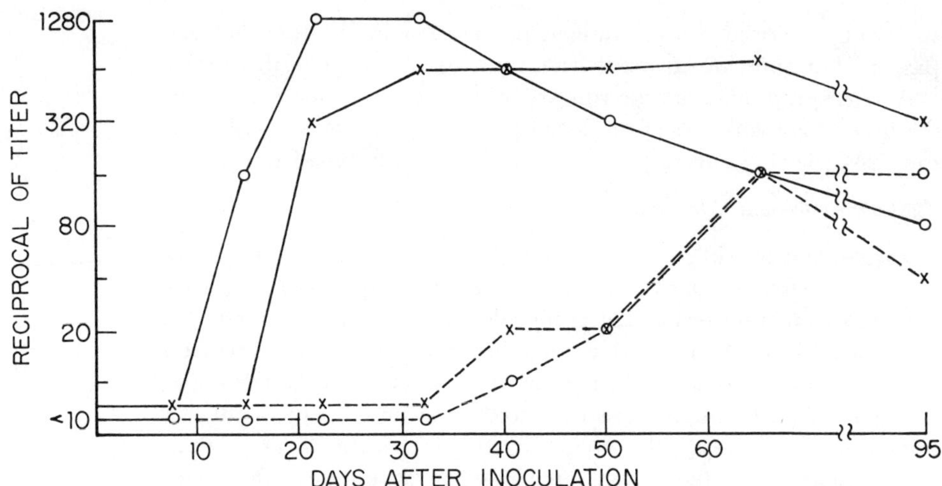

Fig. 4. Phase 1 and phase 2 complement-fixing antibodies in the serum of a guinea pig inoculated with the Nine Mile (Rocky) strain of R. burneti *in phase 1.* ○ – – – ○ *Titers with Nine Mile phase 1 antigen.* ○———○ *Titers with Nine Mile phase 2 antigen.* × – – – × *Titers with Christie phase 1 antigen.* ×———× *Titers with Christie phase 2 antigen.*

from 1 to 14 years after attacks of Q fever, were tested with phase 1 and phase 2 antigens (Table 1). Although most patients had phase 2 antibody only one had phase 1 antibody at 1:10.

One hundred and eleven sera from a flock of naturally infected sheep were tested with a phase 1 antigen from the second yolk sac passage of a strain freshly isolated from the placenta of one of the sheep. Only two of the sera reacted at 1:10, although 32 sera were positive at 1:10 and higher dilutions with antigen prepared from the egg-adapted Henzerling strain.

Identification of Phase 1 and Phase 2 Strains with Early and Late Antisera

It is clear that strains in phase 1 cannot be identified positively as *R. burneti* by testing antigens with stock guinea pig antiserum obtained up to six weeks after inoculation with known strains, or with sera from human patients known to have suffered from Q fever.

Guinea pig serum taken six or more weeks after inoculation containing antibody reacting with phase 1 strains, however, could be used for confirming that the organisms were in fact *R. burneti*. We subsequently discovered that phase 1 antibodies develop in the rabbit more quickly and to higher levels than in the guinea pig; late rabbit antiserum taken six weeks or more after inoculation contained phase 1 antibody in high titer and was especially suitable for identification of phase 1 strains (Fiset, unpublished). Antigens were therefore tested with both early guinea pig serum and late rabbit serum. The tests confirmed that the organism was *R. burneti*, and also allowed the phase to be identified.

Discussion

Our evidence suggests that the variation in serological behavior first observed during egg passage of two English strains may be widely applicable to *R. burneti*. A guinea-pig-adapted line of the Nine Mile strain, obtained from the Rocky Mountain Laboratory, was found to be in phase 1 when first grown in eggs. That is, antigens prepared from early egg passages failed to react with Q fever antisera in complement fixation tests, in marked contrast to the egg-adapted line of the Nine Mile strain routinely used for producing diagnostic antigen. After eight yolk sac passages of the guinea-pig-adapted Nine Mile strain, however, it altered in serological behavior to phase 2, the antigens then reacting satisfactorily with Q fever antisera. This variation of the strain at the eighth passage resembled that found with the Christie (human) strain at the fifth yolk sac passage, or in an earlier experiment between the sixth and eleventh passages, also that occurring with the MI (milk) strain at about the fifth passage, and Herzberg and Urbach's German strains after the 14th or 15th yolk sac passage (6). Similar changes with other strains have also been found by Berge (personal communication). Three additional strains from cows' milk, sheep's placenta, and ticks were also tested by direct inoculation into yolk sacs without intermediate guinea pig passage; all were in phase 1.

It is therefore probable that the strains which are used routinely for preparing stock antigens, and which react so well with Q fever antisera, may all be laboratory variants in phase 2 obtained through multiple yolk sac passage. This view is consistent with the rapid reversion to phase 1 which occurs when these egg-adapted strains are inoculated into either guinea pigs, mice, or hamsters. It should, in fact, be possible to account for some of the previously reported differences between strains as due to variation in the degree of adaptation to growth in yolk sacs; and for the apparent differences in results obtained with the same strain, for example the Dyer strain, when tested in different laboratories (1, 7).

The number of yolk sac passages required for the change to phase 2 varied from 5 to at least 15. This may depend on inherent differences between strains, possibly connected with the source of the strain. The dilution at which the serial yolk sac passages are carried out might also alter the stage at which the variation becomes detectable. If the change is due to the gradual replacement of phase 1 organisms by a phase 2 variant, passage at high dilutions might eliminate the variant at the early stages, while it was still a rarity. Attempts to maintain strains in phase 1 by passage at limiting dilutions have not so far been successful owing to difficulties of titrating the organism in yolk sacs, but the change of the NM (Rocky) strain was certainly less complete when it was passaged at 1:1000 than when passaged at 1:10.

Although complement-fixing antibodies to phase 1 antigens were only occasionally found in low titer in man and sheep, there is a late development of phase 1 antibodies in guinea pigs, reaching a peak some seven to eight weeks after the phase 2 antibodies, and resembling the response found by Smadel and his colleagues (8) and Berge and Lennette (1) to antigens from strains of low sensitivity.

In some of its natural hosts and in laboratory animals, therefore, *R. burneti* exists in a form which is unable to react in complement fixation tests with the antibody produced against it, at least in the early phases of the hosts' immune response. Organisms which react well with this antibody are found only after prolonged growth in yolk sacs, where no such antibody is produced, and on reinoculation into animals they rapidly revert to the original state. It is tempting to postulate that the original organisms in phase 1 have a higher survival value than the phase 2 variant in animals, in the presence of antibody (or in ticks which may ingest antibody), but not in eggs.

It is also possible, however, that the failure of phase 1 strains to react with antibody is only an *in vitro* phenomenon, detectable by complement fixation tests alone. Further studies are now in progress on the antigenic differences between phase 1 and phase 2 organisms and their reactions with antisera *in vivo* as well as *in vitro*. These may throw further light on the biological significance, if any, of phase variation.

Acknowledgments

Thanks are due to Dr. H. R. Cox of Lederle Laboratories, New York, who supplied the egg-adapted Nine Mile strain, and to Dr. D. Lackman of the Rocky Mountain Laboratory, Hamilton, Montana, for the guinea-pig-adapted Nine Mile strain. We are also indebted to Dr. O'Connor of the Commonwealth Serum Laboratories, Melbourne, and to Dr. B. P. Marmion of the Public Health Laboratory Service (Great Britain) for information about the latter strain. We wish to thank Miss Z. Page for valuable laboratory assistance. The work was supported by a grant from the World Health Organization.

M. Schaechter, F. M. Bozeman and J. E. Smadel

Study on the Growth of Rickettsiae: II. Morphologic Observations of Living Rickettsiae in Tissue Culture Cells

With the simplification of techniques for the cultivation of cells *in vitro*, systems became available that were highly conducive to studies on the growth characteristics and on the physiological and morphological behavior of rickettsiae under defined and controlled conditions. Exemplifying the applicability of the cell culture system were the investigations carried out by Schaechter and associates on the mechanisms of rickettsiae replication. They clarified the mode of rickettsial multiplication by observing that single cells of *R. rickettsii* divided by transverse binary fission; this was recorded photomicrographically on three separate occasions. They noted also the mechanism by which rickettsiae escape from cells and the differences in the intracellular behavior between species of rickettsiae. Recently Anacker, Fukushi, Pickens, and Lackman (1) demonstrated numerous examples of binary fission of another rickettsia examined by electron micrographs during the phase of rapid replication: binary fission appeared to be an important replication mode, if not the only one, for *C. burnetii*. The evidence obtained from these studies supports the view that rickettsiae are more closely related to bacteria than to viruses.

Introduction

Morphological studies of intracellular rickettsiae have been limited to light or electron microscopic studies of fixed and stained material. These investigations have yielded useful information on the dimensions of the organisms and on their number and location within the host cells. Moreover, they have engendered hypotheses on the mechanism of rickettsial multiplication. Thus, Wolbach (1) stated that in smears of ticks infected with *Rickettsia rickettsi*, "appearances are found which would indicate that these rods divide by transverse fission." Subsequent authors using light microscopy supported this view (2, 3), as did those who employed electron microscopy (4).

In the present study, phase microscopy of infected tissue culture cells has provided a satisfactory system for morphological observations of living rickettsiae. Several aspects of the intracellular behavior of rickettsiae have been investigated and direct evidence has been obtained that these organisms divide by binary fission.

Materials and Methods

Cell strain. The 14pf strain of fibroblasts used throughout these studies was obtained from Dr. G. O. Gey in April 1953. The strain was derived in culture in 1938 from subcutaneous areolar tissue explanted from a normal rat. These cells characteristically grow as monocellular layers directly on glass (5).

Stock cultures of the 14pf line have been maintained by growing the cells on the wall of a 16- × 150-mm Pyrex tube containing 1 ml of fluid medium composed of the following:

Balanced salt solution (Gey and Gey, n. 21)	50%
Beef embryo extract (1:2 dilution of original)	10%
Horse serum	40%
Phenol red	0.005%
Penicillin	100 units per milliliter
Streptomycin	20 µg per milliliter

All constituents except the antibiotics were obtained from Microbiological Associates, Inc., Bethesda, Maryland. The tubes were stoppered with rubber plugs and rotated at 37° in a commercial roller drum (Wyble Engineering Development Corp.) at 12 revolutions per hour.

The nutrient fluid was renewed every 3 or 4 days and subcultures to new tubes were made every 2 or 3 weeks. At the time of subculture, colonies of cells adherent to the glass were removed with a curved-tip pipette, transferred to a petri dish and cut into fragments about 1 mm in diameter. Three or four of the explants were placed on the wall of a clean, sterile roller tube above the fluid level of the fresh medium. The tube was left standing upright in the incubator for about 20 minutes to allow the fragments to adhere, after which it was placed in the roller drum. A detailed description of these procedures was reported by Ehrmann and Gey (5).

In the present studies, colonies of cells were grown on 11- × 22-mm cover glasses in roller tubes. For this purpose, a cover glass was placed in a tube containing nutrient fluid and, after its surfaces were wet, it was pulled up above the fluid level. Two or three cut fragments of tissue were planted on the cover glass and when the explants had attached, the cover glass was immersed in the fluid medium. The tube was incubated in a roller drum.

Rickettsial strains. Egg-adapted lines of the Karp strain of *R. tsutsugamushi* and the Bitterroot strain of *R. rickettsi* were used in the current work. Tissue cultures of 14pf cells growing on cover glasses were inoculated with semipurified suspensions of rickettsiae obtained from infected yolk sac tissue in the manner described by Bozeman *et al.* (6).

Infection of tissue cultures. The rickettsial suspensions were added in 0.1-ml amounts to 14pf cultures which had been growing on cover glasses for 24 hours. The fluid was replaced the next day with fresh medium, and thereafter every 3 or 4 days. Because *R. rickettsi* is sensitive to the concentrations of penicillin and streptomycin normally employed (Bozeman *et al.*, 1956), the antibiotics were omitted from the medium when this organism was to be studied.

Preparation of chambers for phase microscopy. Chambers containing infected cultures were prepared in the following manner: two lines of paraffin-becswax mixture (1:2) were applied about 18 mm apart on a 1- × 3-inch microscope slide. A cover glass bearing the infected culture was inverted on these lines forming a bridge about 1 mm in depth. The air space between the slide and the cover glass was then filled with nutrient fluid with a capillary pipette and all the edges were sealed with the hot paraffin-beeswax mixture. Because of the highly infectious nature of the material, extreme care was employed during preparation of chambers; furthermore, the completed chamber was swabbed with 70 per cent ethanol before being moved from the contaminated area to the microscope. The chambers were maintained at 35° in a microscope stage incubator. These preparations could be observed for at least 24 hours before obvious damage to the cells was noted. After microscopic observations of the living cells had been completed, the cover glass was removed for fixation and staining of the cells. When *R. tsutsugamushi* was under study, Giemsa stain was employed; cultures infected with *R. rickettsi* were stained by the Macchiavello technique.

Microscopy. A Bausch and Lomb positive phase contrast microscope was used with a 97× (1.25 N.A.) achromatic objective and a 10× Leitz "Periplan" ocular. Illumination was provided by a Bausch and Lomb ribbon filament research lamp with a green filter (Wratten No. 58 or 61). Care was taken to avoid unnecessary exposure of the cultures to light although no harmful effects attributable to illumination were noted. Depending upon the experimental needs, pictures were taken at intervals of 1, 5, 10, or 15 minutes. A Leica camera outfitted with a Leitz Micro Ibso beam splitter and an extension tube was employed. The distance from the ocular to the film was 250 mm. Kodak Microfile film in 35-mm. rolls was used and exposures ranged from 3 to 12 seconds. The film was developed with Kodak Microdol for 12 minutes at 23°.

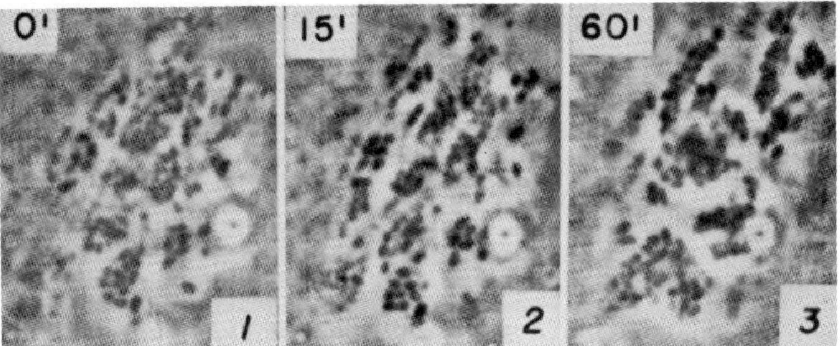

Figs. 1–3. A mass of Rickettsia tsutsugamushi *near the nucleus of a 14pf cell 8 days after infection. Rearrangement of the organisms within the cluster is illustrated over a 60-minute period. The nucleus is out of focus. Time is indicated in the upper left corner of each figure. Phase photomicrographs, magnification 2000 ×.*

Results

General observations. Rickettsiae in living tissue culture cells observed under the phase microscope were readily recognized because of 1) the presence in such infected cells of bacillary structures having the size and shape of rickettsiae, 2) an increase in numbers of these structures as infection progressed, and 3) the direct correlation between the morphology and localization of such structures seen in a given living cell under the phase microscope, and typical rickettsiae seen in the same cell viewed under the ordinary microscope after fixation and staining.

Rickettsiae observed in living cells displayed the typical polymorphism seen in fixed and stained preparations examined by light or electron microscopy. Some were short rods with rounded ends, others were elongated rods, and finally some were diplobacilli. The dimensions of living intracellular *R. tsutsugamushi* and *R. rickettsi,* exclusive of diplobacillary forms, were determined by direct measurement of 50 organisms of each species on photomicrographs of infected cells. The mean and standard deviation for the size of *R. tsutsugamushi* were 1.2 ± 0.35 μ × 0.65 ± 0.03 μ and for *R. rickettsi,* 1.5 ± 0.4 μ × 0.55 ± 0.06 μ. These dimensions are similar to those ordinarily given for these organisms (7).

Rickettsiae could not be recognized with certainty under the phase microscope until the organisms were fairly numerous, usually 3 or 4 days after infection of the tissue culture cells. This was especially true

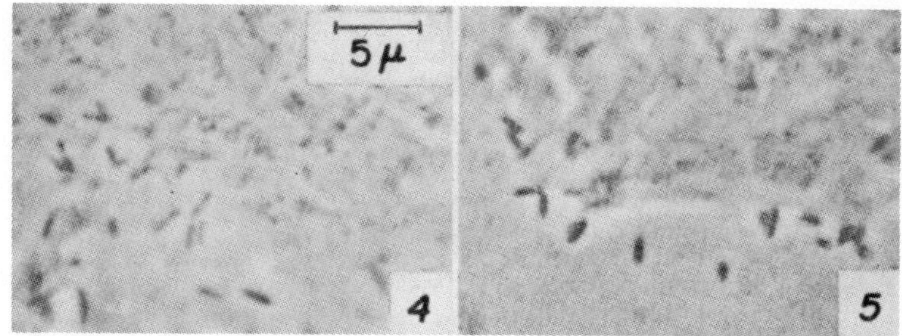

Fig. 4. R. rickettsi *in living 14pf cell 4 days after infection. Fig. 5. Edge of cell showing* R. rickettsi *in microfibrils.*

for *R. tsutsugamushi* which characteristically localized and multiplied in the area adjacent to the nucleus. The identification of small numbers of rickettsiae in the juxtanuclear region was hindered by the density and constant movement of the cellular organelles. When large numbers of organisms were present, as shown in Fig. 1, they displaced cytoplasmic elements from the vicinity of the nucleus and then became recognizable. These large clusters of *R. tsutsugamushi* underwent periodic cycles of aggregation and dispersion. Thus, within a period of 1 hour (Figs. 1, 2, and 3) rickettsiae which were loosely packed, aggregated into small tight clumps composed of variable numbers of organisms and again dispersed into a loose cluster. During the 7 or 8 hours in which a given slide was under observation there was no striking increase in the number of intracellular rickettsiae. However, chambers made with cover slips removed from a given batch of culture tubes on successive days showed a progressive increase in the number of rickettsiae; in some cells the cytoplasm was almost replete with organisms.

Cells infected with *R. rickettsi* contained relatively few organisms, in contrast to cells infected with *R. tsutsugamushi* which often contained hundreds of organisms. Furthermore, *R. rickettsi* was randomly scattered, singly or in relatively small numbers, throughout the cytoplasm with apparently no preferential localization. The latter organism exhibited slow intracytoplasmic movements which had no obvious relation to the displacement of cellular organelles. The frequent presence of *R. rickettsi* in the clear ectoplasmic portion of the cell (Fig. 4) sometimes made it possible to recognize this organism under the phase microscope within 48 hours after cultures were infected. Rickettsiae situated at the periphery of the cell possessed a higher degree of contrast than those

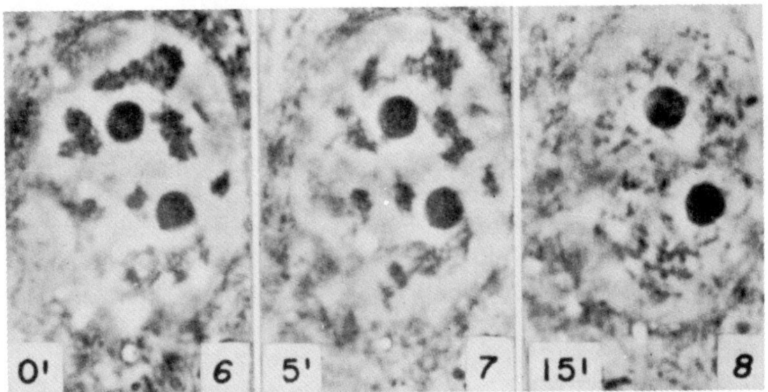

Figs. 6–8. R. rickettsi *in the nucleus of a 14pf cell. The tight clusters of organisms seen in Fig. 6 dispersed into small groups and single organisms after 15 minutes (Fig. 8). Time is indicated in the lower left corner of each figure. Phase photomicrographs, magnification 2000×.*

close to the nucleus, which is probably due to differences in refractive index within the cell.

On a few occasions only, *R. rickettsi* was seen in the nucleus of a 14pf cell (Fig. 6). Here also aggregation and dispersion occurred over short intervals of time. Figures 6 to 8 illustrate the process of redistribution of rickettsiae which was observed in one nucleus during 15 minutes. No distinct spatial relationship between the organisms and the nucleoli was noted. In two instances, intranuclear rickettsiae were observed for a period of 1 hour moving around the periphery of the nucleus, always in the same direction and at seemingly steady rates. Rotation of the nucleoli did not occur during this interval.

Under the conditions used in these experiments not all cells became infected simultaneously. In fact, cells containing no intracellular rickettsiae were often found adjacent to others with numerous organisms. As rickettsial multiplication progressed, more and more cells became infected so that by 5 or 6 days, the majority contained visible organisms.

Rickettsia rickettsi had a greater cytopathogenic effect on 14pf cells than did *R. tsutsugamushi.* Most of the cells in cultures infected with the former displayed severe degenerative changes on the 5th or 6th day even though they usually contained only about 50 discrete organisms. In contrast, most of the cells were stuffed with hundreds of *R. tsutsugamushi*

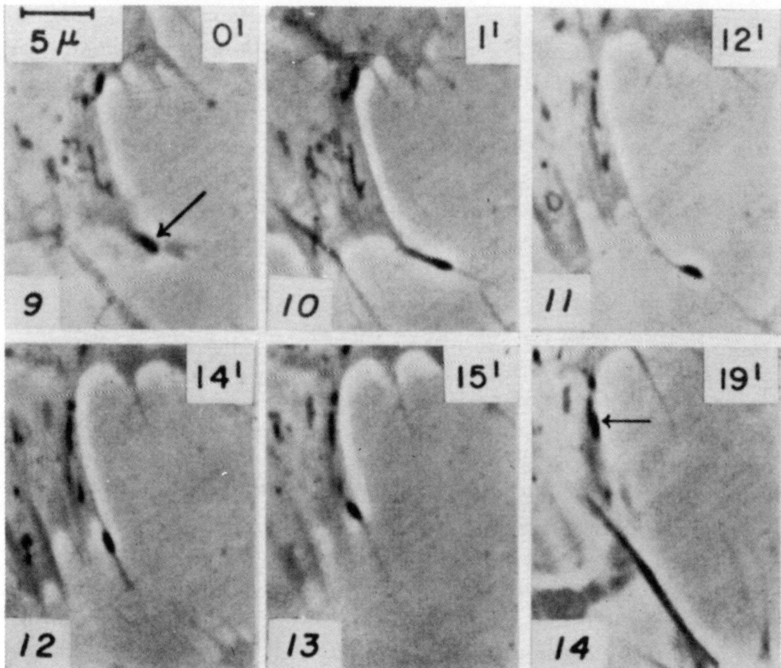

Figs. 9–14. A series of photomicrographs taken over a period of 19 minutes (times indicated in upper right corners) showing a 14pf cell containing a Rickettsia rickettsi *in a microfibril which extrudes and retracts. The organism in Fig. 9 is at the base of the forming fibril; the same organism shown in Fig. 14 has returned to the main body of the cell. Phase photomicrographs, magnification 2000×.*

by the 8th or 9th day, yet only a few showed morphologic abnormalities, i.e., rounding up and disintegration.

Extrusion of rickettsiae from infected cells.   In the course of these studies, rickettsiae were seen to emerge from infected cells by way of long, filamentous microfibrillar structures protruding from the edge or surface of the cell. These fine microfibrils are especially numerous in 14pf cells (8). When rickettsiae were located in an area of the cytoplasm from which a microfibril was being formed, they were often trapped within this structure (Fig. 5). When the microfibril retracted, one of two events happened: the rickettsia was carried back into the cytoplasm of the cell, or the organism was freed from the retracting microfibril and

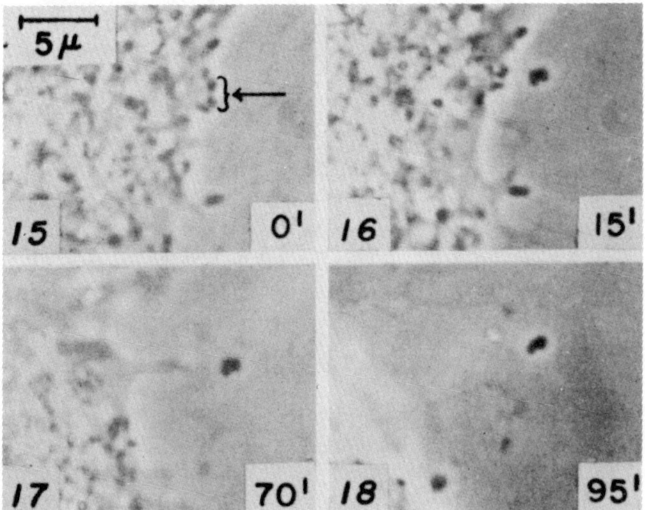

Figs. 15–18. A series of photomicrographs showing a 14pf cell containing two Rickettsia tsutsugamushi in a microfibril. The fibril had begun to retract at the time the picture in Fig. 17 was taken. When photographed 25 minutes later (Fig. 18), the fibril had disappeared, the cell border was out of focus in the lower left corner, and the rickettsiae were in an extracellular position attached to the surface of the glass. The time is indicated in the lower right corner. Phase photomicrograph, magnification 2000 ×.

left in an extracellular position. The former situation, which was the more frequent occurrence, is illustrated with *R. rickettsi* in Figs. 9 through 14. As shown in these photographs, the intrafibrillar rickettsia moved out along the axis of the filament for a period of 12 minutes. Subsequently, the fibril quickly retracted and carried the organism back into the cell. Sometimes organisms which reached the tip of the fibrils were freed into the fluid medium. Immediately before this release occurred, the rickettsia underwent slow lateral movements which gradually became more intense, then it suddenly appeared outside the microfibril and exhibited Brownian motion. Occasionally, organisms were liberated with the retraction of the microfibril and adhered to the glass; such release of a *R. tsutsugamushi* is shown in Figs. 15 through 18.

Division of R. rickettsi *by binary fission.* On three separate occasions, the division of a single *R. rickettsi* by transverse binary fission was

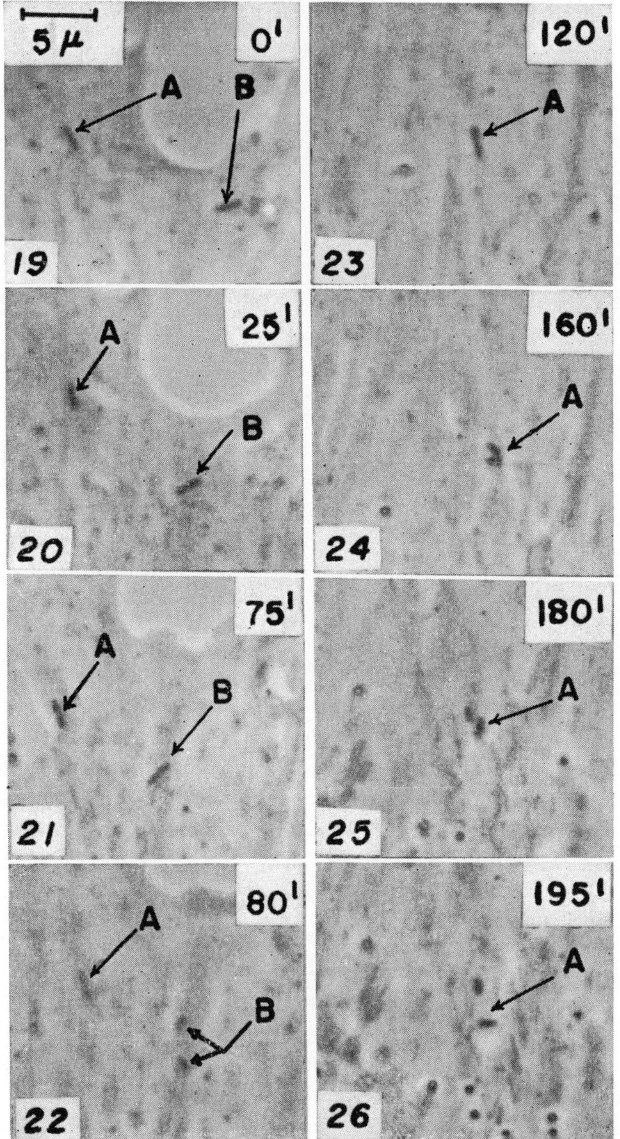

Figs. 19–26. Rickettsia rickettsi *undergoing binary fission. The series of photomicrographs illustrate part of the cytoplasm of a 14pf cell containing two rickettsiae, "A" and "B," each of which divides into two daughter organisms. During the 40-minute period between the photographs shown in Figs. 22 and 23 the daughters of "B" moved away from "A" and could not be included in the same field. The time is indicated in the upper right corner of each figure. Phase photomicrographs, magnification 2000 ×.*

observed and recorded photomicrographically. Figures 19 through 26 represent selected reproductions from a more extensive series of pictures and show the division of two organisms located at the edge of a large cell. The length of the rods and the slight central constriction (which is more prominent in the rickettsia "B") suggest that the organisms were in the later stages of the division cycle when the first photograph was taken. The process is best seen by following the changes in organism "A." It elongated and showed an increasingly pronounced transverse central constriction (Figs. 19 to 22) and, by 120 minutes, had the appearance of a diplobacillus (Fig. 23.) This form remained unchanged until about 159 minutes when the two elements of the diplobacillus separated by sliding past one another (Fig. 24). Subsequently, the daughter rickettsiae moved away in different directions and at 195 minutes were well separated from one another (Fig. 26).

Discussion

Direct microscopic observations of living tissue culture cells infected with *R. rickettsi* revealed that this organism divides by binary fission. On the basis of the mechanism of reproduction, rickettsiae resemble bacteria; they are unlike the smaller mammalian and plant viruses and bacteriophage (9, 10, 11). Although binary fission has been suggested for certain large viruses (cf. Weiss [12], 1955), this hypothesis, like the one proposed earlier for rickettsiae, is based entirely on observation of static material.

The intracellular localization and behavior of *R. tsutsugamushi* was different from that of *R. rickettsi*. The former grew in large clusters in an area adjacent to the nucleus, while the latter remained loosely scattered as individual organisms throughout the cytoplasm. A similar localization of the organisms was observed in stained preparations of infected MB III cells (6). The large clusters of *R. tsutsugamushi* located near the nucleus exhibited periodic cycles of dispersion and aggregation which made it difficult to follow a given organism for a relatively long period of time. We attribute our failure to observe *R. tsutsugamushi* undergo binary fission to this inability to maintain watch on a given organism for many hours. On the other hand, the random distribution of *R. rickettsi* in the cytoplasm and the slow intracytoplasmic movements of single organisms facilitated long term observations and made it possible to record the process of division. What causes the intracellular motion displayed by rickettsiae is unknown. We saw no evidence suggesting intrinsic motility of the organisms and assume that their motion was passive and attributable to the dynamic activities of the living host cell.

During these studies, *R. rickettsi* was occasionally seen in the nucleus of 14pf cells. The intranuclear localization of *R. rickettsi* seems to be dependent to an appreciable extent on the host cells in which they grow. They were frequently found in this structure in tissue cultures prepared from exudates from infected guinea pigs (13), but almost never occurred in infected cultures of mouse MB III cells (6).

Cinephase studies revealed a high degree of mobility of the cytoplasmic processes of living tissue cultures (8). In the present study rickettsiae located close to the edge of the cell frequently became involved in the cell's surface activities. Thus, the coarse fibrous processes and long filamentous microfibrils often contained rickettsiae and as the processes extended they carried the organisms away from the main body of the cell. Upon recession of the cytoplasmic processes the organisms usually were carried back into the cytoplasm, but occasionally the rickettsiae were liberated into the medium.

Although the number of rickettsiae which were lost from cells via microfibrils was considered to be small, this newly recognized means by which organisms are extruded from cells deserves careful consideration since it may play an important role in dissemination of pathogens, particularly between adjacent cells. However, the fact that cells containing large numbers of rickettsiae do undergo cellular disintegration suggests that most organisms are probably released by rupture of the diseased cell. The gradual release of intracellular parasites from infected cells has been suggested by the work of several authors. In stained preparations of tissue cultures of corneal epithelium infected with vaccinia virus, elementary bodies were observed at the tips of what ostensibly were microfibrils (14, 15). A similar phenomenon was found in human carcinoma tissue culture cells which were infected with vaccinia virus, then fixed and treated with fluorescent antibody (16). Results of quantitative studies reported by Dulbecco and Vogt (17) suggest that Western equine encephalomyelitis virus is released from chicken embryo cells either continuously or in small increments. Moreover, other authors have presented evidence for the gradual release from infected cells of influenza virus (18, 19) and vaccinia virus (20).

Marianna R. Bovarnick

Incorporation of Acetate-1-C^{14} into Lipid by Typhus Rickettsiae

The first indication that rickettsiae may be capable of one of the synthetic reactions necessary for growth was reported by Bovarnick, Schneider, and Walter (1) in 1959. They demonstrated that a small but constant amount of methionine-S^{35} is incorporated into rickettsial protein. That the incorporation of a single amino acid represented true protein synthesis was confirmed in subsequent detailed studies, in which glycine-1-C^{14} was also shown to be incorporated into rickettsial protein (2). Glycine incorporation was inhibited by chloramphenicol, a known inhibitor of protein synthesis, and by the omission of a single amino acid from the complex substrate.

In the 1960 paper reprinted here, Bovarnick demonstrated the incorporation of acetate-1-C^{14} by typhus rickettsiae. The acetate-1-C^{14} was found exclusively in the lipid fraction of the cells in contrast to glycine-1-C^{14}, which had been found almost entirely in the protein fraction. Although the amount of acetate incorporated was small, it was definitely greater than that found in control preparations. This implied that rickettsiae are also capable of synthesizing lipids in the course of their metabolic activities. These heuristic findings on the *in vitro* synthesis of rickettsial constituents are significant achievements representing a step toward the eventual cultivation of rickettsiae on artificial media.

Although it has been known for some time that rickettsiae have an independent, if limited, oxidative metabolism (1), evidence of any synthetic activity on the part of these organisms has until recently been lacking. It was noted (2) that they were capable through oxidative phosphorylation of forming ATP,* a compound that appears to be a prerequisite for all known biological syntheses. In spite of this ability it has not yet been possible to detect directly the synthesis of measurable amounts of any substance by viable rickettsiae. However, in the past year Myers, Paretsky, and Downs (3) have found that sonic extracts of *Coxiella burnetii* can form serine from glycine and formaldehyde, and

---

* The following abbreviations are used: GSH, reduced glutathione; DPN and DPNH, the oxidized and reduced forms of diphosphopyridine nucleotide; TPN and TPNH, the oxidized and reduced forms of triphosphopyridine nucleotide; CoA, coenzyme A; ADP and ATP, the di- and triphosphates of adenosine.

Table 1. Composition of Medium

Constituent	Final concentration	Constituent	Final concentration	Constituent	Final concentration
Amino acids	μM	*Vitamins*	μM	*Cofactors*	
DL-Alanine	95	Choline chloride	4.6	DPN	0.38
L-Arginine	48	Folic acid	0.036	DPNH	0.19
L-Asparagine	48	Hemin chloride	0.10	TPN	0.03
L-Cysteine	19	Inositol	3.2	TPNH	0.06
Glycine	48	Biotin	0.32	Coenzyme A	0.035
L-Histidine	19	*p*-Aminobenzoic acid	1.0	Cocarboxylase	0.055
L-Proline	48	*p*-Hydroxybenzoic acid	1.3	GSH	1.0
L-Hydroxyproline	48	Vitamin B_{12}	0.032	ATP	1.0
L-Serine	48	Leucovorin	0.036	Guanosine triphosphate	0.083
L-Threonine	71	DL-α-Lipoic acid	2.0	Uridine triphosphate	0.084
L-Tryptophan	7.1			Cytidine triphosphate	0.085
L-Tyrosine	48		*mg/ml*	Glycerophosphate	0.29
L-Valine	71	Yolk sac protein	0.29	Phosphocholine	0.14
L-Leucine	71			Phosphoethanolamine	0.11
L-Isoleucine	95	*Salts*	*mM*	Phosphoserine	0.11
L-Lysine	71	KCl	105		
L-Methionine	24	K_2HPO_4	3.9	Na-acetate-1-C^{14}	0.008
		KH_2PO_4	1.9	pH7.0–7.2	
L-Phenylalamine	38	$MgCl_2$	0.86		
L-Aspartic acid	48	$MnCl_2$	0.046		
		$CaCl_2$	0.012		
L-Glutamine	5000	$FeCl_3$	0.008		

The medium was sterilized as described by Bovarnick *et al.* (3) and the soluble yolk sac fraction was prepared as described by Bovarnick and Schneider (5).

The acetate-1-C^{14} was obtained from Nuclear-Chicago Corporation with a stated specific activity of 5 mc./mmole. At the concentration used in these experiments the measured activity was 7200 counts:min.:ml.

Bovarnick, Schneider, and Walter (4) and Fujita, Kohno, and Shishido (5) have found that viable preparations of *Rickettsia prowazeki* and *Rickettsia mooseri* can incorporate trace quantities of isotopically labeled amino acids. Some of the conditions necessary for this last process indicate that the incorporation may be due to a small amount of protein synthesis. Recently we have also observed incorporation of acetate into lipid by typhus rickettsiae and, despite difficulties in determining the optimal conditions for incorporation, the data suggest that rickettsiae can carry out a third type of synthetic reaction.

Table 2. Incorporation of Acetate-1-C^{14} by Typhus Rickettsiae

Experiment Number	Time of incubation	Incorporation of acetate-C^{14} by		
		Rickettsiae	Heated rickettsiae[b]	Normal yolk[c] sac particles
	hr		*counts/min*[a]	
I	5	36	I	2
2	5	123	3	3
	24	215		5

[a] The figures for counts per minute represent counts incorporated per mg rickettsial protein or yolk protein.

[b] These rickettsiae were heated for 15 min. at 56°C. before addition to the medium for incubation.

[c] Particles from normal yolk sacs, which had been harvested from uninfected eggs of the same age as the infected eggs, were prepared by the same procedure as used for preparation of the rickettsiae, except that the last cycle of alternate high and low speed centrifugation was omitted to avoid loss of almost all normal yolk sac material. The normal yolk sac particles were suspended in a volume such that their protein content would be approximately the same as that of the rickettsial preparations. The volume was $\frac{1}{3}$ to $\frac{1}{7}$ that used for rickettsiae from an equivalent quantity of starting yolk sac homogenate.

Experimental Methods

The E strain of typhus rickettsiae, grown in the yolk sacs of embryonated eggs, was purified as described elsewhere (2). The incorporation of acetate-C^{14} by these purified rickettsiae was measured as previously described for determination of the uptake of methionine-S^{35} (4). The composition of the basal medium used in these experiments, a modification of the one used in the study of amino acid incorporation and probably much more complicated than necessary, is given in Table 1. Because of the relatively low uptakes observed with acetate, it was necessary to increase the concentration of rickettsiae during incubation to 0.3 mg. protein per ml., and to increase the size of the samples taken for assay to 4 ml. With samples of this size it was not necessary to add carrier rickettsiae before isolation of the labeled rickettsiae for analysis. Uptakes are given as counts:min:mg rickettsial protein and are of the same order of magnitude as the actual counts measured. An uptake of 100 counts/min represents incorporation of 0.11 mμmole acetate.

Table 3. Distribution of Radioactivity in Rickettsiae Labeled with Acetate-1-C^{14} or with Glycine-C^{14}

Fraction	Radioactivity of rickettsiae labeled with			
	Glycine-C^{14}		Acetate-C^{14}	
	Total counts/ min	*Counts: min:mg protein*	*Total counts/ min*	*Counts: min:mg protein*
Initial	1085	199	1320	94
Cold perchloric acid soluble	21		33	
Lipid	6		1110	
Lipid residue	40	226	22	15
Hot perchloric acid soluble	118		70	
Protein	718	197	55	6

The trichloroacetic acid insoluble fraction of rickettsiae that had been incubated for 24 hr. in a medium containing the labeled compound was first isolated as usual, i.e., after heating for 15 min. at 56°C. and addition of carrier glycine or acetate, the mixtures were centrifuged and the precipitates were washed twice with 5 per cent trichloroacetic acid, once with water, then dissolved in 0.003 M KOH. This material represents the initial preparations. A sample of this was removed for counting and protein determination (7) and the remainder was precipitated by addition of perchloric acid to a final concentration of 2.5 per cent. The precipitate was extracted once with 3:1 ethanol-ether at 56°C. for 20 min., once with 1:1 ethanol-ether, and once with ether. The combined alcohol ether extracts were dried, extracted with chloroform, the extract filtered, dried, and counted. The chloroform extract is designated the lipid fraction. The alcohol ether soluble, chloroform insoluble material was dissolved in 0.003 M KOH before drying for counting and is designated the lipid residue. It contained a small amount of protein, possibly from lipoproteins. The alcohol ether insoluble material was extracted twice for 20 min. at 70°C. with 5 per cent perchloric acid to remove nucleic acids, then washed once with water, and finally resuspended in 0.003 M KOH. This is designated the protein fraction. The hot and cold perchloric acid extracts were separately filtered, neutralized with KOH, chilled, centrifuged to remove insoluble $KClO_4$, and concentrated to a small volume.

For preparation of glycine-C^{14} labeled rickettsiae, the organisms were incubated at a concentration of 30 μg rickettsial protein per ml. for 24 hr. at 30°C. in the medium previously described (6), except that glycine-2-C^{14}, with a specific activity of 5 mc/mmole, obtained from Nuclear-Chicago Corporation, was used in place of the glycine-1-C^{14} used earlier.

Results and Discussion

The amount of acetate incorporated after 5 or 24 hr. incubation at 30°C. was very small, at least an order of magnitude lower than the amount of amino acid incorporated by these organisms under similar conditions. In the two experiments given in Table 2 the maximal specific activities attained corresponded to incorporation of 2.4 and 14 μg acetic acid per gram of rickettsial protein, respectively. However, even though low, the observed uptake appeared to be significant, since uptake by heated rickettsiae or by particles from normal yolk sacs was lower by one or two orders of magnitude and probably insignificant.

In an effort to determine the nature of the substances labeled after incorporation of acetate-C^{14}, the labeled rickettsiae were fractionated and the distribution of activity between the different fractions was compared with that found after incorporation of glycine-C^{14} (Table 3). It is quite apparent that after incubation of rickettsiae with acetate-C^{14} the incorporated radioactivity is found almost completely in the lipid, whereas after incubation with glycine-C^{14} it appears chiefly in the protein. It should be mentioned that the reason for the similarity in the initial specific activities of the acetate and glycine labeled rickettsiae is that carrier rickettsiae were added immediately after incubation to those that had incorporated glycine, the ratio of carrier to labeled rickettsiae being about 20:1, but none was added to those that had incorporated acetate. The relatively low recovery of counts in the case of the glycine-C^{14} labeled rickettsiae is probably due to the frequent poor separation of the small precipitates on centrifugation. It was generally necessary to filter all supernatants to obtain completely clear solutions, and recovery of the small amounts of insoluble material, probably largely protein, that was lost on the filters was not attempted.

Although qualitatively the rickettsiae have always been found capable of incorporating labeled acetate, quantitatively the amount of incorporation in different experiments has varied widely. Also the response of the uptake to certain alterations in the conditions of incubation has been variable, partly because the effect of some single constituents of the medium appears to depend upon the presence or absence of others. Since the factors determining this variability have not yet been worked out, detailed presentation of the results does not seem justified, but certain generalizations may be made. Glutamine or glutamate and GSH appear consistently to be needed for good uptake and the reduced pyridine nucleotides usually bring about a 20 to 50 per cent increase in uptake. Many of the other constituents of the medium, i.e., the amino acids other than glutamine, the vitamins, and probably phosphocholine, phosphoethanolamine, phosphoserine, and phosphoglycerate, as well as bicarbonate, which is frequently of importance in lipid synthesis in other systems, appear to be without effect. The response of acetate incorporation to added purine and pyrimidine nucleotides has been particularly variable. The mononucleotides have been consistently without effect, but ATP and the other nucleoside triphosphates have shown effects varying from a 2-fold increase in the amount of acetate incorporated to an 80 per cent decrease. There is some indication that the effect of ATP (and ADP) varies with the concentration of rickettsiae during incubation, also with the concentration of the other nucleoside triphosphates, and that it can be altered by suitable pretreatment of the rickettsiae. The effect of the other nucleoside triphosphates in turn appears to depend at least in part on the concentration of ATP. It is of interest in this connection that one other reaction brought about by typhus rickettsiae, the lysis of sheep erythrocytes, also shows great variation in response to added ATP. The factors bringing about the variations in the case of the hemolytic reaction can be controlled and have been described elsewhere (8).

It is probably not surprising that the uptake of acetate-C^{14} by typhus rickettsiae is small, for glutamate, which they rapidly form from the glutamine present in the medium (F. E. Hahn, unpublished observation), is oxidized by these organisms via the tricarboxylic acid cycle (9, 10, 11, 12). Therefore acetyl-CoA, which in all known systems is a more immediate lipid precursor than acetate itself, is presumably continuously being formed from the unlabeled glutamine as well as from the labeled acetate. It had at first been hoped that this difficulty could be avoided by omitting glutamine and providing ATP and the reduced pyridine nucleotides as substitutes. While a very small uptake was observed under such conditions, much better uptake was obtained in the presence of glutamine, despite the probable dilution of isotopic acetate thereby introduced, probably because glutamate is the best source of energy for whole rickettsiae (13). The extent of the dilution introduced by glutamate oxidation cannot be evaluated, since it is not known whether acetyl-CoA formed during this reaction and that formed from externally added acetate are equivalent as lipid precursors, or whether one or the other is used preferentially. The rate of oxidation of glutamate, about 25 μl O_2:hr:mg rickettsial protein at 30°C. (8) would, if the oxidation were complete, be equivalent to the oxidation of 0.075 μmoles glutamate:hr:ml at the concentration of rickettsiae used in these experiments. Since the oxidation is not usually quite complete (10), the potential rate of acetyl-CoA formation would be lower than this, but still probably sufficient to produce fairly extensive dilution of the acetyl-CoA formed from the added acetate (0.008 μmoles/ml) during the 5- to 24-hr. incubation periods, if there were complete equilibration of acetyl-CoA formed from the two sources. However, equilibration cannot be complete, since decreasing the concentration of rickettsiae, and hence the rate of oxidation of glutamate, has little effect on the amount of labeled acetate incorporated per mg. rickettsial protein. The extent of the dilution must therefore depend on the relative availability and rates of formation of acetyl-CoA from glutamate and from external acetate. Variation in the amount of added labeled acetate incorporated may be produced by any factors that affect the relative utilization of the two sources of acetyl-CoA, as well as by variation in the amount of lipid formed. Because of these complications this system may be inherently a poor one for reliable estimation of the amount of lipid formed from the amount of incorporation and further attempts to improve the quantitative reproducibility of acetate incorporation into lipid by whole viable rickettsiae may not be warranted. The data do nonetheless seem worth recording in that they indicate in a qualitative fashion that rickettsiae are capable of lipid synthesis and that the very simple substrate acetate is one possible precursor for this synthesis.

Summary

Typhus rickettsiae, incubated in a medium similar to that used for demonstration of amino acid incorporation, are capable of incorporating acetate-C^{14}. The amount of acetate incorporated is small but is in marked contrast to the practically negligible uptake of acetate by heated rickettsiae or by particles from normal yolk sac. The incorporated acetate-C^{14} is found exclusively in the lipid fraction of the cells, in contrast to incorporated glycine-C^{14}, which is found almost entirely in the protein fraction.

Acknowledgment

This work was supported by a research grant from the Division of Research Grants of the National Institutes of Health, U. S. Public Health Service (grant no. E-167C7).

J. W. Vinson and H. S. Fuller

Studies on Trench Fever: I. Propagation of Rickettsia-like Microorganisms from a Patient's Blood

The final paper in this collection concerns the recent and provocative studies of Vinson and Fuller on trench fever—a rickettsial disease that was recognized as a clinical entity almost a half century ago. Until the publication of their report in 1961 *R. quintana*, the etiological agent of trench fever, could be cultivated only in man and his body lice, and in some species of monkeys in which a subclinical infection resulted after inoculation. The general difficulty experienced in propagating the rickettsia seriously hampered experimental investigations on this infectious disease. The demonstration by Vinson and Fuller that the rickettsia of trench fever can be cultivated in the yolk sac of the chick embryo and in cell cultures provides a means for obtaining substantial quantities of rickettsiae for research purposes. The distinguishing feature of their research, however, is the cultivation of *R. quintana* on blood agar, the first recorded instance of the successful growth of a rickettsial agent on artificial medium. Recent studies of the fine structure of *R. quintana*, made possible by the ability to cultivate the rickettsia, have revealed the existence of an outer cell wall, a plasma membrane, the presence of both ribonucleic and deoxyribonucleic acids, and evidence that binary fission is the mode of reproduction (1). Added to the accumulated evidence on the marked similarities in structure and function between bacteria and rickettsiae, these new findings strengthen the relation between these two major groups of microorganisms.

That the rickettsia-like microorganism described and cultivated by Vinson and Fuller was the true etiological agent of trench fever was established conclusively in a collaborative study with Dr. Gerardo Varela in Mexico City. Clinical trench fever was produced in volunteers from a culture of rickettsiae propagated on blood agar, and the rickettsiae were reisolated from the patients both on artificial medium and by feeding of lice (2). These results, the induction of the typical clinical disease and the recovery of the infectious agent, fulfilled the requirements of Koch's classic postulates.

The fundamental studies on trench fever assume increasing importance as evidence suggests that *R. quintana* may be distributed on a global scale. Its presence was first recognized only recently in the Western Hemisphere by Varela, Fournier, and Mooser (3). Based on experience in past wars and recent epidemiological reports the *R. quintana* infection appears to exist unrecognized and in ecologic equilibrium throughout world areas, awaiting only natural or manmade disasters to upset the delicate balance and to incite outbreaks of trench fever. The threat of pathogenic rickettsiae to man's health and welfare may be progressively lessened through greater knowledge of their basic behavior patterns and ecologic relations, and the circumstances conducive to disease readily recognized and controlled.

Trench fever was first recognized as a clinical entity during the 1915–1917 epidemic of this disease in Europe (1). Although the disease varied widely in severity, it was characterized by frequent relapses, an extended course and a nonfatal outcome. The etiologic agent, classified with the rickettsiae, was named *Rickettsia quintana* (2). The organism was transmitted from man to man by *Pediculus humanus* var. *corporis* (3). *R. quintana* was shown to multiply extracellularly in the gut of the louse, in which it produced neither apparent pathology nor death (4). All reported attempts to cultivate *R. quintana* on cell-free media, in the chick embryo, in cell culture, or in the usual laboratory animals have been negative (5, 6). Intravenous inoculation of the rhesus monkey with *R. quintana* produced a mild or inapparent infection detectable by a rickettsemia (6, 7). The lack of a convenient method for cultivating the organism has seriously impeded research on the biological characteristics of *R. quintana*.

The present report describes the isolation of a rickettsia-like microorganism from the blood of a case of trench fever and its cultivation in the body louse, on blood agar, in the yolk sac of the developing chick embryo, and in HEP cells grown *in vitro*. In its morphological and tinctorial properties and in its behavior in the louse, the organism is indistinguishable from *R. quintana* described in the literature (4, 8).

Materials and Methods

Strain of R. quintana. These studies were initiated with blood drawn during the acute phase of trench fever experimentally induced in a volunteer by one of the authors (H. S. F.). Lice infected with a strain of *R. quintana* generously supplied by Prof. H. Mooser were fed daily on the volunteer from January 19, 1959, until February 28, when the subject experienced a typical clinical course of trench fever (9). The initial febrile episode lasted from February 28 through March 2, with relapses on March 6 and March 12–13. The patient's blood was infective for lice fed on him until May 20 and thereafter not infective for lice. The blood used as an inoculum for the experiments reported here was drawn on March 27, heparinized, and stored at −70°C. until used.

Louse colony. The louse colony was a laboratory strain of *P. humanus* var. *corporis* maintained on rabbits and known to be free of organisms resembling rickettsiae.

Experimental infection of lice.   Three methods were used for handling and infecting the lice: (a) adult female lice were passed through the decontaminating solutions recommended by Rocha-Lima and Sikora (10), subsequently treated aseptically, and inoculated intrarectally by the Weigl technique (11); (b) newly hatched first nymphal instars were reared aseptically and on molting into adulthood the females were inoculated intrarectally; (c) newly hatched first nymphal instars were fed on a rabbit immediately following the intravenous injection of the rabbit with infectious material, after the method of Snyder and Wheeler (12). Between daily feedings on a rabbit, the lice were kept on strips of sterile bolting silk in sterile glass bottles. Their feces were collected once daily and shell-frozen with or without the addition of phosphate-glutamate-sucrose solution, referred to hereafter as sucrose-PG (13), and stored at $-70°$C. Both infected and control lice were shown to be free of contaminating microorganisms.

HEP cells.   The culture was originally received from Dr. Alice Moore. The strain was derived from a human carcinoma (14). The stock cells were grown as a monolayer in 20 per cent horse serum and 80 per cent maintenance solution, MS (15), with 50 μg. per ml. each of streptomycin and penicillin. After infection they were grown in 10 per cent human plasma (which was somewhat hemolyzed) and 90 per cent MS, without antibiotics. Bacteriological studies, including the Dienes technique (16), showed the cells to be free of microorganisms, including pleuropneumonia-like organisms (PPLO). Cells were infected by layering the inoculum over them. The infected cells were subcultured by scraping the cells off the glass surface, suspending them in the medium by aspiration, and transferring aliquots to new vessels. Cell cultures were incubated at $34°$C.

Chick embryos.   Seven-day-old chick embryos were inoculated into the yolk sac by the standard method (17), using a volume of 0.5 ml. and a dilution of the infectious material dependent upon the number of organisms present. Incubation was at 34 or $35°$C., and the yolk sacs were harvested on the seventh or eighth day post inoculation.

Bacteriological media.   Plates were prepared of blood agar base* with 10 per cent freshly drawn defibrinated horse or human blood. Broth was prepared of tryptose-phosphate broth with 10 per cent freshly

---

* Difco Bacto Blood Agar Base, dehydrated, No. 0045-01, and Difco Bacto Tryptose Phosphate Broth, dehydrated, No. 860, Difco Laboratories, Inc., Detroit, Michigan.

drawn defibrinated human blood. Incubation was at 32 or 34°C., with or without a CO_2 tension of five per cent.

Serology. The fluorescent antibody technique, employing the indirect test, was used. The procedures were those recommended for use with epidemic and murine typhus rickettsiae (18, 19). The antigens included (a) infected yolk sac, (b) infected louse feces, and (c) infected HEP cells. Test sera included the serum specimens from the case of trench fever (pre-infection serum, February 10, 1959; convalescent serum, April 23, 1959), a single serum specimen from a case of trench fever obtained approximately eight years following his attack, and four normal human sera.

The antigens were fixed on glass slides in acetone at -20°C. for two hours, incubated with the undiluted test sera, washed in saline, and incubated with anti-human globulin horse globulin conjugated with fluorescein,† followed by thorough washing in saline. Readings were made in an optical system designed for fluorescent antibody studies.

Experimental Procedures

Microorganisms resembling rickettsiae were propagated from acute phase blood of the trench fever patient in the louse and on cell-free medium. The organism was subsequently cultivated in the yolk sac of the developing chick embryo and in HEP cells grown *in vitro*.

Chart 1 delineates the various manipulations with the patient's blood and the genealogies of the various lines of the microorganism deriving from the blood. The line designations of the organism are used in the text to avoid redundancy (Chart 1). Lines 1 and 4 of the organism, originating directly from the blood of the trench fever patient, were carried in lice and on blood agar, respectively. Lines 2 and 3, derived from the infected louse feces of line 1, were carried in eggs. Lines 2A, 2B, 2C, 2D, and 2E were all derived from line 2 of the organism.

Growth of the Organism in the Louse

Lice were experimentally infected with (a) the blood from the case of trench fever, (b) the organism isolated in the yolk sac of the chick embryo, and (c) the colonial organism isolated on blood agar. All lice were handled aseptically.

(a) Twenty young adult female lice were inoculated intrarectally with blood from the case of trench fever. Twenty control lice were

† The conjugate was obtained commercially from Sylvana Chemical Co., Orange, New Jersey.

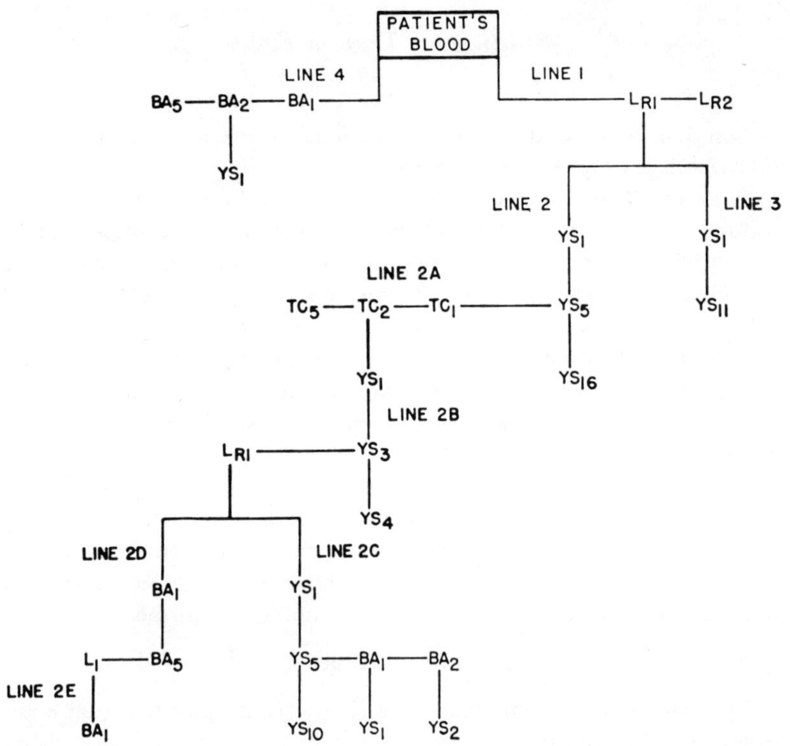

Chart 1. Genealogy of the various lines of the rickettsia-like microorganism derived from the blood of the case of trench fever. Line 1, 2, 3: Line of the organism. L_R: Intra-rectal passage in lice. L: Louse passage effected by feeding lice on rabbit inoculated with the organism. YS: Yolk sac passage. TC: Passage in hep cells. BA: Human blood agar culture. Numerical subscripts: Passage number.

inoculated with saline and another 20 remained uninoculated. *R. quintana* appeared in the feces of the infected lice in scanty numbers on the fifth day following inoculation, in moderate numbers on the sixth day, and subsequently in large numbers until the lice were sacrificed on the twenty-first day post infection. Contaminating microorganisms were not found in the feces of the infected lice. The feces of the control lice remained sterile. The viability of the rickettsiae in the feces of the infected lice was demonstrated by a second intrarectal passage in lice.

(b) Twenty young adult female lice, reared aseptically, were inoculated intrarectally with infectious yolk sac material from Line 2B ($Bl-L_{R1}-YS_5-TC_2-YS_3$, Chart 1). Microorganisms appeared in the louse feces in scanty numbers on the third day post inoculation and in moderate numbers from the fourth to the eighth day, when the lice were sacrificed for histological sectioning. In stained sections the organisms appeared in masses in the lumen of the gut and adjacent to the cuticular border of the epithelial cells lining the gut. None was found intracellularly.

(c) Newly hatched, unfed, first nymphal instars were allowed to feed to repletion on a 1300 gram rabbit which three minutes previously had been inoculated intravenously with four ml. of a heavy suspension of the colonial organism in sucrose-PG. The organisms were from line 2D (Bl—L_{R1}—YS_5—TC_2—YS_3—L_{R1}—BA_5, Chart 1). The typical organisms appeared in the louse feces in scanty numbers on the fourth day and thereafter in moderate, though never profuse in number until the fourteenth day, when the lice were sacrificed for histological sectioning. Stained sections revealed the organisms in masses in the lumen of the gut and deposed on the surface of the epithelial cells lining the gut. None was seen inside cells.

In the feces of the three groups of experimentally infected lice the microorganisms were morphologically and tinctorially characteristic of *R. quintana* described in the literature (4, 5, 8). The histologic picture in the louse gut was identical to that described for the infection of this species with *R. quintana* (4).

Growth of the Organism on Blood Agar

Isolation of the organism on blood agar was accomplished by streaking the various infectious materials on the surface of the agar with a bacteriological loop. Incubation was at 34°C. in a moist atmosphere of five per cent CO_2. Infectious materials from which isolations were made included (a) the blood of the human case of trench fever, (b) yolk sac passage material from lines 3, 2, 2A, 2B, and 2C (Chart 1), and (c) infected louse feces (lines 2D and 2E, Chart 1).

Microorganisms were not isolated from the feces of lice inoculated with saline nor from the first and fifth passage material of the control yolk sac passages initiated with the feces of lice inoculated intrarectally with saline.

On primary isolation on blood agar, the colonies were not visible on the sixth day after streaking but became visible through the dissecting microscope, and sometimes to the naked eye, on the twelfth to fourteenth day. When first visible through the dissecting microscope by reflected light the colonies were convex and transparent, with smooth edges. The colonies were mucoid and were situated on the surface of the agar. The size of the colonies was determined on specimens prepared by the technique advocated by Dienes for the visualization of pleuropneumonia-like organisms (16). Agar blocks containing colonies were cut

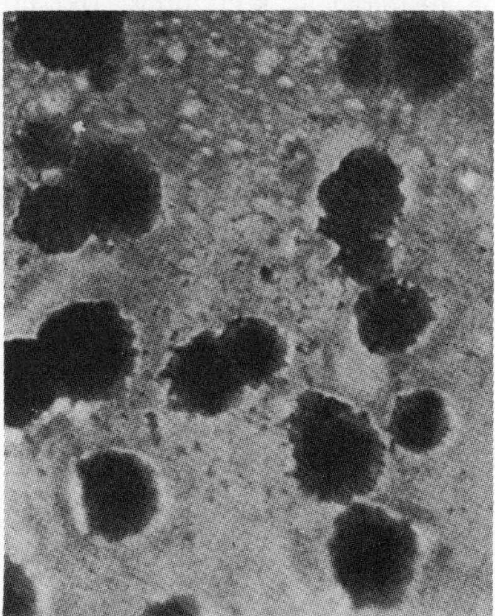

Fig. 1. Microcolonies of the rickettsia-like microorganisms 8 days after inocula-tion on blood agar. The colonies measured from 7.5 to 45 μ in diameter. The colonies in an agar block were stained by the method of Dienes. 200×.

from the culture, placed on a glass slide, and covered with a coverslip impregnated with Dienes' stain. On examination under the oil immersion lens of the compound microscope, individual organisms at the edges of the colonies could be distinguished. The colonies varied from between 7.5 to 45 μ in diameter (Fig. 1).

The colonies increased in size during time and assumed a grayish translucent aspect. The diameter of the largest colonies varied from between 250 to 500 μ. Impression smears made of the colonies by pressing a coverslip on their surface and staining by Macchiavello's method revealed microorganisms morphologically typical of rickettsiae (Fig. 2). On continued cultivation the organisms disintegrated to form blurred masses staining blue by Macchiavello's method.

The organisms were easily subcultured by scraping the colonies into sucrose-PG or by removing agar blocks containing the colonies and emulsifying them in sucrose-PG. On subculture, a heavy suspension of organisms flooded over the surface of the agar produced a profusion of microcolonies after 4 to 6 days' incubation.

That the method is sensitive for the detection of the organism is indicated by the isolations made from the blood of the case of trench fever. One loopful of blood from each of six aliquots of the blood speci-

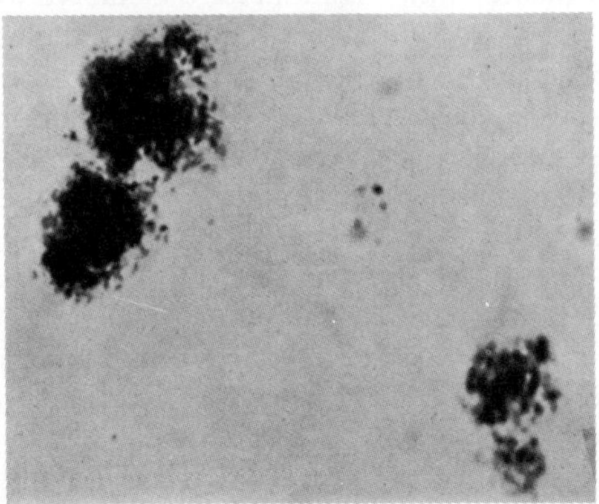

Fig. 2. Impression smear of 3 micro-colonies of the rickettsia-like microorganism grown on blood agar. Macchiavello stain. 1000×.

men (including that used to inoculate lice intrarectally) streaked on the surface of human blood agar resulted in from 20 to 60 microcolonies per plate. The aliquots of blood were streaked concurrently on agar plates prepared from horse blood. A reduction in the number of microcolonies on the horse blood agar suggested that human blood was superior to horse blood for the growth of the organism.

Growth of the Organism in the Yolk Sac of the Chick Embryo

The organism has been propagated in the yolk sac of the chick embryo from infected louse feces, from infected HEP cells cultivated *in vitro*, and from the colonial organism grown on blood agar.

Isolations from infected louse feces. Two isolations of the organism have been made from the feces of lice inoculated intrarectally with blood from the case of trench fever (lines 2 and 3, Chart 1). In both isolations typical organisms appeared in scanty numbers in the first yolk sac passage. Organisms were visible in smears of one of four eggs in line 2 and in two of three eggs in line 3. Line 2 has undergone 16 serial yolk sac passages and line 3, 11. Although the numbers of organisms increased during serial passage, their growth has never equalled that observed with other rickettsiae. The initial passages were made with a 25 per cent suspension of yolk sac in sucrose-PG and the later passages with from 2 to 20 per cent, depending upon the numbers of organisms present in the inocula or the mortality noted in the previous passage.

Increased virulence of the organism for the embryo was reflected in the increased mortality of the embryos during serial passage. In line 2 an inoculum of a 25 per cent suspension of yolk sac caused no deaths in the first four egg passages, while a two per cent suspension caused a mortality of 42 per cent in the sixteenth passage. In line 3 of the organism consistent mortality of the embryo was not observed until the ninth passage.

In both isolates, almost all embryos dying of infection exhibited cutaneous hemorrhage of varying intensity, of the head, legs, and feet. Viable embryos rarely showed this hemorrhagic phenomenon. Increased virulence for the embryo was not accompanied by an increase in the numbers of organisms seen in smears.

Control passages initiated in the yolk sac with the feces of lice inoculated intrarectally with saline remained free of microorganisms throughout a total of six yolk sac passages.

One isolation of the organism was made from the feces of lice which had been inoculated intrarectally with line 2B of the organism (Bl— L_{R1}—YS_5—TC_2—YS_3, Chart 1). The multiplication of the organism of this line (2C) in the yolk sac through a total of 10 passages was greater than that observed in lines 2 and 3. It was not, however, fatal for the embryo.

Isolation from infected HEP cells. The organism was isolated in the yolk sac by the inoculation of heavily infected HEP cells grown *in vitro* (line 2A, Chart 1). The organisms increased in number during a total of four serial passages, and, beginning with the second egg passage, produced a mortality which varied from 20 to 40 per cent.

Isolation of the organism grown on blood agar. The colonial form of the organism, appearing on blood agar after inoculation with several infectious materials, was recovered in the yolk sac of the chick embryo. The colonial organisms were derived from infectious feces, yolk sac, and also directly from the original blood of the trench fever patient, as listed below, and one egg passage was made of each.

(1) Line 2D of the organism (Bl—L_{R1}—YS_5—TC_2—YS_3—L_{R1}— BA_5).

(2) Line 2C of the organism (Bl—L_{R1}—YS_5—TC_2—YS_3—L_{R1}— YS_5—BA_1 and —BA_2).

(3) Line 4 of the organism (Bl—BA_2).

In all isolations in the yolk sac, the organisms appeared in scanty numbers in the first passage. Subsequent serial passages, where these were made, resulted in a moderate increase in the numbers of organisms seen in smears. The pleomorphic microorganisms appearing in all isolations in the yolk sac were morphologically and tinctorially typical of rickettsiae. They stained red by the Macchiavello technique, blue with Giemsa, and light pink by Gram's method. While many of the organisms were intracellular, others were outside cells. It has not been determined whether the latter organisms had multiplied extracellularly or had been released from cells during the course of infection or during the harvesting and smearing procedures.

Growth of the Organism in HEP Cells Cultivated in Vitro

A culture of HEP cells was washed three times with MS and inoculated with 4 ml. of a 50 per cent suspension of infectious yolk sac in sucrose-PG. The inoculum was line 2 of the organism (Bl—L_{R1}—YS_5, Chart 1). After contact for 1.5 hours at 34°C., the yolk sac suspension was aspirated and the cells were washed twice with MS before adding medium. Within 24 hours a moderate number of cells contained single organisms. Proliferation of the organism was not apparent until the ninth day, when many cells contained from 4 to 12 organisms. By the twenty-second day many cells contained, scattered throughout their cytoplasm, knots of organisms in the compact masses reminiscent of those seen in infected louse feces (Fig. 3).

The infected cells were subcultured 22 days following inoculation. Successive subcultures were made at the end of 14, 9, and 29 days, respectively, for a total of four subcultures. The final subculture was harvested at the end of 32 days of growth, at which time the cytoplasm of all cells was replaced by the organism and the cultures were disintegrated. When the growth of the organism became heavy, many organisms could be seen extracellularly, either as single organisms or in the small masses described above. Histological sections of the cultures, which might have provided information as to the possible extracellular growth of the organism, were not made.

Serology and Sensitivity to Antibiotics

Complete studies of the serology and antibiotic sensitivity of the organism will be published separately. Only representative experiments from preliminary studies will be included here.

Serology. The fluorescent antibody technique, employing the indirect method, was used. Antigens consisted of (a) 10 per cent infected yolk sac of line 2C of the organism, (b) infected louse feces (line 1), and (c)

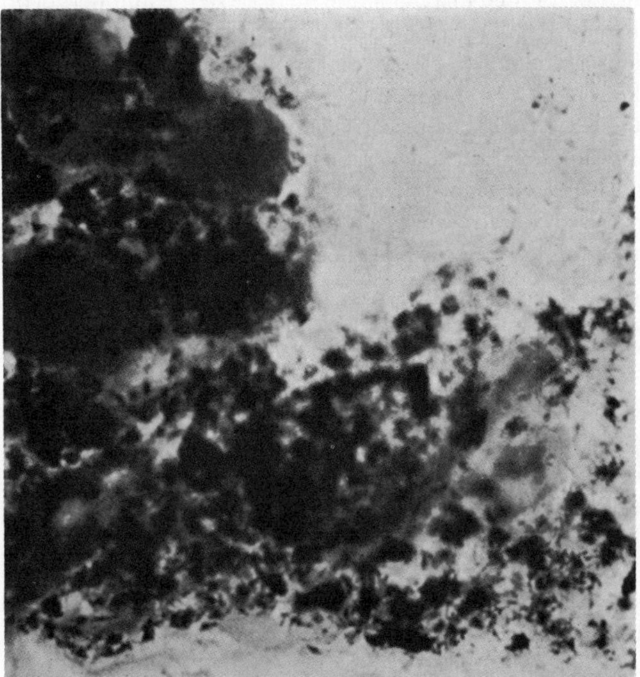

Fig. 3. Heavy infection of the rickettsia-like microorganism in HEP cells. Note the dense knots of the organism both inside and outside cells. Macchiavello stain. 1000 ×.

infected HEP cells (line 2A). The sera consisted of pre-infection and convalescent specimens of the volunteer case of trench fever, a single serum specimen drawn from a man eight years after an attack of trench fever, and four normal human sera.

The four normal sera and the pre-infection serum from the case of trench fever were negative. The trench fever post-infection serum was strongly positive with all antigens. Individual organisms could be seen fluorescing. The serum obtained eight years following an attack of trench fever showed bright fluorescence with the antigen in HEP cells and weak fluorescence with the organism in the louse feces.

While these data suggest a possible relationship of the organism isolated in the louse, in the yolk sac, and in HEP cells to human infection with *R. quintana*, they need confirmation by a wider serological experience.

Sensitivity to Antibiotics. Tests were performed by inoculating the colonial form of the organism into blood broth containing various concentrations of several antibiotics. Smears of the cultures were made daily and were stained by the Macchiavello method. Readings were made against control cultures free of antibiotics. In one experiment penicillin was used in concentrations of 2, 10, and 100 u./ml. and streptomycin in concentrations of 2, 10, and 100 μg./ml. In a second experiment tetracycline hydrochloride was used in concentrations of 2, 20, and 200 μg./ml. Complete inhibition of the growth of the organism was effected by all concentrations of tetracycline; partial to complete inhibition by concentrations of 2, 10, and 100 u. of penicillin/ml.; no inhibition by 2 μg. streptomycin/ml. but partial inhibition by 10 and 100 μg. streptomycin/ml.

Discussion

A rickettsia-like microorganism has been isolated from the acute phase blood of a human case of trench fever directly on blood agar and in the body louse by intrarectal inoculation. The organism has subsequently been propagated in the yolk sac of the chick embryo and in HEP cells cultivated *in vitro*. In view of the failure of all previously reported attempts to propagate *R. quintana* in any of these environments except the louse, it is necessary to examine the evidence for considering a causal relation to exist between the microorganism isolated and trench fever infection in man. Such evidence must (a) exclude the possibility of a contaminant resembling a rickettsia and (b) compare the organism with known strains of *R. quintana*.

Contaminating microorganisms were never seen in the infected or control lice of their feces, nor in yolk passage material initiated with the feces of lice inoculated intrarectally with saline. The HEP cells used for propagating the organism were shown to be free of PPLO. It was necessary to distinguish between PPLO and the rickettsia-like organism which grew on blood agar after plating with infectious materials. The rickettsia-like organism differed completely in its colonial growth: it grew slowly, it remained on the surface of, and did not penetrate into, the agar, and it could be easily subcultured by fishing with a loop or by washing the colonies into sucrose-PG. The colonies themselves, as opposed to colonies formed by PPLO, were composed of separate organisms, typical of rickettsiae, which could be easily differentiated from one another in stained smears.

The volunteer whose blood was used to initiate these studies was infected with an organism considered characteristic of *R. quintana*. It produced a clinical infection typical of trench fever. Blood drawn during the acute phase of the disease, when inoculated into the louse, produced an infection typical of *R. quintana* in this species. Infecting lice with the blood of a suspected case of trench fever and finding *R. quintana* characteristically situated in the louse gut has been the classic method for demonstrating the etiologic agent of trench fever.

Lice infected with the microorganism grown on blood agar or in the yolk sac showed an infection identical to that caused by known strains of *R. quintana* (4, 5, 20). Furthermore, the infection in the lice was indistinguishable from that seen in lice which had fed upon the case of trench fever. In all manipulations made with the microorganism in the yolk sac of the chick embryo, in cells cultivated *in vitro*, and on blood agar, the microorganism has retained the morphological and tinctorial characteristics of a rickettsia.

The fluorescent antibody studies with the pre-infection and convalescent sera of the case of trench fever were suggestive, but they require supporting evidence from wider application and from other serological techniques.

While the rickettsia-like microorganism described in this paper would appear to have a close similarity to *R. quintana*, its identity cannot be definitely established until it can be shown to cause a clinical course of disease typical of trench fever following inoculation of volunteers with a line of the organism distantly removed from its initial isolation.

Summary

A rickettsia-like microorganism has been isolated from acute phase blood of a case of trench fever in the louse and directly on blood agar. It was subsequently propagated in the yolk sac of the chick embryo and in HEP cells grown *in vitro*.

The microorganism was morphologically and tinctorially characteristic of a rickettsia. Lice infected with lines of the organism propagated in the yolk sac or on blood agar showed a picture in the louse gut identical to that described for *R. quintana*.

Preliminary serological studies, using the fluorescent antibody technique, showed that the convalescent serum of the case of trench fever, but not the pre-infection serum, reacted positively with organisms present in infected louse feces, yolk sac, and HEP cells. Under the experimental conditions employed, growth of the colonial organism was completely inhibited by tetracycline and partially inhibited by 10–100 μg./ml. of streptomycin and by 2–100 u./ml. of penicillin.

While the rickettsia-like microorganism isolated in lice, eggs, cell culture, and on blood agar would appear to resemble *R. quintana*, its identity cannot be firmly established until it can be shown to cause typical trench fever in volunteers inoculated with a line of the organism distantly removed from its initial isolation.

Acknowledgments

The authors are grateful to have had, during the course of these studies, the continuing interest and guidance of Dr. J. C. Snyder and Dr. E. S. Murray of the Department of Microbiology, Harvard School of Public Health.

T. A. Stamas rendered technical assistance.

This work was conducted in part with the aid of the Commission on Rickettsial Diseases, Armed Forces Epidemiological Board, Department of the Army, Office of the Surgeon General, Washington 25, D.C., and in part with the aid of the Department of Health, Education, and Welfare, Public Health Service, Rickettsial Disease Training Grant (2E-14[C2]), National Institutes of Health, Bethesda 14, Maryland.

Selected Reading
Notes
Index

Selected Reading

1. *Contributions to Medical Science: H. T. Ricketts, 1870–1910* (Chicago: University of Chicago Press, 1911).

2. S. B. Wolbach, J. L. Todd, and F. W. Palfrey, *The Etiology and Pathology of Typhus* (Cambridge, Mass.: Harvard University Press, 1922).

3. H. Zinsser, *Rats, Lice, and History* (Boston: Little, Brown, 1935).

4. *Virus and Rickettsial Diseases* (Cambridge, Mass.: Harvard University Press, 1940).

5. H. Pinkerton, "The Pathogenic Rickettsiae, with Particular Reference to Their Nature, Biologic Properties, and Classification," *Bacteriological Reviews*, 6 (1942), 37–78.

6. Medical Research Council, Special Report Ser. No. 255 (London: H.M. Stationery Office, 1946).

7. *The Rickettsial Diseases of Man*, ed. F. R. Moulton (Washington, D. C.: American Association for the Advancement of Science, 1948).

8. F. L. Horsfall, Jr., ed., *Diagnosis of Viral and Rickettsial Infections* (New York: Columbia University Press, 1949).

9. F. W. Hartman, F. L. Horsfall, Jr., and J. G. Kidd, eds., *The Dynamics of Viral and Rickettsial Infections* (New York: Blakiston, 1954).

10. B. Babudieri, "Q Fever: A Zoonosis," *Advances in Veterinary Science*, 5 (1959), 81–182.

11. *Symposium on Q Fever*, WRAIR Medical Science Publication No. 6 (Washington, D. C.: U.S. Government Printing Office, 1959).

12. *Symposium on the Spotted Fever Group*, WRAIR Medical Science Publication No. 7 (Washington, D. C.: U.S. Government Printing Office, 1960).

13. P. F. Zdrodovskii and H. M. Golinevich, *The Rickettsial Diseases* (New York: Pergamon, 1960).

14. J. W. Moulder, *The Biochemistry of Intracellular Parasitism* (Chicago: University of Chicago Press, 1962).

15. J. W. Vinson, *Etiology of Trench Fever in Mexico*, Report to Fifth Conference of the Industrial Council for Tropical Health (Boston: Harvard School of Public Health, October 1963).

16. E. H. Lennette and N. J. Schmidt, eds., *Diagnostic Procedures for Viral and Rickettsial Diseases*, 3d ed. (New York: American Public Health Association, 1964).

17. F. L. Horsfall, Jr., and I. Tamm, eds., *Viral and Rickettsial Infections of Man*, 4th ed. (Philadelphia: Lippincott, 1965).

18. J. K. Aikawa, *Rocky Mountain Spotted Fever* (Springfield, Ill.: Charles C. Thomas, 1966).

NOTES

H. T. Ricketts: Further Experiments with the Wood Tick

Preface

1. H. T. Ricketts, "The Study of 'Rocky Mountain Spotted Fever' (Tick Fever?) by Means of Animal Inoculations. A Preliminary Communication," *JAMA*, *47* (1906), 33–36.

2. L. B. Wilson and W. M. Chowning, "Studies in Pyroplasmosis Hominis ('Spotted Fever' or 'Tick Fever') of the Rocky Mountains," *J. Infect. Dis.*, *1* (1904), 31–57.

3. H. T. Ricketts, "The Transmission of Rocky Mountain Spotted Fever by the Bite of the Wood Tick (*Dermacentor occidentalis*)," *JAMA*, *47* (1906), 358. "Observations on the Virus and Means of Transmission of Rocky Mountain Spotted Fever," *J. Infect. Dis.*, *4* (1907), 141–153.

4. W. W. King, "Experimental Transmission of Rocky Mountain Spotted Fever by Means of the Tick: Preliminary Note," *Public Health Reports*, *21* (1906), 863.

5. T. Smith and F. L. Kilbourne, "Investigations into the Nature, Causation and Prevention of Texas or Southern Cattle Fever," Bureau of Animal Industries Bulletin No. 1 (Washington, D. C.: U.S. Dept. of Agriculture, 1893).

6. H. T. Ricketts, "The Role of the Wood Tick (*Dermacentor occidentalis*) in Rocky Mountain Spotted Fever, and the Susceptibility of Local Animals to this Disease. A Preliminary Report," *JAMA*, *49* (1907), 24–27.

7. H. T. Ricketts, "Further Observations on Rocky Mountain Spotted Fever and *Dermacentor occidentalis*," *JAMA*, *47* (1906), 1067–1069.

8. H. T. Ricketts and L. Gomez, "Studies on Immunity in Rocky Mountain Spotted Fever," *J. Infect. Dis.*, *5* (1908), 221–244.

9. H. T. Ricketts, "A Micro-organism which Apparently Has a Specific Relationship to Rocky Mountain Spotted Fever," *JAMA*, *52* (1909), 379–380.

10. R. R. Spencer and R. R. Parker, "Studies on Rocky Mountain Spotted Fever: Infectivity of Fasting and Recently Fed Ticks," *Public Health Reports*, *38* (1923), 333–339.

Nicolle *et al.*: Transmission of Exanthematic Typhus through Body Lice

Preface

1. Matthew Hay, "Typhus Fever and Fleas," *Public Health Reports*, *19* (1907), 772–776.

2. F. P. Mackie, "A Preliminary Note on Bombay Spirillar Fever," *Lancet*, *2* (1907), 832–835.

3. E. Sergent and F. H. Foley, "Fièvre récurrente du sudoranais et pediculus vestimente," *Bull. Soc. Path. Exot.*, *1* (1908), 174–176.

4. C. Nicolle, "Experimental Reproduction of Exanthematic Typhus in the Monkey," *C.R. Acad. Sci.* (Paris), *149* (1909), 157–160.

5 H. T. Ricketts and R. M. Wilder, "The Transmission of the Typhus Fever of Mexico (Tabardillo) by Means of the Louse (*Pediculus vestamenti*)," *JAMA, 54* (1910), 1304–1307.

6. J. F. Anderson and J. Goldberger, "On the Infectivity of Tabardillo or Mexican Typhus for Monkeys and Studies on its Mode of Transmission," *Public Health Reports, 25* (1910), 177–185.

Text

1. C. Nicolle, "Experimental Reproduction of Exanthematic Typhus in the Monkey," *C.R. Acad. Sci., 149* (1909), 157–160.

Ricketts and Wilder: Etiology of the Typhus Fever of Mexico City

Preface

1. H. T. Ricketts and R. M. Wilder, "The Transmission of the Typhus Fever of Mexico (Tabardillo) by Means of the Louse (*Pediculus vestamenti*)," *JAMA, 54* (1910), 1304–1307.

2. H. T. Ricketts and R. M. Wilder, "Further Investigations Regarding the Etiology of Tabardillo, Mexican Typhus Fever," *JAMA, 55* (1910), 309–311.

Text

1. J. F. Anderson and J. Goldberger, "On the Infectivity of Tabardillo or Mexican Typhus for Monkeys and Studies on Its Mode of Transmission," *Public Health Reports, 25* (1910), 177–185.

Conor and Bruch: An Eruptive Fever Observed in Tunisia

Preface

1. *Joint OIHP/WHO Study-Group on African Rickettsioses, Report on the First Session,* WHO Technical Report Ser., No. 23 (Geneva, 1950).

Nathan E. Brill: An Acute Infectious Disease of Unknown Origin

Preface

1. Nathan E. Brill, "A Study of 17 Cases of a Disease Clinically Resembling Typhoid Fever, but without the Widal Reaction . . . ," *N.Y. Med. J., 67* (1898), 48–54; 77–82.

2. J. F. Anderson and J. Goldberger, "The Relation of So-called Brill's Disease to Typhus Fever—An Experimental Demonstration of their Identity," *Public Health Reports, 27* (1912), 149–160.

3. Nathan E. Brill, "A Few Observations of the Symptomatology and Etiology of the Endemic Form of Typhus Fever," *Contributions to Medical and Biological Research, 1* (1919), 347–358.

Text

1. *Médecine éclairée par l'observation et l'ouverture des corps* (Paris, 1804).

2. *Traité de la fièvre entéro-mésentérique* (Paris, 1813).

3. "De la maladie, à laquelle M. Bretonneau a donné le nom de dothiénentérie, ou de dothiénentérité," *Arch. gén. Méd., 10* (1826), Ser. 1, 169. "Notice sur la contagion de la dothiénentérité," *ibid., 21*; also, "de la dothiénentérité," *ibid., 21*.

4. *Recherches sur la maladie connue sous les noms de gastroentérite, fièvre putride, adynamique, etc.* (Paris, 1829).

5. *Leçons de clinique méd.*, I. *Fièvre typhoide* (Paris, 1834).

6. "History of a Fever in the Suburbs of Paisley in 1811," *Edinb. Med. Surg. J., 8* (1812), 134.

7. "Account of an Outbreak of Fever at Newcastle," *Edinb. Med. Surg. J., 14* (1818).

8. "Cases Showing the Frequency of Follicular Ulceration in the Mucous Membrane of the Intestines in Idiopathic Fevers," *London Med. Phys. J.*, 1826.

9. *Reports of Medical Cases*, Vol. I (London, 1827).

10. "Observations on the Epidemic Fever, Now Prevalent Among the Lower Orders in Edinburgh," *Edinb. Med. Surg. J., 28* (1827).

11. "Report of Cases Treated in Edinburgh Infirmary in 1832–33," *Edinb. Med. Surg. J., 41* (1834); also *Elements of the Practice of Physic*, I. *Fevers* (Edinburgh, 1837).

12. "On Epidemic Gastric Fever," *Cyclop. Pract. Med., 2* (1833), 233.

13. "Observations on Petechial Fevers and Petechial Eruptions," *Edinb. Med. Surg. J., 44* (1835).

14. "Observations on Continued Fever in the Glasgow Hospitals," *Edinb. Med. Surg. J., 45* (1836); also "Letter on Typhus Fever," *Dublin J. Med. Sci., 10* (1836).

15. "Études clin. sur les fièvres typhoïdes," *Gaz. méd.*, 1839.

16. *Ueber den ansteckenden Typhus* (Vienna, 1810).

17. "On the Typhus Fever Which Occurred at Philadelphia in 1836, Showing the Distinction between It and Dothinenteritis," *Am. J. Med. Sci., 19* and *20*, February and August, 1837.

18. *Z. Hyg.*, vol. *21*.

19. *Proc. Roy. Soc.*, vol. *59*.

20. *Bull. méd.*, 1896.

21. N. E. Brill, *N. Y. Med. J.*, January 8, 1898, and January 15, 1898.

22. *Am. J. Med. Sci.*, August 1908, p. 190.

23. *The Principles and Practice of Medicine*, by Wm. Osler, M.D. 6th ed. (1906), p. 91.

24. *A Treatise on the Continued Fevers of Great Britain*, 2nd ed. (London, 1873).

25. *Der Unterleibstyphus, Spec. und Ther.* (Vienna, 1902; also, American edition, with additions by Wm. Osler, Philadelphia, 1902).

26. N. E. Brill, "Paratyphoid Fever," *Med. Rec.*, November 29, 1902.

H. da Rocha-Lima: On the Etiology of Typhus Fever

Preface

1. A. Gaviño and J. Girard, "Nota Preliminar Sobre, Ciertos Cuerpos Encontrados en la Sangre de los Individuos Etacados de Tifo, Mexico City," *Publicaciones del Instituto Bacteriologia Nacional*, No. 2, May 20 (1910).

2. C. Hegler and S. von Prowazek, "Untersuchungen über Fleckfieber," *Berl. klin. Wschr.*, *1* (1913), 2035.

3. S. von Prowazek, "Ätiologische Untersuchungen über den Flecktyphus in Serbien 1913 und Hamburg 1914," *Beitr. klin. Infekt.*, *4* (1914), 5–31.

4. H. da Rocha-Lima, "Beobachtungen bei Flecktyphuslausen," *Arch. Schiffs- u. Tropenhyg.*, *20*, No. 2 (1916), 17–31.

5. S. B. Wolbach, J. L. Todd, and F. W. Palfrey, *The Etiology and Pathology of Typhus* (Cambridge, Mass.: Harvard University Press, 1922).

Weil and Felix: On Serological Diagnosis of Spotted Fever

Preface

1. J. W. Wilson, "The Etiology of Typhus Fever," *J. Hyg.* (Lond.), *10* (1910), 155–176.

2. A. Felix, "Die Serodiagnostik des Fleckfiebers," *Wien. klin. Wschr.*, *29* (1916), 873–877.

3. A. Felix and R. M. Pitt, "A New Antigen of *B*. Typhosus: Its Relation to Virulence and to Active and Passive Immunization," *Lancet*, *227* (1934), 186–191.

4. M. R. Castaneda, "The Antigenic Relationship between Proteus X-19 and Typhus Rickettsia II. A Study of the Common Antigenic Factor," *J. Exp. Med.*, *60* (1934), 119–125.

5. A. Felix, "The Typhus Group of Fevers, Classification, Laboratory Diagnosis, Prophylactic Inoculation, and Specific Serum Treatment," *British Med. J.*, *2* (1942), 597–601.

6. N. Fletcher and J. E. Lesslar, "Tropical Typhus in the Federated Malay States," *Bull. Inst. Med. Res. Fed. Malay States*, No. 2 of 1925, 1–88.

Text

1. Weil and Spaet, *Wien. klin. Wschr.*, No. 8 (1915).

M. H. Neill: Experimental Typhus Fever in Guinea Pigs

Preface

1. H. Mooser, "Experiments Relating to the Pathology and the Etiology of Mexican Typhus (Tabardillo)," *J. Infect. Dis.*, *43* (1928), 241–272.

2. H. Plotz *et al.*, "Morphological Structure of Rickettsiae," *J. Exp. Med.*, *77* (1943), 355–358.

Text

1. Olitsky, Denzer, and Husk, *JAMA*, *68*, No. 16 (1917), 1167.

2. Ricketts, *JAMA*, *47* (1906), 33.

3. Lecount, *J. Infect. Dis.*, *8* (1911), 421.

4. Wolbach, *J. Med. Res.*, *34* (1916), 122.

5. Frankel, *Münch. med. Wschr.*, *61* (1914), 57.

6. Aschoff, *Med. Klin.* (1915), 798.

7. Poindecker, *Münch. med. Wschr.*, *63*, No. 5 (1916), 176.

Kenneth F. Maxcy: Typhus Fever in the United States

Preface

1. J. E. Paullin, "Typhus Fever with a Report of Cases," *Sth. Med. J.*, *6* (1913), 36–43.

2. F. S. Hone, "A Series of Cases Closely Resembling Typhus Fever," *Med. J. Austral.* (Sidney), *1* (1922), 1–13.

3. F. T. Wheatland, "Fever Resembling a Mild Form of Typhus Fever," *Med. J. Austral.*, *1* (1926), 261–266.

4. K. F. Maxcy, "Clinical Observations on Endemic Typhus (Brill's Disease) in the United States," *Public Health Reports*, *41* (1926), 1213–1220.

5. R. E. Dyer, A. Rumreich, and L. F. Badger, "Typhus Fever. A Virus of the Typhus Type Derived from Fleas Collected from Wild Rats," *Public Health Reports*, *46* (1931), 334–338.

6. H. Mooser, M. R. Castaneda, and H. Zinsser, "Rats as Carriers of Mexican Typhus Fever," *JAMA*, *97* (1931), 231–232.

7. J. L. Monteiro, "Estudos Sobre o Typho Exantematico de Sao Paulo," *Mem. Inst. Butantan*, *6* (1931), 1–135.

8. H. Mooser and M. R. Castaneda, "Multiplication of Virus of Mexican Typhus Fever in Fleas," *J. Exp. Med.*, *55* (1932), 307–323.

9. H. Zinsser and M. R. Castaneda, "Studies on Typhus Fever. IX. On the Serum Reactions of Mexican and European Typhus Rickettsia," *J. Exp. Med.*, *56* (1932), 455–467.

10. H. Mooser, "Essai sur L'Histoire Naturelle du Typhus Exanthematique," *Arch. Inst. Pasteur Tunis*, *21* (1932), 1–19.

11. Y. Biraud and S. Deutschman, "Typhus and Typhus-Like Rickettsia Infections," *Epidemiological Reports* (Geneva: League of Nations *15*, 1936), 90–160.

Nigg and Landsteiner: Studies on the Cultivation of the Typhus Fever Rickettsia

Preface

1. C. Nigg and K. Landsteiner, "Growth of Rickettsia of Typhus Fever (Mexican Type) in the Presence of Living Tissue," *Proc. Soc. Exp. Biol. Med.*, *28* (1930), 3–5.

2. K. Sato, "Dauerkultur des Fleckfiebervirus," *Deutsche med. Wschr.*, *57* (1931), 892–893; and "Die Morphologie des in Vitro Kultivierten Fleckfiebervirus," *Deutsche med. Wschr.*, *57* (1931), 1409–1410.

3. H. Pinkerton and G. M. Hass, "Typhus Fever; Behavior of *Ricksettsia prowazeki* in Tissue Cultures," *J. Exp. Med.*, *54* (1931), 307–314.

Text

1. C. Nigg and K. Landsteiner, *Proc. Soc. Exp. Biol. Med.*, *28* (1930), 3.

2. M. H. Kuczynski, *Berl. klin. Wschr.*, *2* (1921), 1489.

3. A. A. Krontowski and I. W. Hach, *Münch. med. Wschr.*, *70* (1923), 144; *Klin. Wschr.*, *2* (1924), 1625; *Arch. Zellforsch.*, *3* (1926–27), 297; *Z. Immun.-Forschung*, *54* (1927–28), 237.

4. S. B. Wolbach and M. J. Schlesinger, *J. Med. Res.*, *44* (1923–24), 231.

5. E. Rix, *Z. Hyg. Infect.-Kr.*, *108* (1927–28), 103.

6. H. Zinsser and A. P. Batchelder, *J. Exp. Med.*, *51* (1930), 847.

7. H. Zinsser and M. R. Castaneda, *J. Immun.*, *21* (1931), 403.

8. K. Sato, *Deutsche med. Wschr.*, *57* (1931), 892, 1409.

9. H. Pinkerton and G. M. Hass, *J. Exp. Med.*, *54* (1931) 307.

10. H. Pinkerton, *J. Exp. Med.*, *54* (1931), 181.

11. T. M. Rivers, E. Haagen, and R. S. Muckenfuss, *J. Exp. Med.*, *50* (1929), 665; cf. A. Carrel and T. M. Rivers, *C. R. Soc. Biol.*, *96* (1927), 848.

12. H. B. Maitland and M. C. Maitland, *Lancet*, *2* (1928), 596.

13. T. M. Rivers, E. Haagen, and R. S. Muckenfuss, *J. Exp. Med.*, *50* (1929), 181.

14. M. R. Castaneda, *J. Infect. Dis.*, *47* (1930), 416.

15. C. P. Li and T. M. Rivers, *J. Exp. Med.*, *52* (1930), 465.

16. T. M. Rivers, *J. Exp. Med.*, *54* (1931), 453.

17. G. Pincus and A. Fischer, *J. Exp. Med.*, *54* (1931), 323.

18. G. H. Eagles and D. McClean, *Brit. J. Exp. Path.*, *11* (1930), 337; *ibid.*, *12* (1931), 97.

19. T. M. Rivers, *Physiol. Rev.*, in press.

20. H. H. Dale, *Nature*, *128* (1931), 599.

21. C. Hallauer, *Z. Hyg. Infekt.-Kr.*, *113* (1931), 61.

22. K. Landsteiner and M. Berliner, *Z. Bakt.*, Abt. I, Orig., *67* (1912–13), 165.

Hans Zinsser: Varieties of Typhus Virus

Preface

1. J. F. Anderson and J. Goldberger, *Collected Studies on Typhus*, Hygienic Laboratory Bull. No. 86 (Washington, D. C.: U.S. Public Health Service, 1912).

2. E. S. Murray *et al.*, "Brill's Disease, Clinical and Laboratory Diagnosis," *JAMA*, *142* (1950), 1059–1066.

3. E. S. Murray and J. C. Snyder, "Brill's Disease: Etiology," *Amer. J. Hyg.*, *53* (1951), 22–32.

4. W. H. Price, "Studies on Interepidemic Survival of Louse-Borne Epidemic Typhus Fever," *J. Bact.*, *69* (1955), 106–107.

5. W. Loeffler and H. Mooser, "Ein Weiterer Fall von Brill-Zinsserscher Krankheit in Zurich (Spater Ruckfall bei Klassischem Fleckfieber)," *Schweiz. med. Wschr.*, *82* (1952), 493–495.

Text

1. M. H. Neill, *Public Health Reports*, *32* (1917), 1105.

2. H. Mooser, *J. Infect. Dis.*, *43* (1928), 241, 261.

3. K. F. Maxcy, *Public Health Reports*, *41* (1926), 2967.

4. R. E. Dyer, A. Rumreich, and L. F. Badger, *Public Health Reports*, *46* (1931), 334.

5. H. Mooser, M. R. Castaneda, and H. Zinsser, *JAMA*, *97* (1931), 231.

6. H. Zinsser and M. R. Castaneda, *J. Exp. Med.*, *56* (1932), 455.

7. *Ibid.*, *57* (1933), 381.

8. *Ibid.*, 391.

9. C. Nicolle and J. Laigret, *Arch. Inst. Pasteur Tunis*, *21* (1933), 357.

10. C. Nigg and K. Landsteiner, *Proc. Soc. Exp. Biol. Med.*, *23* (1930), 3.

11. H. Mooser, G. Varela, and H. Pilz, *J. Exp. Med.*, *59* (1934), 137.

12. M. R. Castaneda, *J. Exp. Med.*, *52* (1930), 195.

13. R. I. Lee, *Boston Med. Surg. J. 168* (1913), 122.

14. A. C. Ernstene and J. E. F. Riseman, *New Eng. J. Med.*, *209* (1933), 542.

E. H. Derrick: "Q Fever," a New Fever Entity

Preface

1. F. M. Burnet and M. Freeman, "Experimental Studies on the Virus of 'Q' Fever," *Med. J. Austral.*, *2* (1937), 299–305.

2. E. H. Derrick, "*Rickettsia burnetii*: The Cause of 'Q' Fever," *Med. J. Austral.*, *1* (1939), 14.

3. G. E. Davis and H. R. Cox, "A Filter-Passing Infectious Agent Isolated from Ticks: I. Isolation from *Dermacentor andersoni*, Reactions in Animals, and Filtration Experiments," *Public Health Reports*, *53* (1938), 2259–2267.

4. H. R. Cox, "Studies of a Filter-Passing Infectious Agent Isolated from Ticks. V. Further Attempts to Cultivate in Cell-Free Media. Suggested Classification," *Public Health Reports*, *54* (1939), 1822–1827.

5. R. E. Dyer, "Filter-Passing Infectious Agent Isolated from Ticks. Human Infection," *Public Health Reports*, *53* (1938), 2277–2282; "Similarity of Australian 'Q' Fever and a Disease Caused by an Infectious Agent Isolated from Ticks in Montana," *Public Health Reports*, *54* (1939), 1229–1237.

6. H. R. Cox, "*Rickettsia diaporica* and American Q Fever," *Amer. J. of Trop. Med.*, *20* (1940), 463–469.

7. F. M. Burnet and M. Freeman, "Studies of X Strain (Dyer) of *Rickettsia burnetii*; Chorioallantoic Membrane Infections," *J. Immunol.*, *40* (1941), 405–419.

8. C. B. Philip, "Comments on Name of Q Fever Organism," *Public Health Reports*, *63* (1948), 58.

9. F. C. Robbins *et al.*, "'Q' Fever in Mediterranean Area; Report of Its Occurrence in Allied Troops; Clinical Features of the Disease," *Amer. J. Hyg.*, *44* (1946), 6–22, 23–50, 51–63, 64–71.

10. B. Babudieri, "Q Fever: A Zoonosis," *Advanc. Vet. Sci.*, *5* (1959), 81–182.

Text

1. Manson's *Tropical Diseases*, 10th ed., p. 200.

2. M. Nagayo, T. Tamiya, T. Mitamura, and K. Sato, "On the Virus of Tsutsugamushi Disease and Its Demonstration by a New Method," *Jap. J. Exp. Med.*, Aug. 20, 1930, p. 309 [quoted in the Annual Report of the Institute for Medical Research, Federated Malay States (1931), 33].

3. R. Lewthwaite, "Clinical and Epidemiological Observations on Tropical Typhus in the Federated Malay States," *Bull. Inst. Med. Res. Fed. Malay States*, No. 1 (1930).

4. A. Pijper and H. Dau, "Die fleckfieberartigen Krankheiten des südlichen Afrika," *Z. Bakt.*, *133* (November 20, 1934), 7.

Herald R. Cox: Use of Yolk Sac as Medium for Growing Rickettsiae

Preface

1. H. R. Cox, "Cultivation of Rickettsiae of the Rocky Mountain Spotted Fever, Typhus and Q Fever Groups in the Embryonic Tissues of Developing Chicks," *Science, 94* (1941), 399–403.

Text

1. R. R. Spencer and R. R. Parker, "Variations in the Behavior of the Virus," in *Studies on Rocky Mountain Spotted Fever*, Hygienic Laboratory Bull. No. 154 (Washington, D. C.: U.S. Public Health Service, 1930), 49.

2. W. L. Bradford and R. Titsler, "Experimental Gonococcal Infection in the Chick Embryo," *Proc. Soc. Exp. Biol. Med., 34* (1936), 241.

3. W. Barykine, in collaboration with A. Kompaneez, A. Botcharowa, and H. Bauer, "Nouvelle methode de culture du virus du typhus exanthématique," *Bull. Off. Int. Hyg. Publ., 30* (1938), 326.

4. H. B. Maitland and M. C. Maitland, "Cultivation of Vaccinia Virus without Tissue Culture," *Lancet, 2* (1928), 596.

5. C. P. Li and T. M. Rivers, "Cultivation of Vaccine Virus," *J. Exp. Med., 52* (1930), 465.

6. T. M. Rivers, "Cultivation of Vaccine Virus for Jennerian Prophylaxis in Man," *J. Exp. Med., 54* (1931), 453.

7. A. M. Woodruff and E. W. Goodpasture, "The Susceptibility of the Chorio-allantoic Membrane of Chick Embryos to Infection with the Fowl-pox Virus," *Amer. J. Path., 7* (1931), 209.

Lewthwaite and Savoor: Rickettsia Diseases of Malaya

Preface

1. T. A. Palm, "Some Account of a Disease Called Shima-Mushi or Island Insect Disease by the Natives of Japan Peculiar (it is believed) to that Country and Hitherto Not Described," (Letter to Rev. John Lowe), *Edinb. Med. J., 24*, Pt. I (1878), 128.

2. E. Baelz and Kawakami, "Das Japanische Fluss-oder Ueberschwemmungsfieber, eine Acute Infectionskrankheit," *Virchows Arch. path. Anat., 78* (1879), 373.

3. F. G. Blake *et al.*, "Studies on Tsutsugamushi Disease (Scrub Typhus, Mite-Borne Typhus) in New Guinea and Adjacent Islands: Epidemiology, Clinical Observations, and Etiology in the Dobadura Area," *Amer. J. Hyg., 41* (1945), 243–373.

4. P. M. Asburn and C. F. Craig, "A Comparative Study of Tsutsugamushi Disease and Spotted or Tick Fever of Montana," *Boston Med. Sur. J., 159* (1908), 749–761.

5. T. Kitashima and M. Miyajima, "Studien über die Tsutsugamushi-Krankheit," *Kitasato Arch. Exp. Med., 2* (1918), 91 and 237.

6. M. Nagayo *et al.*, "Sur le virus de la maladie de Tsutsugamushi," *C. R. Soc. Biol., 104* (1930), 637–641.

7. N. Ogata, "Aetiologie der Tsutsugamushikrankheit; *Rickettsia tsutsugamushi*," *Z. Bakt., 122* (1931), 249–253.

8. W. Fletcher, J. F. Lesslar, and R. Lewthwaite, "The Aetiology of the Tsutsu-gamushi Disease and Tropical Typhus in the Federated Malay States," *Trans. Roy. Soc. Trop. Med. Hyg., 23* (1929), 57–70, Part II.

9. R. Lewthwaite and S. R. Savoor, "The Typhus Group of Diseases in Malaya. Part II. The Study of the Virus of the Urban Type in Laboratory Animals," *Brit. J. Exp. Path., 17* (1936), 23–34.

Text

1. W. Fletcher and J. E. Lesslar, *Bull. Inst. Med. Res. Fed. Malay States*, No. 2 (1925).

2. J. Gray, B. A. Peters, and I. G. Davies, *Lancet, 1* (1938), 490.

3. R. Lewthwaite and S. R. Savoor, *Brit. J. Exp. Path., 17* (1936), 461.

4. M. L. Unwin, *Med. J. Austral., 2* (1935), 303.

5. J. W. Wolff, *J. Hyg.* (Cambridge), *31* (1931), 352.

6. S. B. Wolbach *et al.*, *The Etiology and Pathology of Typhus* (Cambridge, Mass.: Harvard University Press, 1922).

7. W. Fletcher and J. W. Field, *Bull. Inst. Med. Res. Fed. Malay States*, No. 1 (1927).

8. W. Fletcher and J. E. Lesslar, *Bull. Inst. Med. Res. Fed. Malay States*, No. 1 (1926).

9. A. Felix and M. Rhodes, *J. Hyg.* (Cambridge, *31* (1931), 225.

10. R. Lewthwaite and S. R. Savoor, *Rep. Inst. Med. Res. Fed. Malay States* (1936).

11. R. Lewthwaite and S. R. Savoor, *Rep. Inst. Med. Res. Fed. Malay States* (1939).

12. R. Lewthwaite, *J. Path. Bact., 42* (1936), 23.

13. R. Lewthwaite, *Bull. Inst. Med. Res. Fed. Malay States*, No. 1 (1930).

14. B. A. R. Gater, *Trans. Far-East Assn. Trop. Med., 2* (1930), 132.

15. R. Lewthwaite and S. R. Savoor, *Brit. J. Exp. Path., 17* (1936), 309.

16. W. Fletcher and R. Lewthwaite, *Trans. Roy. Soc. Trop. Med. Hyg., 22* (1928), 161.

17. L. Anigstein, *Stud. Inst. Med. Res. Fed. Malay States* (1933).

18. C. Nicolle, *Arch. Inst. Pasteur d'Afrique Nord, 21* (1933), 349.

19. R. Lewthwaite and S. R. Savoor, *Brit. J. Exp. Path., 17* (1936), 208.

20. R. Lewthwaite, *Bull. Inst. Med. Res. Fed. Malay States*, No. 3 (1930).

21. R. Lewthwaite and S. R. Savoor, *Brit. J. Exp. Path., 17* (1936), 1.

22. H. Zinsser *et al.*, *J. Exp. Med., 53* (1931), 333.

23. M. Nagayo *et al.*, *Jap. J. Exp. Med., 9* (1931), 87.

24. R. Lewthwaite and S. R. Savoor, *Brit. J. Exp. Path., 17* (1936), 448.

25. E. Weil and A. Felix, *Z. Immun.-Forsch., 31* (1921), 457.

26. A. Felix, *Trans. Roy. Soc. Trop. Med. Hyg., 26* (1933), 365.

27. J. W. Wolff and W. Kouwenaar, *Geneesk Tijdschrift Ned.-Ind., 76* (1336), 272.

28. R. Kawamura, Y. Imagawa, and T. Ito, *Kitasato Arch., 12* (1935), 26.

29. P. Lepine, *Trans. Roy. Soc. Trop. Med. Hyg., 29* (1936), 577.

30. R. Lewthwaite and S. R. Savoor, *Trans. Roy. Soc. Trop. Med. Hyg., 29* (1936), 561.

31. J. W. Megaw, *Rep. Inst. Med. Res. Fed. Malay States* (1936), 579.

Gildemeister and Haagen: Typhus Fever Studies

Preface

1. N. H. Topping *et al.*, *Studies of Typhus Fever*, Nat. Inst. Health Bull. No. 183 (Washington, D. C., 1945).

2. J. E. Smadel *et al.*, "A Toxic Substance Associated with the Gilliam Strain of *R. orientalis*," *Proc. Soc. Exp. Biol. Med.*, *62* (1964), 138–140.

3. E. J. Bell and E. G. Pickens, "A Toxic Substance Associated with the Rickettsias of the Spotted Fever Group," *J. Immunol.*, *70* (1953), 461–472.

4. J. Craige *et al.*, "The Serological Relationships of the Rickettsiae of Epidemic and Murine Typhus," *Canad. J. Res.*, *24*, Sec. E (1946), 84–103.

5. H. L. Hamilton, "Specificity of the Toxic Factors Associated with the Epidemic and the Murine Strains of Typhus Ricksettsiae," *Amer. J. Trop. Med.*, *25* (1945), 391–395.

6. E. J. Bell and H. G. Stoenner, "Immunologic Relationships among the Spotted Fever Group of Rickettsias Determined by Toxin Neutralization Tests in Mice with Convalescent Animal Serums," *J. Immunol.*, *84* (1960), 171–182.

7. D. H. Clarke and J. P. Fox, "The Phenomenon of *In Vitro* Hemolysis Produced by the Rickettsiae of Typhus Fever, with a Note on the Mechanism of Rickettsial Toxicity in Mice," *J. Exp. Med.*, *88* (1948), 25–41.

8. P. Y. Paterson, C. L. Wisseman, and J. E. Smadel, "Studies of Rickettsial Toxins. I. Role of Hemolysis in Fatal Toxemia of Rabbits and Rats," *J. Immunol.*, *72* (1954), 12–23.

9. F. A. Neva and J. C. Snyder, "Studies on the Toxicity of Typhus Rickettsiae. III. Observations on the Mechanism of Toxic Death in White Mice and White Rats," *J. Infect. Dis.*, *97* (1955), 73–87.

10. S. E. Greisman and C. L. Wisseman, "Studies of Rickettsial Toxins. IV. Cardiovascular Functional Abnormalities Induced by *Rickettsia mooseri* Toxin in the White Rat," *J. Immunol.*, *81* (1958), 345–354.

Bibliographical References

1. H. R. Cox, *Public Health Reports*, *53* (1938), 2241.

2. R. Otto and R. Wohlrab, *Fleckfiebergruppe. Handbuch der Viruskrankheiten*, II (Jena, 1939), 528; *Arbeits Institut Experimentaler Therapie*, No. 38 (Frankfurt, 1939). *Z. Hyg.*, *122* (1939), 2.

Plotz *et al.*: Morphological Structure of Rickettsiae.

Preface

1. S. L. Wissig *et al.*, "Electron Microscopic Observations on Intracellular Rickettsiae," *Amer. J. Path.*, *32* (1956), 1117–1133.

2. M. G. P. Stoker, K. M. Smith, and P. Fiset, "Internal Structure of *Rickettsia burnetii* as Shown by Electron Microscopy of Thin Sections," *J. Gen. Microbiol.*, *15* (1956), 632–635.

3. M. Schaechter *et al.*, "Morphological, Chemical, and Serological Studies of the Cell Walls of *Rickettsia mooseri*," *J. Bact.*, *74* (1957), 822–829.

4. A. C. Allison and H. R. Perkins, "Presence of Cell Walls Like Those of Bacteria in Rickettsiae," *Nature*, *188* (1960), 796–798.

Text

1. H. Pinkerton, *Bact. Rev.*, *6* (1942), 37.

2. V. K. Zworykin, J. Hillier, and A. W. Vance, Trans. *Elect. Eng.*, *60* (1941), 157.

3. H. R. Cox, *Science*, *94* (1941), 399.

4. H. Zinssser, H. Plotz, and J. F. Enders, *Science, 91* (1940), 51.

5. R. H. Green, T. F. Anderson, and J. E. Smadel, *J. Exp. Med., 75* (1942), 651.

6. Macchiavello, cited by Zinsser, "Immunity in Rickettsial Disease," in *Virus and Rickettsial Diseases*, Harvard Symposium (Cambridge, Mass.: Harvard University Press, 1940), p. 896.

7. S. B. Wolbach, *J. Med. Res., 41* (1919), 1.

8. H. Pinkerton and G. M. Hass, *J. Exp. Med., 56* (1932), 151.

9. S. Mudd, K. Polevitzky, and T. F. Anderson, *Arch. Path., 34* (1942), 199.

10. R. R. Spencer and R. R. Parker, Hygienic Laboratory Bull. No. 154 (U.S. Public Health Service, 1930).

Greiff *et al.*: Effect of Enzyme Inhibitors and Activators.

Preface

1. J. C. Snyder, J. Maier, and C. R. Anderson, Report to the Division of Medical Sciences (Washington, D. C.: National Research Council, December 26, 1942).

2. D. Greiff, "Biology of the Rickettsiae," in *Rickettsial Diseases of Man* (Washington, D. C.: AAAS, 1948), 51–63.

3. H. L. Hamilton, "Effect of P-Aminobenzoic Acid on Growth of Rickettsiae and Elementary Bodies with Observations on Mode of Action," *Proc. Soc. Exp. Biol. Med., 59* (1945), 220–226.

4. E. S. Murray, C. J. D. Zarafonetis, and J. C. Snyder, "Further Report on Effect of Para-Aminobenzoic Acid in Experimental Tsutsugamushi Disease (Scrub Typhus)," *Proc. Soc. Exp. Biol. Med., 60* (1945), 80–84.

5. A. Yeomans *et al.*, "Therapeutic Effect of Para-Aminobenzoic Acid in Louse-Borne Typhus Fever," *JAMA, 126* (1944), 349–356.

6. J. C. Snyder and B. Davis, "Reversal of Rickettsiostatic Effect of P-Aminobenzoic Acid by P-Hydroxybenzoic Acid," *Fed. Proc., 10* (1951), 419.

7. N. Takemori and M. Kitaoka, "Reversal of P-Aminobenzoic Acid Inhibition of Growth of Rickettsiae by P-Hydroxybenzoic Acid in Agar-Slant Tissue Culture," *Science, 116* (1952), 710—711.

8. J. E. Smadel and E. B. Jackson, "Chloromycetin, Antibiotic with Chemotherapeutic Activity in Experimental Rickettsial and Viral Infections," *Science, 106* (1947), 418–419.

9. S. C. Wong and H. R. Cox, "Action of Aureomycin against Experimental Rickettsial and Viral Infections," *Ann. N. Y. Acad. Sci., 51* (1948), 290–305.

10. J. C. Snyder *et al.*, "Experimental Studies on Anti-Rickettsial Properties of Terramycin," *Ann. N. Y. Acad. Sci., 53* (1950), 362–374.

11. Y. Hara and T. Abe, "Influence of Chemotherapy on Mortality Rates of Tsutsugamushi Disease in Northern Japan, and Some Other Statistical Information," *Amer. J. Trop. Med. Hyg., 5* (1956), 218–223.

Text

1. H. Pinkerton, *Arch. Zellforsch., 15* (1934), 425.

2. H. Zinsser and E. B. Schoenbach, *J. Exp. Med., 66* (1937), 207.

3. H. Pinkerton and O. A. Bessey, *Science, 89* (1939), 368.

4. H. Pinkerton, *Bact. Rev.*, *6* (1942), 37.

5. C. Foster *et al.*, *J. Exp. Med.*, *79* (1944), 221.

6. D. Greiff and H. Pinkerton, *Proc. Soc. Exp. Biol. Med.*, *55* (1944), 116.

7. V. Moragues and H. Pinkerton, *J. Exp. Med.*, *79* (1944), 35.

8. V. Moragues and H. Pinkerton, *ibid.*, p. 41.

9. V. Moragues and H. Pinkerton, *ibid.*, p. 431.

10. J. Ungar, *Nature*, *152* (1943), 245.

11. O. L. Peterson, *Proc. Soc. Exp. Biol. Med.* *55* (1944), 155.

12. A. F. Dyer, *Arch. Path. Pharm.*, *170* (1933), 39.

13. O. Bessey and H. Pinkerton, unpublished observations.

14. Unpublished observations by the authors.

Topping and Shear: Studies of Typhus Fever Vaccines

Preface

1. H. Plotz, "Complement Fixation in Rickettsial Diseases," *Science*, *97* (1943), 20–21.

2. J. S. Colter, "The Preparation of a Soluble Immunizing Antigen from Q Fever Rickettsiae," *J. Immunol.*, *76* (1956), 270–274.

3. H. Plotz *et al.*, "The Serological Pattern in Typhus Fever. I. Epidemic," *Amer. J. Hyg.*, *47* (1948), 150–165.

Huebner *et al.*: Rickettsialpox

Preface

1. L. N. Sussman, "Kew Garden's Spotted Fever," *N. Y. Medicine*, *2* (1946), 27–28.

2. M. Greenberg *et al.*, "Rickettsialpox—A Newly Recognized Rickettsial Disease. II. Clinical Observations," *JAMA*, *133* (1947), 901–906.

3. R. J. Huebner, W. L. Jellison, and C. Pomerantz, "Rickettsialpox—A Newly Recognized Rickettsial Disease. IV. Isolation of a Rickettsia Apparently Identical with the Causative Agent of Rickettsialpox from *Allodermanyssus sanguineus*, a Rodent Mite," *Public Health Reports*, *61* (1946), 1677–1682.

4. R. J. Huebner, W. L. Jellison, and C. Armstrong, "Rickettsialpox—A Newly Recognized Rickettsial Disease. V. Recovery of *Rickettsia akari* from a House Mouse (*Mus musculus*)," *Public Health Reports*, *62* (1947), 777–780.

5. M. Greenberg, O. Pellitteri, and W. L. Jellison, "Rickettsialpox—A Newly Recognized Rickettsial Disease. III. Epidemiological Findings," *Amer. J. Pub. Health*, *37* (1947), 860–868.

6. L. R. Hershberger and R. J. Huebner, "A Report on the Histopathology of the Cutaneous Lesions of a Case of Rickettsialpox," *Public Health Reports*, *62* (1947), 1740–1742.

7. Jackson *et al.*, "Recovery of *Rickettsia akari* from the Korean Vole *Microtus fortis pelliceus*," *Amer. J. Hyg.*, *66* (1957), 301–307.

Text

1. L. N. Sussman, "Kew Garden's Spotted Fever," *N. Y. Medicine, 2* (August 5, 1946), 27–28.
2. N. H. Topping and C. C. Shepard, "The Preparation of Antigens from Yolk Sacs Infected with Rickettsiae," *Public Health Reports, 61* (May 17, 1946), 701–707.
3. P. Durand, "La reaction de Weil-Félix dans la fièvre boutonneuse," *Arch. l'Inst. Pasteur Tunis, 20* (March 1932), 395–421.
4. R. J. Huebner, unpublished data.
5. L. F. Badger, "Rocky Mountain Spotted Fever and Boutonneuse Fever, a Study of Their Immunological Relationships," *Public Health Reports, 48* (May 12, 1933), 507–511.
6. B. Shankman, "Report on an Outbreak of Endemic Febrile Illness, Not Yet Identified, Occurring in New York City," *N. Y. St. J. Med., 46* (October 1, 1946), 2156–2159.

Bovarnick and Snyder: Respiration of Typhus Rickettsiae

Preface

1. C. L. Wisseman *et al.*, "Metabolic Studies of Rickettsiae. I. The Effects of Antimicrobial Substances and Enzyme Inhibitors on the Oxidation of Glutamate by Purified Rickettsiae," *J. Immunol., 67* (1951), 123–136.
2. A. Karp, "An Immunological Purification of Typhus Rickettsiae," *J. Bact., 67* (1954), 450–455.
3. C. L. Wisseman *et al.*, "Metabolic Studies of Rickettsiae. II. Studies on the Pathway of Glutamate Oxidation by Purified Suspensions of *Rickettsia mooseri*," *J. Immunol., 68* (1952), 251–264.
4. R. A. Ormsbee and M. G. Peacock, "Metabolic Activity in *Coxiella burnetii*," *J. Bact., 88* (1964), 1205–1210.
5. M. R. Bovarnick and J. C. Miller, "Oxidation and Transamination of Glutamate by Typhus Rickettsiae," *J. Biol. Chem., 184* (1950), 661–676.
6. M. R. Bovarnick, "Phosphorylation Accompanying the Oxidation of Glutamate by the Madrid E Strain of Typhus Rickettsiae," *J. Biol. Chem., 220* (1956), 353–361.
7. D. Paretsky *et al.*, "Studies on the Physiology of Rickettsiae. I. Some Enzyme Systems of *Coxiella burnetii*," *J. Infect. Dis., 103* (1958), 6–11.

Text

1. D. J. Bauer, *Brit. J. Exp. Path., 28* (1947), 440.
2. I. A. Bengtson, N. H. Topping, and R. G. Henderson, Nat. Inst. Health Bull. No. 183 (1945), 25.
3. G. Clavero and F. Perez Gallardo, *Revista de Sanidad e Higiene Publica, 18* (1944), 547.
4. H. R. Cox, *Science, 94* (1941), 399.
5. F. Perez Gallardo and J. P. Fox, *Amer. J. Hyg., 48* (1948), 6.
6. F. Fulton and A. M. Begg, Great Britain Medical Research Council, Special Report Ser., No. 255 (1946), 163.

7. H. A. Lardy, in W. W. Umbreit, R. H. Burris, and J. F. Stauffer, *Manometric Techniques* (Minneapolis: Burgess Pub. Co., 1945).

8. H. R. Morgan, D. A. Stevens, and J. C. Snyder, *Proc. Soc. Exp. Biol. Med.*, *64* (1947), 342.

9. N. Nelson, *J. Biol. Chem.*, *153* (1944), 375.

10. E. Racker and I. Krimsky, *J. Exp. Med.*, *84* (1946), 191; *85* (1947), 715.

11. L. J. Reed and H. Muench, *Amer. J. Hyg.*, *27* (1938), 493.

12. C. C. Shepard and N. H. Topping, *J. Immunol.*, *55* (1947), 97.

Ris and Fox: The Cytology of Rickettsiae

Preface

1. W. H. Price, "A Quantitative Analysis of the Factors Involved in the Variations in Virulence of Rickettsiae," *Science*, *118* (1943), 49–52.

2. Z. A. Cohn *et al.*, "Unstable Nucleic Acids of *Rickettsia mooseri*," *Science*, *127* (1958), 282–283.

Text

1. C. F. Robinow, Addendum in R. J. Dubos, *The Bacterial Cell* (Cambridge, Mass.: The Harvard University Press, 1945).

2. A. Boivin, in Cold Spring Harbor Symposia on Quantitative Biology, Cold Spring Harbor, Long Island Biological Association (1947) *12*, 7.

3. H. Pinkerton, *Bact. Rev.*, *6* (1942), 37.

4. H. Plotz, J. E. Smadel, T. F. Anderson, and L. A. Chambers, *J. Exp. Med.*, *77* (1943), 355.

5. V. I. Tovarnickij, M. K. Krontovskaja, and N. V. Ceburkina, *Nature*, *158* (1946), 912.

6. S. S. Cohen, *Fed. Proc.*, *5* (1946), 129.

7. A. E. Mirsky and A. W. Pollister, *J. Gen. Physiol.*, *30* (1946), 117.

8. J. Brachet, *C. R. Soc. Biol.*, *133* (1940), 88.

9. T. Caspersson *et al.*, *Nord. Med.*, *28* (1945), 2636.

10. J. Callot and R. Vendrely, *C. R. Soc. Biol.*, *142* (1948), 396.

11. R. Tulasne and R. Vendrely, *C. R. Soc. Biol.*, *141* (1947), 674.

12. R. Vendrely and J. Lipardy, *C. R. Acad. Sci.*, *223* (1946), 342.

13. C. F. Robinow, *Proc. Roy. Soc.* (Lond.) [B], *130* (1942), 299.

14. J. S. Rafalko, *Stain Technol.*, *21* (1946), 91.

Ley *et al.*: Immunization against Scrub Typhus

Preface

1. J. P. Fox, "The Relative Infectibility of Laboratory Animals and Chick Embryos with Rickettsiae of Murine or Epidemic Typhus," *Amer. J. Hyg.*, *49* (1949), 313–320.

2. H. S. Fuller, "Studies of Human Body Lice, *Pediculus humanus corporis*. II. Quantitative Comparisons of the Susceptibility of Human Body Lice and Cotton Rats to Experimental Infection with Epidemic Typhus Rickettsiae," *Amer. J. Hyg.*, *58* (1953), 188–206.

3. W. H. Price *et al.*, "Ecologic Studies on the Interepidemic Survival of Louse-Borne Epidemic Typhus Fever," *Amer. J. Hyg.*, *67* (1958), 154–178.

4. W. D. Tigertt and A. S. Benenson, "Studies on Q Fever in Man," *Trans. Assn. Amer. Phycns.*, *69* (1956), 98–104.

Text

1. H. L. Ley, Jr., *et al.*, "Immunization against Scrub Typhus. IV. Living Karp Vaccine and Chemoprophylaxis in Volunteers," *Amer. J. Hyg.*, *56* (1952), 303–312.

2. J. E. Smadel *et al.*, "Immunization against Scrub Typhus: Duration of Immunity in Volunteers Following Combined Living Vaccine and Chemoprophylaxis," *Amer. J. Trop. Med. Hyg.*, *1* (1952), 87–99.

3. J. E. Smadel *et al.*, "Immunity in Scrub Typhus: Resistance to Induced Reinfection," *Arch. Path.*, *50* (1950), 847–861.

4. E. B. Jackson and J. E. Smadel, "Immunization against Scrub Typhus. II. Preparation of Lyophilized Living Vaccine," *Amer. J. Hyg.*, *53* (1951), 326–331.

5. L. J. Reed and H. Muench, "A Simple Method of Estimating Fifty Per Cent End-points," *Amer. J. Hyg.*, *27* (1938), 493–497.

6. M. Pizzi, "Sampling Variation of the Fifty Per Cent End-point, Determined by the Reed-Muench (Behrens) Method," *Hum. Biol.*, *22* (1950), 151–190.

7. M. F. Boyd and S. F. Kitchen, "On Attempts to Hyperimmunize Convalescents from Vivax Malaria," *Amer. J. Trop. Med.*, *23* (1943), 209–225.

8. N. B. McCullough and C. W. Eisele, "Experimental Human Salmonellosis. I. Pathogenicity of Strains of *Salmonella meleagridis* and *Salmonella anatum* Obtained from Spray-dried Whole Egg," *J. Infect. Dis.*, *88* (1951), 278–289.

9. N. B. McCullough and C. W. Eisele, "Experimental Human Salmonellosis. III. Pathogenicity of Strains of *Salmonella newport*, *Salmonella derby*, and *Salmonella bareilly* Obtained from Spray-dried Whole Egg," *J. Infect. Dis.*, *89* (1951), 209–213.

10. N. B. McCullough and C. W. Eisele, "Experimental Human Salmonellosis. IV. Pathogenicity of Strains of *Salmonella pullorum* Obtained from Spray-dried Whole Egg," *J. Infect. Dis.*, *89* (1951), 259–265.

11. H. J. Shaughnessy *et al.*, "Experimental Human Bacillary Dysentery: Polyvalent Dysentery Vaccine in Its Prevention," *JAMA*, *132* (1946), 362–368.

12. H. Koprowski, G. A. Jervis, and T. W. Norton, "Immune Responses in Human Volunteers upon Oral Administration of a Rodent-adapted Strain of Poliomyelitis Virus," *Amer. J. Hyg.*, *55* (1952), 108–126.

13. C. M. Southam and A. E. Moore, "West Nile, Ilheus, and Bunyamwera Virus Infections in Man," *Amer. J. Trop. Med.*, *31* (1951), 724–741.

14. C. Nicolle and E. Conseil, "Vaccinations préventives par voie digestive chez l'homme dans la dysenterie bacillaire et la fièvre mediterranéenne," *Arch. Inst. Pasteur*, *36* (1922), 579–613.

15. P. Morales-Otero, "Brucella Abortus in Porto Rico," *Puerto Rico J. Pub. Hlth*, *6* (1930), 3–88.

16. R. Kawamura *et al.*, "On the Prevention of Tsutsugamushi Disease, Including a New Method of Fever Therapy," *Kitasato Arch.*, *14* (1937), 75–98.

17. B. Kreis, "La maladie d'Armstrong: chorioméningite lymphocytaire: une nouvelle entité morbide?" Thesis for the Doctorate in Medicine (Paris: Librairie J. B. Bailliére, 1937).

18. A. A. Smorodintsev, "Etiology of Hemorrhagic Nephroso-Nephritis," *Moscow Medgiz* (1944), 28–38 (in Russian).

19. G. Blanc *et al.*, "Quelques données sur la Q fever experimentale," *Bull. Acad. Méd.* (Paris), *132* (1948), 243–250.

20. A. B. Sabin, "Research on Dengue during World War II," *Amer. J. Trop. Med. Hyg.*, *1* (1952), 30–50.

Gilford and Price: Virulent-Avirulent Conversions

Preface

1. M. R. Bovarnick and E. G. Allen, "Reversible Inactivation of Typhus Rickettsiae; Inactivation by Freezing," *J. Gen. Physiol.*, *38* (1954), 169–179.

2. M. R. Bovarnick and E. G. Allen, "Reversible Inactivation of Typhus Rickettsiae at 0°C," *J. Bact.*, *73* (1957), 56–62.

3. M. R. Bovarnick and E. G. Allen, "Reversible Inactivation of the Toxicity and Hemolytic Activity of Typhus Rickettsiae by Starvation," *J. Bact.*, *74* (1957), 637–645.

4. R. R. Spencer and R. R. Parker, "Studies on Rocky Mountain Spotted Fever. Infection by Other Means than Tick Bite," *Hygienic Laboratory Bull. No. 154* (Washington, D. C.: U.S. Public Health Service, 1930), 60–63.

Text

1. W. H. Price, *Science*, *118* (1953), 49–52.

2. W. H. Price, in *Dynamics of Virus and Rickettsial Infections*, ed. Hartman, Horsfall, and Kidd (New York: Blakiston Co., 1954), 164–183.

3. R. R. Spencer and R. R. Parker, *Hygienic Laboratory Bull.* Report No. 154 (1930), 1–116.

4. M. R. Bovarnick, J. C. Miller, and J. C. Snyder, *J. Bact.*, *59* (1950), 509–522.

5. J. C. Snyder and B. D. Davis, *Fed. Proc.*, *10* (1951), 419.

6. W. H. Price, *Am. J. Hyg.*, *58* (1953), 248–268.

7. M. R. Bovarnick and E. G. Allen, *J. Gen. Physiol.*, *38* (1954), 169–179.

Stoker and Fiset: Phase Variation of *Rickettsia burneti*

Preface

1. R. A. Ormsbee, E. G. Pickens, and D. B. Lackman, "An Antigenic Analysis of Three Strains of *Coxiella burnetii*," *Amer. J. Hyg.*, *79* (1964), 154–162.

2. R. A. Ormsbee *et al.*, "The Influence of Phase on the Protective Potency of Q Fever Vaccine," *J. Immunol.*, *92* (1964), 404–412.

Text

1. T. O. Berge and E. H. Lennette, "Q Fever. A Study of Serological Relationship among Strains of *Coxiella burneti* (Derrick)," *Amer. J. Hyg.*, *57* (1953), 144–169.

2. G. Cheney and W. A. Geib, "The Identification of Q Fever in Panama," *Amer. J. Hyg.*, *44* (1946), 158–172.

3. R. R. A. Coombs and M. G. P. Stoker, "Detection of Q Fever Antibodies by the Antiglobulin Sensitization Test," *Lancet, 11* (1951), 15–22.

4. H. R. Cox and E. J. Bell, "The Cultivation of *Rickettsia diaporica* in Tissue Culture and in the Tissues of Developing Chick Embryos," *Public Health Reports, 54* (1939), 2171–2178.

5. G. E. Davis and H. R. Cox, "A Filter-passing Infectious Agent Isolated from Ticks. I. Isolation from *Dermacentor andersoni*, Reactions in Animals, and Filtration Experiments," *Public Health Reports, 53* (1938), 2259–2267.

6. K. Herzberg and H. Urbach, "Untersuchungen mit Europäischen Q-Fieber-Antigenen. I. Mitteilung," *Z. Immun.-Forschung, 108* (1951), 376–388.

7. F. C. Robbins *et al.*, "Q Fever in the Mediterranean Area: Report of Its Occurrence in Allied Troops. III. The Etiological Agent," *Amer. J. Hyg., 44* (1946), 51–63.

8. J. E. Smadel, M. J. Snyder, and F. C. Robbins, "Vaccination against Q Fever," *Amer. J. Hyg., 47* (1948), 71–81.

9. M. G. P. Stoker, "Q Fever in Great Britain. The Causative Agent," *Lancet, 11* (1950), 616–621.

10. M. G. P. Stoker, "Variation in Complement-fixing Activity of *Rickettsia burneti* during Egg Adaptation," *J. Hyg., 51* (1953), 311–321.

11. M. G. P. Stoker, Z. Page, and B. P. Marmion, "Problems in the Diagnosis of Q Fever by Complement Fixation Tests," *WHO Bull.* (1955).

12. N. H. Topping, C. C. Shepard, and R. J. Huebner, "Q Fever: An Immunological Comparison of Strains," *Amer. J. Hyg., 44* (1946), 173–182.

13. R. C. Williams and R. C. Backus, "Macromolecular Weights Determined by Direct Particle Counting. I. The Weight of the Bushy Stunt Virus Particle," *J. Amer. Chem. Soc., 71* (1949), 4052–4057.

Schaechter *et al.*: Study on the Growth of Rickettsiae

Preface

1. R. L. Anacker *et al.*, "Electron Microscopic Observations of the Development of *Coxiella burnetii* in the Chick Yolk Sac," *J. Bact., 88* (1964), 1130–1138.

Text

1. S. B. Wolbach, "Studies on Rocky Mountain Spotted Fever," *J. Med. Res., 41* (1919), 1–197.

2. A. Bacot, J. A. Arkwright, and E. E. Atkin, "An Hereditary Rickettsia-like Parasite of the Bedbug (*Cimex lectularius*)," *Parasitology, 13* (1921), 27–36.

3. H. Sikora, "Zur Morphologie der Rickettsien," *Z. Hyg. Infekt.-krankh., 124* (1942–1943), 250–270.

4. S. L. Wissig, L. G. Caro, E. B. Jackson, and J. E. Smadel, "Electron Microscopic Observations of Intracellular Rickettsiae," *Amer. J. Path., 32* (1956), 1117–1133.

5. R. L. Ehrmann and G. O. Gey, "The Use of Cell Colonies on Glass for Evaluating Nutrition and Growth in Roller-tube Cultures," *J. Nat. Cancer Inst., 13* (1953), 1099–1121.

6. F. M. Bozeman, H. E. Hopps, J. X. Danauskas, E. B. Jackson, and J. E. Smadel, "Study on the Growth of Rickettsiae. I. A Tissue Culture System for the Quantitative Estimations of *Rickettsia tsutsugamushi*," *J. Immunol., 76* (1956), 475–488.

7. R. S. Breed, E. G. D. Murray and A. P. Hitchens, *Bergey's Manual of Determinative Bacteriology*, 6th ed. (Baltimore, Md.: Williams and Wilkins, 1948), 1083–1099.

8. G. O. Gey, P. Shapras, and E. Borysko, "Activities and Responses of Living Cells and Their Components as Recorded by Cinephase Microscopy and Electron Microscopy," *Ann. N. Y. Acad. Sci.*, *58* (1954), 1089–1109.

9. W. W. Ackermann and T. Francis, Jr., "Characteristics of Viral Development in Isolated Animal Tissues," *Advanc. Virus Res.*, *2* (1954), 81–108.

10. S. S. Cohen, "Comparative Biochemistry and Virology," *Advanc. Virus Res.*, *3* (1955), 1–48.

11. E. A. Evans, Jr., "Bacteriophage as Nucleoprotein," *Fed. Proc.*, *15* (1956), 827–832.

12. E. Weiss, "The Nature of the Psittacosis-Lymphogranuloma Group of Micro-organisms," *Ann. Rev. Microbiol.*, *9* (1955), 227–252.

13. H. Pinkerton and G. M. Hass, "Spotted Fever. I. Intranuclear Rickettsiae in Spotted Fever Studied in Tissue Culture," *J. Exp. Med.*, *56* (1932), 151–156.

14. J. O. W. Bland and C. F. Robinow, "The Inclusion Bodies of Vaccinia and Their Relationship to Elementary Bodies Studied in Cultures of the Rabbit's Cornea," *J. Path. Bact.*, *48* (1939), 381–403.

15. C. F. Robinow, "A Note on the Stalked Forms of Viruses," *J. Gen. Microbiol.*, *4* (1950), 242–243.

16. W. F. Noyes and B. K. Watson, "Studies on the Increase of Vaccine Virus in Cultured Human Cells by Means of the Fluorescent Antibody Technique," *J. Exp. Med.*, *102* (1955), 237–242.

17. R. Dulbecco and M. Vogt, "One-step Growth Curve of Western Equine Encephalomyelitis Virus on Chicken Embryo Cells Grown *in Vitro* and Analysis of Virus Yields from Single Cells," *J. Exp. Med.*, *99* (1954), 183–199.

18. H. J. F. Cairns, "Quantitative Aspects of Influenza Virus Multiplication. III. Average Liberation Time," *J. Immunol.*, *69* (1952), 168–173.

19. W. Henle, "Multiplication of Influenza Virus in the Entodermal Cells of the Allantois of the Chick Embryo," *Advanc. Virus Res.*, *1* (1953), 141–227.

20. H. B. Maitland and B. M. Tobin, "The Growth of Vaccinia Virus in the Chorio-allantois of the Developing Chick Embryo and the Production of Complement-fixing Antigen and Haemagglutinin," *J. Hyg.*, *54* (1956), 102–113.

21. G. O. and M. K. Gey, "The Maintenance of Human Normal Cells and Tumor Cells in Continuous Culture. I. Preliminary Report: Cultivation of Mesoblastic Tumors and Normal Tissue, and Notes on Methods of Cultivation," *Amer. J. Cancer* 27 (1936), 45–76.

M. R. Bovarnick: Incorporation of Acetate-1-C^{14} into Lipid by Typhus Rickettsiae

Preface

1. M. R. Bovarnick, L. Schneider, and H. Walter, "The Incorporation of Labeled Methionine by Typhus Rickettsiae," *Biochim. Biophys. Acta*, *33* (1959), 414–422.

2. M. R. Bovarnick and L. Schneider, "The Incorporation of Glycine-1-C^{14} by Typhus Rickettsiae," *J. Biol. Chem.*, *235* (1960), 1727–1731.

Text

1. M. R. Bovarnick and J. C. Snyder, "Respiration of Typhus Rickettsiae," *J. Exp. Med.*, *89* (1949), 561–565.

2. M. R. Bovarnick, "Phosphorylation Accompanying the Oxidation of Glutamate by Typhus Rickettsiae," *J. Biol. Chem.*, *220* (1956), 353–361.

3. W. F. Myers, D. Paretsky, and C. M. Downs, "Physiology of Rickettsiae, Transformylation and Oxidative Phosphorylation with *Coxiella burnetii*," *Bact. Proc.* (1959), 122.

4. M. R. Bovarnick, L. Schneider, and H. Walter, "The Incorporation of Labeled Methionine by Typhus Rickettsiae," *Biochim. Biophys. Acta*, *33* (1959), 414–422.

5. K. Fujita, S. Kohno, and A. Shishido, "The Incorporation of Methionine into Purified Rickettsiae," *Jap. J. Med. Sci. Biol.*, *12* (1959), 387–390.

6. M. R. Bovarnick and L. Schneider, "The Incorporation of Glycine-C^{14} by Typhus Rickettsiae," *J. Biol. Chem.*, *235* (1960), 1727–1731.

7. O. H. Lowry, N. J. Rosebrough, A. L. Farr, and R. J. Randall, "Protein Measurement with the Folin Reagent," *J. Biol. Chem.*, *193* (1951), 265–275.

8. M. R. Bovarnick and L. Schneider, "Role of Adenosine Triphosphate in the Hemolysis of Sheep Erythrocytes by Typhus Rickettsiae," *J. Bact.*, *80* (1960), 344–354.

9. C. L. Wisseman, Jr., F. E. Hahn, E. B. Jackson, F. M. Bozeman, and J. E. Smadel, "Metabolic Studies of Rickettsiae. II. Studies on the Pathway of Glutamate Oxidation by Purified Suspensions of *Rickettsia mooseri*," *J. Immunol.*, *68* (1952), 251–264.

10. M. R. Bovarnick and J. C. Miller, "Oxidation and Transamination of Glutamate by Typhus Rickettsiae," *J. Biol. Chem.*, *184* (1950), 661–676.

11. W. H. Price, "A Quantitative Analysis of the Factors Involved in the Variations in Virulence of Rickettsiae," *Science*, *118* (1953), 49–52.

12. D. Paretsky, C. M. Downs, R. A. Consigli, and B. K. Joyce, "Studies on the Physiology of Rickettsiae. I. Some Enzyme Systems of *Coxiella burnetii*," *J. Infect. Dis.*, *103* (1958), 6–11.

13. M. R. Bovarnick and E. G. Allen, "Reversible Inactivation of the Toxicity and Hemolytic Activity of Typhus Rickettsiae by Starvation," *J. Bact.*, *74* (1957), 637–645.

Vinson and Fuller: Studies on Trench Fever

Preface

1. S. Ito and J. W. Vinson, "Fine Structure of *Rickettsia quintana* Cultivated in Vitro and in the Louse," *J. Bact.*, *89* (1965), 481–495.

2. J. W. Vinson, "Etiology of Trench Fever in Mexico," *Industry and Tropical Health*, *5* (1964), 109–114.

3. G. Varela, R. Fournier, and H. Mooser, "Presencia de *Rickettsia quintana* en piojos *Pediculus humanus* de la Ciudad de México. Inoculactión experimental," *Rev. Inst. Salub. Enferm. Trop.*, *14* (1954), 39–42.

Text

1. H. F. Swift, "Trench Fever," *Arch. Int. Med.*, *26* (1920), 76–98.

2. A. Schminke, "Histopathologischer Befund in Roseolen der Haut bei wolhynischem Fieber," *Münch. Med. Wschr.*, *64* (1917), 961.

3. *Trench Fever*. Report of Commission, Medical Research Committee, Am. Red Cross (Oxford University Press, 1918).

4. S. B. Wolbach, J. L. Todd, and F. W. Palfrey, *The Etiology and Pathology of Typhus* (Cambridge, Mass.: Harvard University Press, 1922).

5. H. Mooser, A. Leeman, S. H. Chao, and H. U. Gubler, "Beobachtunger an Fünftagefieber. I. Mitteilung," *Schweiz. Z. Path.*, *11* (1948), 513–522.

6. H. Mooser and F. Weyer, "Experimental Infections of *Macacus rhesus* with *Rickettsia quintana* (Trench Fever)," *Proc. Soc. Exp. Biol. Med.*, *83* (1953), 699–701.

7. H. Mooser and F. Weyer, "Die Infektion des Rhesusaffen mit Fünftagefieber (*Rickettsia quintana*)," *Z. Tropenmed. Parasit.*, *4* (1953), 513–539.

8. J. A. Arkwright, A. Bacot, and F. M. Duncan, "The Association of Rickettsia with Trench Fever," *J. Hyg.*, *18* (1919), 76–94.

9. H. S. Fuller, unpublished experiments.

10. H. da Rocha-Lima and H. Sikora, "Methoden zur Untersuchung von Läusen als Infektionsträger," in Abderhalden's *Handbuch der biologischen Arbeitsmethoden*, XII, Pt. I (1925), 769–814.

11. R. Weigl, "Untersuchungen und Experimente an Fleckfieberlausen. Die Technik der Rickettsial-Forschung," *Beitr. z. Klin. Infekt.-krank.*, *8* (1920), 353–376.

12. J. C. Snyder and C. M. Wheeler, "The Experimental Infection of the Human Body Louse, *Pediculus humanus corporis*, with Murine and Epidemic Louse-borne Typhus Strains," *J. Exp. Med.*, *82* (1945), 1–20.

13. M. R. Bovarnick, J. C. Miller, and J. C. Snyder, "The Influence of Certain Salts, Amino Acids, Sugars, and Proteins on the Stability of Rickettsiae," *J. Bact.*, *59* (1950), 509–522.

14. A. E. Moore, L. Sabachewsky, and H. W. Toolan, "Culture Characteristics of Four Permanent Lines of Human Cancer Cells," *Cancer Res.*, *15* (1955), 598–602.

15. W. F. Scherer, "The Utilization of a Pure Strain of Mammalian Cells (Earle) for Cultivation of Viruses *in Vitro*. I. Multiplication of Pseudo-Rabies and Herpes Simplex Viruses," *Amer. J. Path.*, *29* (1953), 113–138.

16. L. Dienes, "L Organisms of Klieneberger and *Streptobacillus moniliformis*," *J. Infect. Dis.*, *65* (1939), 24–42.

17. J. E. Smadel, "Rickettsial Diseases," in *Diagnostic Procedures for Virus and Rickettsial Diseases*, 2d ed. (New York: Amer. Public Health Association, 1956).

18. W. B. Cherry, M. Goldman, and T. R. Carski, *Fluorescent Antibody Techniques in the Diagnosis of Communicable Diseases* (Washington, D. C.: U.S. Government Printing Office, 1960).

19. R. A. Goldwasser and C. C. Shepard, "Fluorescent Antibody Methods in the Differentiation of Murine and Epidemic Typhus Sera: Specificity Changes Resulting from Previous Immunization," *J. Immunol.*, *82* (1959), 373–380.

20. F. Weyer, "Eigenschaften und systematische Stellug der *Rickettsia quintana* mit Bemerkungen zur Systematik und Nomenklatur der Rickettsien," *Z. Tropenmed. Parasit.*, *6* (1955), 2–18.

Index

(Page numbers in italics refer to citations in the Notes.)